The International Library of Psychology

INFANT SPEECH

Founded by C. K. Ogden

The International Library of Psychology

DEVELOPMENTAL PSYCHOLOGY
In 32 Volumes

I	The Child's Discovery of Death	*Anthony*
II	The Psychology of the Infant	*Bernfeld*
III	The Psychology of Special Abilities and Disabilities	*Bronner*
IV	The Child and His Family	*Bühler*
V	From Birth to Maturity	*Bühler*
VI	The Mental Development of the Child	*Bühler*
VII	The Psychology of Children's Drawings	*Eng*
VIII	Educational Psychology	*Fox*
IX	A Study of Imagination in Early Childhood	*Griffiths*
X	Understanding Children's Play	*Hartley et al*
XI	Intellectual Growth in Young Children	*Isaacs*
XII	Conversations with Children	*Katz*
XIII	The Growth of the Mind	*Koffka*
XIV	The Child's Unconscious Mind	*Lay*
XV	Infant Speech	*Lewis*
XVI	The Growth of Reason	*Lorimer*
XVII	The Growing Child and its Problems	*Miller*
XVIII	The Child's Conception of Physical Causality	*Piaget*
XIX	The Child's Conception of Geometry	*Piaget et al*
XX	The Construction of Reality in the Child	*Piaget*
XXI	The Early Growth of Logic in the Child	*Inhelder et al*
XXII	The Growth of Logical Thinking from Childhood to Adolescence	*Inhelder et al*
XXIII	Judgement and Reasoning in the Child	*Piaget*
XXIV	The Moral Judgment of the Child	*Piaget*
XXV	Play, Dreams and Imitation in Childhood	*Piaget*
XXVI	The Psychology of Intelligence	*Piaget*
XXVII	Mental Health and Infant Development, V1	*Soddy*
XXVIII	Mental Health and Infant Development, V2	*Soddy*
XXIX	Modern Psychology and Education	*Sturt*
XXX	The Dynamics of Education	*Taba*
XXXI	Education Psychology	*Thorndike*
XXXII	The Principles of Teaching	*Thorndike*

INFANT SPEECH

A Study of the Beginnings of Language

M M LEWIS

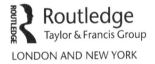

Routledge
Taylor & Francis Group

LONDON AND NEW YORK

First published in 1936 by
Routledge, Trench, Trubner & Co., Ltd.
2 Park Square, Milton Park, Abingdon, Oxfordshire OX14 4RN
711 Third Avenue, New York, NY 10017

First issued in paperback 2014

Routledge is an imprint of the Taylor and Francis Group, an informa business

British Library Cataloguing in Publication Data
A CIP catalogue record for this book
is available from the British Library

Infant Speech
ISBN 0415-20995-1
Developmental Psychology: 32 Volumes
ISBN 0415-21128-X
The International Library of Psychology: 204 Volumes
ISBN 0415-19132-7

ISBN 13: 978-1-138-87514-2 (pbk)
ISBN 13: 978-0-415-20995-3 (hbk)

CONTENTS

CHAP.   PAGE

PREFACE   xi

I INTRODUCTION   1
   Object of the work. Sources of the data. Arrangement of
   the work.

II SOME CHARACTERISTICS OF LANGUAGE . . .   5
   Language as an activity. Language and speech. The
   main features of speech. The patterns of the spoken language. The speaker, the listener, and the situation.
   Bühler: the threefold nature of speech. (i) Expression
   and the emotive function of language. (ii) Representation
   and reference. (iii) Evocation and communication. The relation between function and form. The fundamental nature
   of these functions.

SECTION I. THE BEGINNINGS

III EARLY UTTERANCE   21
   The child's earliest cries. The differentiation of expressive utterance. Records of observations. Discomfort-cries:
   vowels and early consonants. Comfort-sounds: vowels and
   early consonants. The front consonants. Phonetic features
   of the child's earliest sounds: the earlier discomfort cries;
   the earlier comfort-sounds; the front consonants: front
   consonants expressive of discomfort; front consonants
   expressive of comfort.

IV EARLY RESPONSE TO SPEECH   38
   The child's first response to sounds. The child's first
   response to the human voice. Divergent theories of this
   response. The further development of response to speech.
   The two factors: affect and situation. Theories of the
   nature of training.

SECTION II. TWO IMPORTANT FEATURES
OF THE CHILD'S SPEECH

V BABBLING   55
   Babbling and expression. Development of babbling.
   I. The beginning of babbling. Babbling in isolated and repeated sounds. II. Babbling as play. The source of play
   movements; their goal. III. The incentive in babbling.
   IV. Babbling as a form of art; characteristics of language
   with an æsthetic intention: (i) the experience symbolised,
   (ii) the language that symbolises the experience. Presence
   of these characteristics in babbling.

CHAP.   PAGE

VI IMITATION 70
The data. Three stages of development. *Stage I.* The
data. (i) the importance of attention to the speaker, (ii) the
effect of the human voice, (iii) the form of the child's response. The nature of these responses : (i) the innate tendency to respond vocally to speech, (ii) the expressive response to expression, (iii) the effect of babbling. *Stage II.*
The data. Imitation and the growth of meaning. Effects
of the growth of meaning. *Stage III.* The data. The
growth of awareness. (i) the imitation of familiar sounds,
(ii) the response to intonational form, (iii) metalalia or
delayed imitation, (iv) the imitation of new sound-groups,
(v) echolalia.

*SECTION III. THE FIRST ACQUISITION
OF CONVENTIONAL SPEECH*

VII THE BEGINNING OF COMPREHENSION OF CONVENTIONAL
SPEECH 105
The onset of comprehension. The nature of this comprehension. The persistence of tendencies already observed :
(i) the maturation of purposive movements, (ii) response
to the intonational patterns of speech. Adult speech
as a stimulus. The process of training.

VIII THE BEGINNING OF MEANINGFUL USE OF CONVEN-
TIONAL SPEECH 124
The occurrence of the child's earliest conventional words.
The form of these words. Their meaning. The process
of stabilisation : (i) expression as a factor, (ii) babbling as
a factor, (iii) imitation as a factor, (iv) training as a
factor. The concurrence of these factors.

IX THE NATURE OF THIS PROGRESS 143
The growth of objective reference. Our judgment of the
change. The data. The general course of development :
response and utterance. The process of development :
(i) response to a word ; (ii) the growth of utterance : (*a*) the
child's primitive cries, (*b*) conventional words, (iii) mutual
effect of utterance and response, (iv) the child's resistance to
change, (v) what is referred to at this stage ? Summary of
the process.

*SECTION IV. THE APPROACH TO THE
CONCEPTUAL USE OF SPEECH*

X THE MASTERY OF CONVENTIONAL FORMS. . . 167
The data. Characteristics of child's language when conventional words are acquired. Relation between the child's
speech and adult language. Characteristics of the middle
period : (i) Elision, (ii) Substitution, (iii) Assimilation :
(*a*) general, (*b*) special. Uniformity of children's language.
The parallel with Verbal Aphasia.

CONTENTS

CHAP.   PAGE

XI   THE EXPANSION OF MEANING   189
Occurrence of expansion. Extension as the growth of
generalisation. I. The early wide use of sounds. II.
The kinds of similarity among situations : Objective
similarity : (i) of the situation as a whole, (ii) of particular
features, (iii) shifting from feature to feature. The affective aspect of extension. Functional similarity (i) in the
child's own activity, (ii) in the activity of others. III. The
place of the word in the child's behaviour. Wide range
of responses to conventional words. The wide application of spoken words : (i) the natural features of the acquired word, (ii) its conventional features. Declarative
extension. Manipulative extension.

XII FURTHER PROGRESS IN CONVENTIONAL USE   .   .   210
The child's own discrimination. Personal and social
factors. The process as observed. Objective discrimination. The affective aspect. The functional aspect.
The instrumental aspect. The conventional nature of
conceptual thinking. Genesis of conceptual thinking.
Stern's account. Spearman's account.

APPENDICES :

I   THE SOUNDS UTTERED SPONTANEOUSLY BY CHILDREN
IN THE COURSE OF THEIR FIRST YEAR.   .   .   233

II   SOUNDS UTTERED IN IMMEDIATE IMITATION DURING THE
FIRST YEAR   243

III THE DEVELOPMENT OF FORM   253

IV   RESPONSE AND UTTERANCE   300

V   THE APPROACH TO CONVENTIONAL USAGE   .   .   314

REFERENCES   323

INDEX   329

KEY TO PHONETIC SYMBOLS

(Symbols of International Phonetic Association, with words in which they normally occur)

SE. = Southern English ; Fr. = French ; Ger. = German.

VOWELS

a	Fr. l*a*.		ɔ	SE. h*o*g.
ɑ	SE. f*a*ther.		ø	Fr. p*eu*.
e	SE. p*e*n.		u	SE. l*oo*k.
ɛ	Fr. p*è*re.		ai	SE. l*i*ke.
æ	SE. m*a*n.		ei	SE. p*a*ne.
ə	Fr. l*e*.		ou	SE. h*o*pe.
i	SE. p*i*n.		au	SE. n*ow*.
i:	SE. k*ee*n.		:	lengthening.
o	Fr. p*au*se.		~	nasalisation.
ʌ	SE. b*u*t.			

CONSONANTS

ç	Ger. i*ch*.		ŋ	SE. thi*ng*.
ð	SE. *th*en.		s	SE. *s*ing.
j	SE. *y*our.		ʃ	SE. *sh*ip.
g	(velar fricative ; see p. 31).		θ	SE. *th*ought.
ɲ	Fr. oi*gn*on.		ʒ	SE. plea*s*ure.
			x	Ger. do*ch*.

Other consonants approximately as in SE.

SEMI-CONSONANTS

ɥ	Fr. p*ui*s.		ŭ	(consonantal *u* ; see p. 27).

PREFACE

THIS book began in an attempt to make clear to myself the manner in which speech begins in children. When I first became interested in the growth of language, I was impressed, as anyone must be, by the wealth of the material that had accumulated. It did not occur to me that any part of the subject remained to be examined. But as I read on, I found myself often coming back to the same question : How are those characteristics of speech, which we usually see flowering during the course of a child's second year, related to his earlier experience and behaviour ? I realised then, that apart from one or two pioneers such as Preyer, writers were surprisingly silent on this topic.

But I am no longer surprised. The sounds that a child makes during his first few months are so elusive and apparently so remote from anything that might be called language that any observer—however interested in speech—might well be pardoned for waiting until the noises become, at any rate, a little more obviously human. To persist in making observations one must be interested in the variety of human sounds merely as sounds, one must have faith in the continuity of growth, and in addition, perhaps, one must have something of that insensitiveness to ridicule which is found at its highest in the truly devoted parent.

Before I had the opportunity of making the observations which I discuss in this book, I had become familiar with the work of such men as Preyer, Meumann and Stern. These made me feel the importance of close attention to the child's actual sounds, while an interest in phonetics had given me some practice in attempting to record unfamiliar speech. At the same time, an acquaintance with recent discussions of the nature of language convinced me of the necessity of recording the details of the child's behaviour while he was making sounds and responding to those made by others. If, then, there is any central theme in the book, it is this : I have tried to show that a coherent account of the child's linguistic growth may be given by considering at every stage the relation between his general behaviour and his behaviour as a speaker and listener.

While thinking about these topics, I was fortunate in being able to discuss them with others. Thus, part of Chapter XI was given as a paper at the Aberdeen meeting of the British Association in 1934, and part of Chapter XII at the Norwich meeting in 1935, and much of Chapter X was summarised before the Second International Congress of Phonetic Sciences in London in 1935. The greater part of the work in its original form was approved as a thesis for the degree of Ph.D. in the University of London. While preparing this thesis, I had the inestimable advantage of constant discussions with Dr. J. C. Flugel; to him I owe a debt of gratitude I cannot easily express. Finally, I will mention my wife, although I will not attempt to thank her in this place : she has given me help and encouragement since I first began to think about the speech of children.

INFANT SPEECH

Chapter i

INTRODUCTION

THE object of the present work is to give an ordered account
of the early stages of the development of language in children,
based upon the published records and my own observations.
The standard work on this topic is, of course, C. and W. Stern's
Die Kindersprache, a book which, when it was published in 1907,
summarised in a masterly fashion the observations which had
been so plentiful during the preceding twenty or thirty years.
After nearly another thirty years, this book still remains the
indispensable guide of all who study the subject, and will, there
is little doubt, prove to be the foundation of much further work.

Since Stern's book was published, observations have perhaps
not been so plentiful as they were in the preceding generation,
so that its fourth edition in 1928 had little need of revision on
this account. But if this period has been poor in observations,
it has been rich in other work which has thrown new light upon
our subject. In particular, the development of the mechanical
reproduction of the human voice has given a fresh impetus to
the study of phonetics ; unfortunate victims of the War made
possible the remarkable work of Head on aphasia ; while a
general increase of interest in the conditions of communal life
has brought with it a closer study of the social functions of
language. All this is making a vast difference to the manner
in which we must approach the study of children's language,
but—it is not unfair to say—it has received little recognition
in the last edition of *Die Kindersprache*.

It is, therefore, possible for us to supplement that work. In
the first place, we can make a much fuller analysis of the earliest
stages of development. The first few months of the child's life
form a period whose importance is being increasingly recognised : but the beginnings of language at this time have

received little attention from the Sterns. As Grégoire points out (AP 375), neither their observations nor their general conclusions have much to tell us of the child before his ninth month. Further, Stern himself—and it is to him that we owe the theoretical sections of *Die Kindersprache*—shows little or no interest in phonetics : yet a phonetic analysis of the rudiments of speech is essential if we are to understand the true nature of its development. I hope that my own observations and conclusions will be found to have some value in making clear the earliest stages of language in the child.

Secondly, I have given fuller attention to the bearing of recent linguistic work upon our subject. The recognition of the essential characters of language in human life—characters which tend to be obscured in the highly-developed written language of civilised societies—makes it possible to discern the rudiments of speech in the earliest sounds that the child utters. Further, recent linguistic study has also laid stress upon the effect of the accompanying situation in determining the particular use of speech at any given moment ; so that an examination of the situations in which a child makes sounds or responds to the speech of others gives us a further clue to the beginnings of his linguistic growth. The continuity of his development becomes clear. Where Stern tends to describe the various characteristics of the child's early stages as isolated topics, regarding everything before the moment when he begins to use conventional speech as a mere preparation for that achievement, we may now trace a progressive development up to and beyond this point right from the very beginning.

Sources of the Data.—The study of children relies upon sources of two kinds for its data : the continued observations of individual children, and the statistical results derived from the examination of a large number of children with regard to particular points. It is evident that in both cases the validity of any conclusions will depend either upon the control of the circumstances in which the observations are made ; or—in the absence of this—on as full a record as possible of the uncontrolled circumstances. Unfortunately, a good deal of the early work on children's language satisfied neither of these conditions.

The effect of this in the study of individual children is seen in the weakness of those " anecdotal " records in which isolated incidents were noted without any relation to the course of the child's development. The parallel to this among statistical studies is to be found in those voluminous lists of vocabulary—often presented with an entire absence of background—the uselessness of which has become a byword. Stern found himself unable to make much use of either of these groups of data.

But by each method of observation results of value may certainly be achieved. In statistical work this has been shown by the studies of children which have issued from the school of Charlotte Bühler : Stern makes some reference to this work, and I have been able to use it more fully, both that which was available when the last edition of *Die Kindersprache* appeared, and that which has been done since.

To a large extent, however, I have relied upon a source which for long has been under a cloud : the detailed observation of a particular child. It is true that the recital of isolated anecdotes —as was the custom forty years ago—can furnish us with results of little importance ; but careful observations extending over a long period of a child's life may be of the highest value, provided that due attention is given not only to the actual sounds that he makes and to those to which he responds, but also to the circumstances in which these events occur. These observations will not enable us to formulate statistical conclusions, such as the time when children in general first begin to behave in a particular way, or the extent of a normal vocabulary at any particular age ; but they certainly give us the greatest insight into the processes of development, by enabling us to relate the child's linguistic behaviour at any one moment both to his earlier behaviour and to the concurrent events. I have drawn therefore upon the work of Preyer, Deville, Ament, Guillaume, Hoyer, Valentine and Stern himself wherever the necessary conditions of observation are satisfied ; and to these I have added my own regular observations of a boy K, who was born in October 1929, and whose physical development has been normal. It will be seen that I used a recognised phonetic script to record his sounds, and that I also made full notes both of the conditions of their utterance and of his responses to the speech of others.

Arrangement of the Work.—I have tried to present a systematic account of the usual course of development ; but since there are many factors at work, to study each one and yet keep all in view is only possible if we consider this development as a series of successive stages. As will be seen from the summary of the chapters, I have begun with an introductory section in which I describe my view of the nature of language, based on recent work on the subject ; in the next section I deal with the beginnings, first of utterance, then of response to speech ; in Section III I discuss in detail two fundamental processes, babbling and imitation ; in Section IV I pass on to the first acquisition of conventional language, which leads on in the last section to a study of the beginning of the conceptual use of speech. Throughout I have attempted to present each stage in relation to the whole course of development, while all the material upon which I have drawn is given, together with my own records, in the Appendices.

CHAPTER II

SOME CHARACTERISTICS OF LANGUAGE

THE student of children's language will inevitably be guided in some measure by fundamental assumptions concerning the nature of language in general ; and as it is best that these should be clearly formulated at the outset, I propose in the present chapter to outline briefly what seem to me the acceptable views that emerge from recent work.

During the last few years there has been a marked increase of interest in the nature of language and—in spite of some divergence of opinion on questions of detail—one idea has received marked emphasis : that language is a form of activity, a mode of human behaviour, perhaps the most important. This emphasis on activity, one might hazard, is one aspect of the growing tendency in recent years to look at the mind with the eye of the biologist, to see thought as a form of behaviour : and, recognising the close relation between thought and language, to see the latter also as a form of behaviour.

The change of attitude towards language may be illustrated by reminding ourselves of the controversy aroused by Max Müller's famous *Lectures* in 1887. It is important to notice that the criticisms directed against his dictum " No thoughts without words " were not concerned to deny the connection between thought and words. It was felt, rather, that he had either gone too far or not far enough.

The former point—that Müller had gone too far—was taken up by such men as Galton and Romanes.[1] Although prepared to accept the basic assertion that words are the " signs " of thoughts, they were also concerned to show that a good deal of mental activity might go on without the intermediary of words. In brief, Müller was making too much of the dependence of thought upon language.

The contrasting criticism, that Müller had not gone far enough, came from across the Atlantic. Whitney, without mincing matters, assured his colleague Müller that he had

[1] Appendix to Müller ST 1, 13.

missed the point (MM 26) : on the one hand thought is quite possible without words, on the other hand language has a far wider function than providing " signs " for " thoughts ". Language plays a fundamental part in all human activity : it is man's chief instrument. To quote what he had said nearly twenty years since : " The human capacity to which the production of language is most directly due is the power of intelligently . . . adapting means to ends " (LG 303).

It is the view here expressed by Whitney which has become the leading idea in the study of language during recent years. And it is essentially a biological view—it brings immediately into the foreground the main function of language in human life as the mediator between man and man. Language comes into its own, as one of the chief of human activities.

In America, in particular, we find this idea taken up and developed by a line of writers. Dewey, in a series of publications extending from the time of Müller up to our own day (PI, published 1894 ; CT, published 1931), has repeatedly insisted that language is an instrument, a mode of activity, whereby human behaviour in society is initiated and fostered. In the same way, Watson's Behaviouristic advance upon Müller —" No thoughts, *only* words "—becomes possible by insisting that language is the prime instrument of human behaviour. And this Behaviouristic attitude towards language, in one form or another, influences a great deal of American writing to-day : it permeates such recent work as that of Markey (SP), Lorimer (GR) and De Laguna (S), all of whom acknowledge the influence of Dewey.

A similar emphasis is to be found in recent work by European writers. In France it is represented by what we may regard as the standard work on language—Delacroix's *Le Langage et la Pensée* ; in Switzerland by De Saussure (LG), in Austria and Germany by K. Bühler (TS and KP) and Cassirer (CS) ; and in England by Head (A), Malinowski (MM) and Gardiner (SL).

Now it is noteworthy that these writers, almost without exception, have been driven to the recognition of the instrumental function of language through the study of primitive communities, of aphasics, or of children. For it is only when we confine ourselves to language in its complete and sophisticated form—the system that is to be found preserved in books— that we are likely to lose sight of its essential nature. Where we see it in a primitive form, or impaired, the fact of its instrumental function is forcibly brought home to us. Certainly, the student of children can be in no doubt; when he observes the rudimentary beginnings of speech in an infant it is not the acquisition of a " system of signs " that he sees, but the growth of a mode of action which rapidly becomes an important instrument for the child within his limited communal life.

In brief, if we compare Max Müller's dictum with the trend of recent linguistic study, we find this very significant change : that words are regarded, not as the signs of thoughts, but as the symbols of behaviour. Language is recognised to be that particular form of behaviour whose function it is to take the place of any other behaviour.

Language and Speech.—This change of emphasis has made modern writers more conscious of the distinction between language as behaviour and as a human institution, preserved in literature and codified in grammars and dictionaries. In French, the distinction is marked by a difference of terms— *langue* for the institution, *langage* for the activity—a point well brought out by De Saussure (LG 27) and adopted from him by Delacroix (LP 54). English writers find themselves in a difficulty here, and Gardiner (SL 62) therefore suggests that the word " language " should be used in the sense of the French *langue*, while " speech " is reserved for the name of the activity.

In dealing with children we find ourselves almost unwittingly adopting this distinction, particularly as one ambiguity in the use of the word " speech " does not arise—the child has no written language. We can say that we study the child by observing how his speech advances to the acquisition of adult language, influenced as he is at every point by adult speech.

However the distinction between the activity and the institution may be marked, it is certainly an important one. The linguist, who—in the past at any rate—has been concerned mainly with language as an institution, is likely to say that the infant has no language. But although this may be true, the infant certainly has speech : his cries rapidly become an instrument mediating between himself and his social environment. It may safely be said that failure to recognise that these early cries are rudimentary speech has been one of the main defects of the study of the child's linguistic development.

Our problem then is this : at the outset we find the child engaged in uttering cries, and somewhat later engaged in responding to the speech of others. By what process does this rudimentary linguistic activity become transformed into the use and comprehension of conventional language ? This is a fundamental problem of education, a very important instance of that process whereby the child's innate endowment of propensities and abilities becomes transformed by social life into an accepted mode of behaviour.

The Main Features of Speech.—To say that speech is an instrument, a tool, helps us at once to distinguish its main features. We can ask about any instrument, of what material it is made, how it works, and what purpose it serves.

Speech is made up of written or spoken patterns ; it works by mediating between the speaker and the listener ; and it subserves all the ultimate purposes of human activity—practical, scientific, æsthetic and religious alike. These ultimate purposes we are not called upon to discuss here ; we have to confine ourselves to the other two aspects of speech as an instrument—the material of which it is made, and how it works.

The Patterns of the Spoken Language.—It is sometimes asserted—as by De Saussure and Sapir—that the material of which language consists has nothing whatever to do with its functions : that phonetics can give no help to the linguist. De Saussure (LG 37) goes so far as to say that the vocal organs have no more to do with language itself than a telegraph machine has to do with the Morse alphabet. If he really means this, he is undoubtedly wrong, but perhaps he means no more than Sapir when he points out (L 21) that the mere sounds of speech are not the essential fact of language.

Of course, it is true that sounds are not the only possible material for a language ; it is none the less true that language has become what we know it to be to-day because it is made up of sounds. Even apart from the fact that vestiges of its "natural" origin remain embedded in every conventional language, to the student of the development of speech in children some attention to linguistic form is indispensable. For the forms of the child's primitive cries reveal their physiological basis, and thus help us to understand their functions in his life. Further, as the child grows, these changes in the form of his speech run parallel to changes in function, and indicate the progress of his development in relation to the adult language.

The most important feature of the form of language for our

special topic here is one to which increasing recognition has been given in recent linguistic studies : the fact that a speech-sound has not an absolute value, once and for all, but that its effectiveness in action depends upon its relationship to the other sounds with which it forms a *pattern*. According to such linguists as De Saussure (LG 171) and Sapir (L 56), speech is not, therefore, merely a series of sounds each of which can be defined by its pitch and mode of articulation : speech is, rather, composed of a succession of patterns.

These patterns are of two kinds, which may be called the *phonetic* and the *intonational*. By phonetic pattern I mean the mere succession of sounds, such as might be indicated in phonetic script for such a sentence as *Who is this man?* (**hu iz ðis mæn**). When I utter this sentence I probably do not make exactly the same sounds as you do, but we understand each other ; partly, no doubt, because our different individual sounds fall within certain limits, but still more because the general phonetic pattern of our sentences remains the same. Intermingled with this phonetic pattern there is the intonational [1] pattern, by which I mean the pattern of rhythm, stress and pitch. Thus while the phonetic pattern of a given unit of speech may remain constant there will still be variations of intonational form according to the meaning. In the sentence *Who is this man?* the word *man* is a phonetic pattern having a definite intonational pattern according to the conditions under which the sentence is spoken.

The spoken language may be said, then, to consist of an intermingling of phonetic and intonational patterns ; and the child's development is a process of learning to practise these patterns of activity.

What is the relation between these patterns and the meaning ; in other words, what part is played by each of these characteristics of form in promoting the effectiveness of language as a means of mediating between man and man ? Before we can answer this question we have to consider briefly how language obtains this effectiveness—that is to say, how it works.

The Speaker, the Listener, and the Situation.—Taking language as we find it at work, we may say that essentially it is a means whereby one man brings another into relation with a given

---

[1] Though this is perhaps not quite satisfactory, I think it is nearer to current usage than Beach's term *tonetic* (cited by Palmer EI 3) or Gardiner's term *elocutional* (SL 200).

situation. We have a speaker, a listener, and something spoken about—a situation.

This analysis, only too obvious though it may be, is worth making, because in the past the emphasis on language in relation to the speaker has been so strong that its other functions—in relation to a situation and a listener—have almost been forgotten. To say that words are the signs of thoughts is true, but it loses more than half its truth when we forget that thoughts are our means of dealing with the world around us, and words the means by which we get others to help us to do so. It has become necessary, therefore, for recent writers to remind us of this—De Saussure (LG 129), Ogden and Richards (MM 11), and Dewey (CT 203)—while a professed linguist like Gardiner finds it worth while to write a whole book in order to make this one assertion (SL 126). Gardiner goes so far as to say that the nature of speech cannot be understood unless we consider the situations in which acts of speech occur. Certainly, nothing could be truer of children's language; it is one of the main themes of the chapters which follow to show that the chief clue to understanding the development of the child's speech lies in considering the situations in which it is used.

Our problem, then, resolves itself into this : in what manner does language work as a means of mediation between speaker and listener with regard to a situation ? We may take as a basis for discussion the analysis made by K. Bühler (TS), which is of double interest to us here as coming from one who is both a student of children and a linguist.

Bühler : the Threefold Nature of Speech.—Bühler points out that three functions are present in every act of speech : Expression (*Kundgabe*), Evocation (*Auslösung*) and Representation (*Darstellung*). On a given occasion one or the other may be dominant : but when any of the three is absent, the activity cannot be regarded as language.

I think that, subject to some modification, this analysis is not only fundamentally sound, but particularly illuminating for the study of children's speech. What is the nature of each of these three functions ?

(i) *Expression and the Emotive Function of Language.*—As a translation of *Kundgabe*, Bühler sanctions the use of *expression*, a word which, however, introduces a difficulty, for it has at least three different meanings. First there is the common meaning—given, for instance by the Oxford Dictionary : " To express is to reveal or manifest by external tokens." In this way the term covers the complete function of language ; Head, for instance, defines language as " symbolical formulation and expression ".

Two narrower meanings of the word belong to special theories. Of these the first is associated with Croce, the other with Darwin.

For Croce (A 11), the word *expression* is to be used only for the work of an artist, the process whereby his intuition is given a form. Expression here is equivalent to æsthetic symbolisation, although the symbols need not appear in overt behaviour, but may exist solely in the mind of the artist.[1] This meaning of the term has found acceptance only among professed followers of Croce, such as Vivante and Vossler.

Darwin's use of the word, as put forward in his work on *The Expression of the Emotions*, is limited in another way ; it names those forms of overt behaviour which not only reveal an affective state but are also innately bound up with that state, and one of the chief forms of expression consists in uttering cries. What, however, Bühler maintains is that the expressive function of language in adult life is something more than Darwinian expression. Let us therefore, he says, call this fully-fledged function not expression (*Ausdruck*) but *Kundgabe* ; it is a pity, then, that he allows this latter term also to be translated " expression ", and does not adopt either " emotional " (suggested by Hughlings Jackson) or " emotive " (suggested by Ogden and Richards).

What do we mean by this emotive function of language ? To answer the question we have to make a brief survey of the history of the theory of expression. We find that this comes into the modern study of language by two routes, both of which derive something from Herbert Spencer's *Essay on Music* (1857). On one side we have Hughlings Jackson, leading to Head's great work on aphasia, on the other Darwin, leading to the modern view of expression in general psychology.

Hughlings Jackson, in one of the papers rescued for us by Head, pointed out in 1866 (B 44) that aphasia is only rightly to be understood if a clear distinction is made between the emotional and propositional functions of language, a distinction, he tells us, which he owed to Spencer's *Essay*. The expression

---

[1] Thus what Croce calls expression would be regarded by most people as the absence of expression !

of emotion, he adds, is innately determined; in the civilised adult it lies buried beneath the acquired habits of propositional language.

A little later, in 1873, Darwin put forward the same idea in another form, with emphasis upon the innate character of the expression of emotion and an attempt to trace its evolution. Acknowledging his debt (EE 86) to Spencer's *Essay* for the special notion that speech arises as a form of expression, he adds that the general theory of innate expression had been suggested several times in the course of the century, since the publication of Bell's work, *The Anatomy of Expression*, in 1806. Bell had maintained that there was an innate connection between those muscular movements, which we call expressive, and the changes of respiration which characterise an emotional state (AE 83). Darwin extended the notion, to include a wider range of bodily reactions; for instance, when a creature is in pain, glandular and muscular activity occurs, which shows itself as the movements and gestures expressive of pain; this characteristic activity is to be regarded as innate.

Darwin's view is the foundation of the modern view of expression. Among the physiologists, for instance, we find Cannon, a recognised authority on the nature of bodily change in affective states, accepting Darwin's account of expressive movements and two out of his three principles explaining their origin (BC 43). Among the psychologists, Darwin's view has been adopted, in the essentials, by all the divergent schools alike—by McDougall, by the Gestalt School, by the psychoanalysts, by the Reflexologists and by the Behaviorists.[1]

We may then take these two points as fully accepted, first that fully-fledged adult language is emotive, secondly that affective states of the individual find innate forms of expression, some of which are vocal. The question which now arises is whether there is any connection between the emotive use of fully-fledged language and these innate forms of vocal expression.

Bühler's answer is definitely, None. Not only is *Kundgabe* in adult language something more than mere *Ausdruck*, but in the development of the individual, articulate speech is quite distinct from expressive cries (TS 1).

Now there can be no doubt that the emotive use of language in adult life is not the same thing as Darwinian expression—

[1] McDougall OP 322; Koffka GM 131, 398; Bernfeld PI 19; Bekhterev ER 276; Watson PB 338; Landis EE 498.

this is asserted by one writer after another, for instance Whitney (SL 438) and Sapir (L 7), among the linguists, Croce (A 95) among the philosophers, and Stout (MP 546) among the psychologists.

But does this necessarily mean that there is no connection at all between the emotive use of complete adult language and the innate vocal expression of childhood? At an early age the child utters sounds expressive of emotion; later he uses words expressive of emotion; what is the relation between these two acts? Two alternatives are possible: either—as Bühler maintains (TS 1)—there comes a moment in the child's life when he suddenly acquires emotive adult language which has no connection with his earlier expressive cries, or—as I hope to show in the pages that follow—there is a continuous process of development from the earliest expressive cry to the full use of emotive speech.

(ii) *Representation and Reference*.—Bühler's notion of *Darstellung* is beset with difficulty, both in its original form and when translated as *representation*. For one way of representing a thing is to make something else stand for it, take its place: language certainly does this to some extent. But language also points things out for us, a fact that Bühler recognises by asserting that Darstellung includes the function of *hinweisen*. Thus he is really emphasising what everybody recognises, that words are signs, for a sign may sometimes take the place of a thing and sometimes point it out.

When, however, we have said this we have certainly not said all; words, in acting as signs, have something more than the two functions we have just described, and a good deal of recent discussion has been concerned in elucidating just what it is that they do. Among English psychologists nobody has put the matter so clearly as Stout, whose statement in his *Analytic Psychology* remains after forty years one of the most penetrating studies of language, although largely unacknowledged by subsequent writers on this theme.

A word, he agrees (AP II 193), is certainly a sign, but signs may be of three kinds: suggestive signs, substitute signs and expressive signs. A word is not merely a suggestive sign, like a number on a door, a means of pointing out the thing to us. Nor is a word a substitute sign which, like an algebraical symbol, stands instead of a thing, and " so long as it fulfils its *representative* function, renders useless all *reference* to that which it represents ".[1] A word is, rather, an expressive sign, that is, " an instrument for thinking about the meaning which it expresses ". Thus Stout distinguishes very clearly between representation and reference, and decides that words have undoubtedly the latter function, their use being to foster our reference to things.

It may safely be said that nothing is so fundamental to a true understanding of the nature of language as this distinction which Stout introduces so quietly into his analysis. It is the theme of pages of discussion by one writer after another.

Thus a good deal of recent German work has been summarised by Dempe who, in his critical amplification of Bühler, points out (WS 84) that the relation between a word and its meaning is always something more than mere association ; the word must be interpreted (aufgefasst). We pass from a word to its meaning by an act of interpretation. This is exactly Stout's view that words enable us to " think about " their meaning.

In recent American work again, we find precisely the same point made by Lorimer, who shows (GR 84) that Dewey and Whitehead have this in common, that both insist upon the referential function of language : Dewey when he urges that language serves as the means of organising our thought about things, and Whitehead when he tells us that " symbolic reference "—the essential character of language—is a process of functioning in which a transition is made from a symbol to its meaning.

What clearly emerges from these discussions is that the main use of language is not " representative " but " referential " ; it is by means of words that we refer to things. To cite Ogden and Richards, from whom we have adopted this term " referential " ; a word is not a sign of a thing, it is a symbol of an act of reference (MM 205).

The most cogent support for this distinction comes from the study of aphasia ; this is, indeed, Head's great contribution to the theory of language. Inspired by the work of Hughlings Jackson, he has pointed out the great significance of the fact that aphasics, as a rule, are not defective in the power of matching a word with a thing : what suffers is the more recently acquired and more complex process of " symbolic formulation and expression : a mode of behaviour in which

[1] Italics mine.

some verbal or other symbol plays a part between the initiation and the execution of an act " (A 211).

The full implication of this for the study of language has been taken up by Cassirer. Symbolisation—of which speech is the most important type—is a means, he points out (CS 321), through which we deal with phenomena by grouping them together, relating them to each other, instead of taking each one as it comes. This is true of the whole range of thinking, from perception onwards. The normal person, for instance, sees a number of diverse colours as gradations of red ; this only becomes possible by the use of some such symbol as the word " red ". But the aphasic, whose power of symbolisation has become defective, can no longer carry out this grouping ; on seeing a given red he says " blood ", thus linking it with a single particular object, rather than relating it to other reds.

All civilised life, says Cassirer, depends upon behaviour of this kind. The main difference, indeed, between human and animal life is this, that the animal tends to live on the plane of the immediate—he deals directly with the world around him ; whereas man, using language, substitutes the mediate behaviour of symbolisation. The aphasic, then, may be regarded as having retrogressed from civilised thinking towards a more primitive immediacy of behaviour.

Thus we see that on all sides—among linguists, psychologists and pathologists—there is a growing recognition of the referential function of language as that process in which we make use of the special behaviour of speech instead of more immediate intercourse with things : so that if words represent at all, they represent, not things, but our behaviour with regard to things. And in studying children we shall find that their progress consists not in learning words as names labelling or representing things but in the growth of power to use vocal behaviour as a means of supplementing—and in the end, replacing—other behaviour.

(iii) *Evocation and Communication.*—The third essential feature of language is that it arouses a response in the listener. This has two important effects upon the speaker's use of words : he directs them so that they will evoke a response from another, and he himself responds to them as he speaks them. It has been the object of a good deal of recent work to emphasise this idea that the evocative function plays an important part in making language what it is : not that language consists of words which have emotive and referential functions and are then communicated, but that by the very act of communication language becomes more effectively emotive and referential.

The place of language in social life has long been understood ; as Ward puts it (PP 287), " without language we should be mutually exclusive and impenetrable ". What, however, is now being emphasised is the converse : the effect of social life upon language. The point touched on by Whitney in 1867 (SL 438)—that the ideas of speech and of community are inseparable—has since then been reiterated in a variety of ways and with increasing emphasis, largely under the influence of such work as that of Durkheim and Lévy-Bruhl on the social origin of individual human behaviour.

Among those who maintain the importance of society in determining the nature of language are De Saussure (LG 24), Delacroix (LD 63), and De Laguna (L 139) ; the last of these attempting to demonstrate that the evolution of language has been determined more by the need to communicate than by any other factor, and urging that this need permeates all the aspects of language ; that is, its evocative function determines its emotive and referential features. The latter point, again, is the special theme of Hocart (PL) and Malinowski (MM), both of whom show that the conceptual use of words arises out of communal needs in dealing with environment ; and it is taken up by Gardiner (SL) in discussing our everyday speech, and by Piaget (LP) in dealing with the development of logical thinking in children over the age of three. In the chapters which follow I hope to show what effect this function of evocation has upon the very beginnings of growth of speech.

Further, the fact that each person responds to language when he himself speaks has a far-reaching effect upon the growth of its meaning for him. This has been made the subject of special study by Markey, who sets out to show (SP 123) that responses of this kind constitute an important influence in determining the growth of language as an instrument in thinking. Certainly, the young children with whom we are here concerned are helped enormously by the fact that adults take over their sounds and stabilise the function of these as language, so that the child learns language by responding to his own sounds—as spoken both by himself and by others.

The Relation between Function and Form.—To come now to

the relation between the functions of language and its forms : it is commonly held that the emotive function of language is expressed in its intonational form, while its referential function appears in its phonetic form. Thus the phonetic pattern in the word *man* is a means of causing reference to a particular object, while the tone in which it is said expresses the affective attitude of the speaker and evokes some such attitude in the listener. But while in the main this is undoubtedly true, we must recognise that the parallel between function and form is by no means absolute : the phonetic pattern, for instance, may be emotive, as in the phrase *I'm sorry* ; the intonational pattern may be referential, as when we say *tiny* in a thin high-pitched voice. This intercrossing of functions and forms is, in fact, one of the means by which the child passes from his own expressive utterance to the fully-fledged referential speech of adults.

The Fundamental Nature of these Functions.—There can be no doubt that the analysis of Bühler's, which we have found to be implied in the work of many other writers, does reveal the three essential factors present in every act of speech : the emotive, the referential and the evocative. But while Bühler maintains that the child's own spontaneous utterance is merely expressive, and that at a given moment he begins to adopt adult language which has these three characters, it will be part of our task to show, in the following pages, that they must arise gradually and inevitably in the growth of a normal child, living in society. Certainly, the child's earliest cries are merely expressive, but as soon as he begins to turn his attention— while uttering them—to the situation and to his hearers, the change towards speech also begins. For as he turns his attention to the situation his cries gradually become linked up with this, and thus in some measure representative of it. And as others respond to the child's cries, these become evocative ; at the same time, since his cries are representative of the situation for the child's hearers, they tend to become increasingly representative for him also. Throughout all this the child will tend to use his cries more and more as an aid to the rest of his behaviour, and even as a substitute for it : this means that he is beginning to use it referentially. Gradually the child's utterance changes from a merely expressive cry into speech which is emotive, referential and evocative ; the process occurring partly as the child's hold upon his material and social environment grows, and partly because he is surrounded by speakers of emotive, referential and evocative language.

The details of this process, and the other contributory factors, are discussed in the chapters which follow.

SECTION I
THE BEGINNINGS

CHAPTER III

EARLY UTTERANCE

THE Child's Earliest Cries.—There is no need to point out that language is not imposed upon a silent creature. Whatever else a child may lack, it is certainly not the power of making a noise. No doubt the very first cry that we hear is merely a sign that the child has begun to breathe. The centres which control respiration are stimulated. As the child breathes, the passage of air through the vocal organs produces a characteristic sound which has the phonetic quality of α or ε.

But within a very few hours, the child's cry may be taken as a sign of discomfort ; he is silent only when, as Stern suggests, he is in a state of indifference (KSp 152). We may say that the child's utterance has already become " expressive " of his condition, in Darwin's sense of the word. And to this extent Darwin is generally followed : that the child's cry of discomfort is an innately-determined expression of that state. For us, therefore, it may stand as a first principle.

The further question now arises whether this innate vocal equipment becomes differentiated as the affective states of the child become differentiated. Is each affective state, as it develops, characterised by a specific cry ?

The Differentiation of Expressive Utterance.—Stern (KSp 152) summarising a good deal of earlier work as well as his own observations, concludes that an innate differentiation of affective states may arise within the child's first three months, with a corresponding differentiation of utterance. Immediately after birth, he tells us, the infant moves between two general affective conditions : a state of discomfort, manifested by the characteristic expressive cry, and a state of indifference, manifested by silence. Later, a further differentiation appears ; the child now expresses discomfort and comfort, each by a characteristic utterance, and a state of indifference as before by silence.

This statement is fully corroborated by other observers not mentioned by Stern, for instance, by Bekhterev (PO 426) and by Bridges (GT 516). The latter in her study of fifty children found that soon after birth any strong stimulus produces a state of undifferentiated excitement ; within a short time, sometimes only a few hours, the child's responses begin to be differentiated into the two states of distress and delight, each state being accompanied by specific vocalisation—crying in the former case and soft gurgling noises in the latter.

Are we able to go beyond this, and trace differences of utterance according to the different kinds of discomfort or comfort which the child experiences ? Stern's view (KSp 153) is that after a few weeks it is possible to distinguish the cry of hunger from that of other discomforts ; in this he is in agreement with Preyer (MC 101), Major (FS 284), O'Shea (LD 2), Hoyer (LK 364) and C. Bühler (FY 36). But most of these observers do not tell us what are the differences of utterance corresponding to the different states : Hoyer says only that the cry of general discomfort is more nasalised than the cry of hunger ; Bühler that the latter is often interspersed with sucking-movements. It is of course very difficult to observe either the different cries or the different affective states of a new-born child, so that the remark of Hoyer (LK 365) that on the whole no close correspondence is to be recorded within the first few months must probably be accepted, at any rate so long as observations are carried out by the unaided human eye and ear.

For the present we have to content ourselves with observing the broad differences between sounds expressing comfort and those expressing discomfort. But even here we are in something of a difficulty ; very few of the available records are sufficiently detailed to help us.

Records of Observations.—It might seem surprising that although a great deal has been written on this topic, there are scarcely any published accounts of the earliest sounds made by a child, systematically recorded together with a sufficient statement of the accompanying circumstances. Most observers begin their detailed record at the point where the child first understands and uses conventional language, and mention only a few occasional observations during the previous months. This is true, for instance, of Stern's own work (KSp), as well as of most of the literature named in his bibliography.

The fact is that if an observer is merely keeping a general record of a child's speech he is unlikely to detail either the child's earliest sounds or the circumstances in which they are made. For in the first place it is difficult to identify these sounds as the vowels and consonants of conventional language, and difficult to record them even if one uses a phonetic script. In addition, the circumstances in which the sounds occur will often not seem sufficiently striking to warrant a record. The child, to most observers, begins to be interesting when he shows some understanding of our words, and when his utterances begin to resemble our speech.

But the development of a child's language is only to be fully understood in the light of his earliest utterances, and for this we need not only a list of his speech-sounds, but a statement of the circumstances in which they have occurred. In consulting many of the publications mentioned by Stern, I have been able to find only one, that of Preyer, in which the record is full enough to be of much service to us. From the observations of the Sterns and the Hoyers it is possible to piece together briefer accounts of three more children. In Appendix I I have tabulated these four accounts together with my own record of K.

I feel that I need not apologise for giving my own observations at length, in view of the meagreness of most available accounts. I used the script of the International Phonetic Association, noting each sound by means of the symbol which seemed to represent it most nearly. This means that I have certainly omitted many of the vaguer gurglings and babblings, and probably also that where I have recorded " no new sounds " it was because I was unable to discriminate differences which actually existed.

It will be noted that Appendix I includes only sounds uttered spontaneously ; those made in immediate imitation are given in Appendix II.

In all five cases I have set down the records in two divisions, distinguishing between sounds made in a state of comfort and those made in a state of discomfort. It is evident from their remarks that observers find no difficulty in making this distinction. The circumstances, the child's features, posture and movements and the intonation of his utterance all contribute to give the onlooker an unfailing impression of the child's state. Charlotte Bühler (FY) and Gesell (IG) have, for instance, given very full descriptions of children's expressive movements in their earliest months, Gesell's account being accompanied by detailed photographs, although again neither of these observers has recorded the corresponding utterance in sufficient detail.

From the five records in Appendix I and the general remarks of these and other observers, we can draw up the following summary of the child's development :

TABLE I

THE CHILD'S EARLY SPONTANEOUS UTTERANCE

	Sounds uttered in discomfort.	Sounds uttered in comfort.
I. Vowels . . .	(i) Onset : immediately after birth. (ii) Limited mainly to sounds ɑ, a, ɛ, e. (iii) Often nasalised.	(i) Onset : when the discomfort cries have already begun to appear. (ii) A wider range, much less well-defined in quality. (iii) Very rarely nasalised.
II. Early consonants.	The semi-consonant ŭ appears early, followed by h, l and ŋ.	The back consonants g, x, g, k, r.
III. Later consonants.	The front consonants, almost exclusively nasal : labial m dental n	The front consonants, both nasal and oral : labial nasal m ; oral, p, b dental nasal n; oral, t, d.

(For the key to the phonetic symbols, see page viii, and for a classification of consonants, Appendix III, p. 259.)

Comparison of this with the actual records shows that there are some differences of detail, particularly with regard to the first appearance of nasal consonants. Thus Preyer and Hoyer find that the consonant m occurs in the third month, while Stern does not report its occurrence until the ninth. These are differences which we may put down to the difficulty of observing and recording children's early sounds. But there is no question of the general agreement concerning the order in which the successive characteristic groups of sounds appear, as may be seen from the following brief survey of the statements made by different observers.

Discomfort cries (I and II) : *Vowels and Early Consonants.*— Stern (KSp 152) tells us as a matter of common acceptance, that the characteristic earliest utterance of the child is a rhythmical succession of vocalic cries, ranging from e to ɑ,

interspersed perhaps with the semi-vocalic consonants ŭ or
h (ŭe, he). Among the observations not cited by him, those
of Blanton (BI) made on "a large number of children," fully
bear out his view.

At an early stage, we have pointed out, these vowels sometimes take on a nasal quality. This, as we shall see, is a matter
of some importance, although Stern does not mention it. The
fact is that a nasalised vowel might easily be recorded as though
it were an oral vowel preceded by a nasal consonant ; thus
Blanton (BI 458) tells us that nga (phonetically ŋɛ) is heard
from some children at birth. But as it is not easy to utter this
combination without nasalising the vowel, it is fairly certain
that as soon as a child is recorded as having uttered the nasal
consonant, he has also uttered a nasalised vowel.

There is no question but that nasalisation generally occurs
at an early stage. It is specially mentioned by the Hoyers,
who noticed it at the end of their son's first week (LK 364) ;
Lorimer concludes, from a summary of the published records,
that early nasalisation is of common occurrence (GR 39). I
myself observed nasalised vowels during K's sixth week
(see Appendix I, p. 240).

With regard to the consonants uttered at this stage (ŭ, h, l
and ŋ) ; we have just mentioned that Stern (KSp 152) and
Blanton (BI 458) record the semi-consonants ŭ and h among
the earliest cries ; l occurred in Preyer's son in the third
month (MC 103), in K in the first month ; and ŋ is noted by
Blanton as occurring in the first week, by Preyer in the
third month, by myself in the second month.

Comfort-sounds (I and II) : Vowels and Early Consonants.—
The five records in Appendix I show that when the child is in
a state of comfort he tends to utter vowels of less determinate
character than when he is uncomfortable. They cover a wider
range than the e- to -ɑ discomfort-cries and are rarely nasalised.

As for the consonants, Stern's summary of the published
records brings out these points (KSp 153–5) :

(i) The characteristic back consonants (g, x, g, k, r) appear
when the ŭe, ŭa, discomfort-series are already well established.

(ii) They appear before the occurrence of labials and dentals.

(iii) They occur characteristically in states of comfort. It
is evident that in these back consonants we have a definite
form of utterance, with well-marked characteristics.

The Front Consonants (III).—To turn now to the front consonants : many observers have noted the occurrence of the characteristic labial and dental consonants. In Stern's summaries of the records we find that they appear after the back consonants (KSp 153–5), and that the nasals (**m, n**) occur chiefly in states of discomfort (KSp 355). As to the occurrence of the oral labials and dentals (**p, b, t, d**) he is not so explicit ; but it is evident from our five records, which include two of his own, that they occur almost exclusively in states of comfort. Thus here again we have a well-defined group, with characteristic differences corresponding to states of discomfort and comfort.

It must be noted, however, that the differentiation is certainly not absolutely strict. For instance, while the back consonants **g** and **x** and the labial **b** occur characteristically in states of comfort, they also occur occasionally in states of discomfort. Similarly **m** and **n** occur fairly frequently in states of comfort in the course of the child's second half-year. But a survey of the observations in Appendix I and also of the general remarks that we have just cited shows that the summary given above does represent the main characteristic tendencies of the child's early utterance.

In brief we can say this. The new-born child in a state of discomfort utters vowel-like cries, ranging from **e** to **a,** and frequently nasalised. Soon the semi-consonant **ŭ** intervenes, followed by **h, l,** and **ŋ.** Finally the nasal front consonants **m** and **n** appear. Contrasting with these are the sounds he utters when comfortable. At first these are non-nasalised vowels, of indeterminate quality, interspersed with the back consonants **g, g, x, k,** and **r.** Then front consonants appear, mainly non-nasal, **p, b, t** and **d,** together with the corresponding nasals **m** and **n.**

What light does this analysis throw upon the expressive character of the child's early sounds ? The answer lies in considering their phonetic nature, that is, in noticing which movements of the vocal organs are required to make them.

Phonetic Features of the Child's Earliest Sounds.—We may first of all be allowed to recall that phonetically there is no clear line of division between vowels and consonants. If in the course of utterance we contract some part of the vocal apparatus so that complete or partial closure results, the sound produced has the quality of a consonant ; in the absence of such closure the sound has the quality of a vowel. Evidently there will be instances of sounds which will seem partly vocalic, partly consonantal, in character. For example, if when uttering the vowel **u** we contract the lips still further, the sound takes on the quality of a consonant (**ŭ**) ; in this way we may speak of the child's **ŭ** in **ŭe** as semi-vocalic.

The child's earliest sounds, as we have seen, are vocalic ; consonants begin to appear in his utterance when the contractions at different points of the vocal apparatus become more definite. We may regard this as one instance of that increase in definiteness which marks all the child's motor activities. During a period, therefore, which extends over several months, it is not always easy to decide whether a given sound is vocalic or consonantal.

With this reservation, we may examine the phonetic characteristics of the child's utterance, and consider the relation between the specific sounds and the effective states which they express.

The Earlier Discomfort Cries.—We begin with the principle that there is an innate tendency for a child to vocalise when in discomfort. If he were merely to open his mouth widely and phonate, the sound would be heard as **a** ; and this does occasionally occur, as our summary shows. We might call this the primary open vowel, for when we produce this sound **a,** the tongue is in a more or less relaxed position, resting on the floor of the mouth, and the lips are also in a medium position between the extreme rounding which occurs in **u** and the extreme stretching which occurs in **i.**

But many of the earliest cries of the child are not simply produced by opening the mouth as widely as possible. He is in discomfort, and as Darwin has pointed out (EE 151), the mouth of a child in such circumstances tends to take on " an oblong, almost squarish outline ", the upper lip being raised by the contraction of the muscles round the eye—a reflex mechanism, as he thought, to protect the eyeball from becoming engorged by the increase of blood pressure in the head and face. Darwin himself was not inclined to lay much stress on this explanation, but of the accuracy of the observation there can be no doubt—clear instances are given in the photographs of crying children in his book.

Let us notice what happens to the open sound **a** when the mouth is drawn into this oblong shape ; it inevitably changes its quality and becomes **a**—precisely the sound which is most characteristic of the child's earliest cries. This possibility, that the shape of the mouth—itself due to expressive muscular contractions—might give rise to expressive differences of speech, occurred to Darwin (EE 92), although he did not attempt to apply it to the cry of the child. Following up the clue given by him, we can say that the characteristic form of the child's cry **a** may certainly be called expressive, for it is the direct vocal manifestation of the contractions which occur in a state of discomfort.

We are not saying here that the muscular contractions are the " cause " and the sound **a** the " effect ". What we are pointing out rather is this : that specific contractions are the innate accompaniment of a state of discomfort, that vocalisation is another accompaniment of this state, and that when vocalisation and the contractions occur simultaneously, we hear the sound **a.**

With this clue before us, let us now look at the other sounds which we have found to be characteristic of the child's earliest cries. First we have the further narrowing of the primary open sound **α** in the direction of **ɛ** and **e.** Now it is interesting to notice that these sounds may be produced if the *pitch* of the voice is raised while uttering **a.**[1] And, as we are again reminded by Darwin (EE 88), shrillness is an expressive characteristic of the cries of animals when in pain. Thus **e** and **ɛ** may also be regarded as expressive in nature : they are the vocalic modifications which result from the expressive raising of pitch during a state of discomfort.

A further marked characteristic of utterance at this stage is nasalisation. This too we may show to have an expressive basis. For nasalisation in speech occurs very frequently when we wish to produce a greater volume of sound ; it is well known that some public speakers tend unconsciously to nasalise their speech in the effort to increase its carrying power. The volume of sound is certainly increased by nasalisation : Paget, working with his artificial resonators, found (HS 215) that the addition of a nasal cavity (the equivalent of nasalisation in human speech) invariably had this effect.

We may reasonably suppose that nasalisation occurs in the child's utterance, as he tries to scream his loudest under the stress of hunger or other discomfort. If this is so, nasalisa-

---

[1] This has been demonstrated experimentally by Engelhardt and Gehrcke (VT) by means of gramophone records played at varying speeds.

tion may well be regarded as expressive in the Darwinian sense, in that it is a quality taken on by the child's cries as he tries—unconsciously—to increase their volume. This is a point of some importance when we come to consider the nasal consonants which appear later.

We pass now to the group of sounds ŭ, l, ŋ, h which commonly occur interspersed among the child's early vocalic cries: ŭ and h from the outset, the others later. Phonetically, these four sounds may all be characterised in this way: they occur during the utterance of a vowel if the vocal organs are momentarily either allowed to relax or to contract. The child does not utter one prolonged vowel; he produces a series of rhythmical cries: for instance, ŭe-ŭe-ŭe . . . or le-le-le . . . , the one vowel e in fact being broken up into a series of cries, as the mouth partially contracts for a moment before letting out the next bellow. The contraction however is not usually sharp enough to produce the effect of a definite consonant.

Now there are, roughly speaking, four points in the vocal apparatus at which a vocalic cry might be modified: the lips, the front of the tongue against the hard palate, the back of the tongue against the soft palate, and the vocal chords. The first of these modifications would give the quality of ŭ, the second that of l, the third that of g, or with nasalisation ŋ, the fourth that of h. For if the lips partially contract while a vowel is being uttered, the semi-consonantal ŭ will tend to appear; the vowel, a or e or whatever it may be, takes on for the moment the character of ŭ. Again, if the tip or blade of the tongue [1] happens to touch the hard palate—while the sides of the tongue are still lowered to allow the breath to pass out—l results. This, as Jones points out (PE 22), may happen during the utterance of any vowel, the main part of the tongue being still in position for that vowel. Again, during the utterance of the nasalised vowels which tend to appear in crying, the back of the tongue is raised and the uvula correspondingly relaxed so that the breath may pass out through the nasal passage. If now the back of the tongue is contracted further towards the soft palate, ŋ results. Finally, if the vocal chords, which are being held close together during the production of a vowel, are relaxed for a moment,

[1] Jespersen (ND 194) noticed that in children of this age l is formed by the blade of the tongue, and not as in adults by the tip. In other words, the sound is produced rather less definitely by the infant, the contact being made vaguely by the fore part of the tongue.

h appears ; to cite Jones again, " **h** is the fricative sound heard as the air passes through the open glottis, the other organs being in position for the following vowel " (PE 33). In other words, **h** is the sound heard if the voice is momentarily withheld in the act of uttering any vowel.

Each of these four semi-consonants is therefore expressive. The child's vocal organs function rhythmically ; as Wundt points out (VP 287), we may regard this as an instance of the rhythm which characterises the utterance of all animals. The child, in fact, utters not one prolonged cry, but a series of cries, and as the vocal apparatus is contracted or relaxed at the beginning of each successive cry, the listener hears a modified sound which is consonantal in quality. Then, according to the place at which the modification takes place, it is heard as something approaching ŭ, l, ŋ, or h.

Thus we are able to show that all the chief characteristics of the child's discomfort cries—vocalic and consonantal— are expressive, in the accepted Darwinian sense of this term.

The Earlier Comfort-sounds.—Let us pass to the comfort-sounds. Here again we begin with the principle that there is an innate tendency for the child to vocalise when in a state of comfort, although this vocalisation makes its appearance only when the expression of discomfort is already well established. But why should the sounds uttered in comfort take the form of the back consonants ɡ, x, g, k, and " guttural " r ?

The first point to notice is that all these five consonants are produced at the same spot in the mouth—by raising the back of the tongue so that it comes into contact with, or approaches, the soft palate (velum). The difference between the pair of spirants, ɡ and x, and the corresponding stops g, k is merely that the former pair is uttered during narrowing by a continuous emission of breath, the latter pair by a full closure followed by an explosion of breath. Further, in the first pair, x differs from ɡ only in being unvoiced, i.e. there is little or no vibration of the vocal chords in its production ; in the second pair, k differs from g precisely in the same way. And " guttural " r is produced at the same point of the mouth, or slightly farther back, by a rapid series of broken contacts between the back of the tongue and the termination of the soft palate—the uvula. In the case of the child, this r may be regarded as a rolled form of the sound ɡ.

This voiced spirant ɡ is the most characteristic sound of the group. It is a sound which—as made by the child—does not happen to occur in any European language, with the result that different observers have resorted to different signs in recording its occurrence in children's cries. It is the sound indicated by Stern (KSp 153) as *rr* in *erre*, for he tells us of this, that it resembles both guttural *r* and *ch* as in *doch*—a good description of the spirant ɡ. This is the sound, he adds, that is the earliest comfort-sound to be noted by the majority of observers—the sound recorded by Preyer in *örrö, arra* (see Appendix I). To this we may add further that from Hoyer's account it must be the sound recorded by him as ɡ̈, and that Guillaume (IE 44) must mean to indicate this same sound when he tells us that among the earliest comfort-sounds of his son *gh* was most marked.

Why should the raising of the back of the tongue towards the soft palate occur in a state of comfort ? One answer—that of Grégoire (AP 376)—is that when the child is lying comfortably on his back, his tongue naturally lolls against his soft palate, producing the characteristic sounds. But we can perhaps suggest a more exact answer. Under what conditions do these sounds appear ? On this point, observers are fully agreed. The normal child during his first weeks, manifests pleasure, if at all, mainly after feeding : when he is lying satisfied in his mother's arms. It is then that " smiles " and gurgling noises appear, not very easily distinguishable at first from belchings, gruntings and signs of "wind". In the case of K, observed by me, the first certain instance of ɡ occurred when he was just six weeks old, lying on his back very comfortable after a feed. A few faint utterances of this sound appeared interspersed among grunting noises, accompanied by those face and lip movements which are regarded as signs of "wind".

This is a possible clue to the origin of back consonants in states of comfort. The movements which take place in the back of the child's mouth as he expels "wind" are, if accompanied by phonation, heard by us as guttural gruntings, some of which approximate to ɡ. A notion of this kind may have been in the mind of Kussmaul, when he named these back consonants "Vomitiv-Lauten".[1]

There is, however, a further condition which determines the child's utterance in a state of comfort after a feed. Some

[1] Mentioned by Gutzmann (SK) without detailed reference.

swallowing movements are likely to occur, partly because of the excess of saliva which will have remained in the mouth, partly perhaps as the persistence of reflex movements of those organs which have been working rhythmically throughout the period of feeding. Now the movement of swallowing involves just that approximation of the back of the tongue to the soft palate which, if made during phonation, would be heard as sounds of the g-type.

It is clear then that the production of this back consonant g probably arises directly out of the movements intimately connected with the business of feeding in which the child has just been engaged. If we are willing to accept the principle that there is an innate tendency in the child to utter a cry expressive of his state of satisfaction, then the facts we have mentioned help to show why the cry should take on the form of this specific back consonant g. It is the vocal manifestation of the fact that the child is making guttural movements expressive of satiety while uttering a cry of satisfaction. As for the sounds x, k, g and uvular r, these are all either voiced or unvoiced variations of g, and have the same expressive origin ; they arise as movements inherently connected with the state of satiety which they manifest.

Do these back consonants express other states of comfort in addition to satiety ? On this point the published records are not quite clear, the observer usually indicating no more than the fact that the child was making the sounds in a state of comfort. In my own observations (Appendix I, pp. 239–43), I certainly noticed that throughout the child's earlier months, whenever he used back consonants with the characteristic intonation expressing comfort, it was immediately after a feed. But Preyer, Stern and Hoyer all give cases of the occurrence of these consonants as expressive of contentment without mentioning definitely that this was a state of satiety : and a curious instance of the wider function of the expressive back consonants occurs in an early account of the blind deaf-mute Laura Bridgman given by Lieber in 1851. " Frequently I have heard Laura expressing a feeling of satisfaction by a subdued tone, somewhat between chuckling and a slight groaning." He adds quaintly, " I would have said *grunting*, as more accurately expressing the sound, had I not felt reluctant to use this word in connexion with that amiable and delicate being " (Lieber, LB 10).

It is clear that a transition of this kind might readily occur, so that sounds expressive of satiety would ultimately become expressive of other states of satisfaction. In the child's earliest weeks, as Charlotte Bühler points out (FY 62), the *only* time when he expresses satisfaction at all is when he is satiated, immediately after feeding ; when he is not asleep, he is either crying, taking food, or resting peacefully after feeding : only in this last state does he express satisfaction. As time goes on, the periods of waking satiety grow longer: the child begins to notice—with apparent pleasure—the things about him, and then to play. And because these periods of contentment are extensions of his states of satiety, the guttural sounds which expressed his satisfaction after feeding will tend to become expressive of his comfort in general.

The Front Consonants.—We come finally to those consonants which are so important in relation to the first " words " uttered by the child : the nasals **m, n,** the dentals **t, d,** and the labials **p, b.** What are the physiological conditions of their formation ; are they to be regarded as expressive ?

The first point to notice is that **m** falls into a group with the labials **p, b** ; **n** into a group with the dentals **t, d.** The three consonants of each group are formed by contact at the same part of the mouth. In the labial group, **m, p, b,** the lips are brought together ; but for **m** the uvula is lowered towards the back of the tongue so that the breath passes out through the nose in a continuous stream, the difference between **p** and **b** being only that the former is unvoiced. In the same way, in the dental group, all three consonants **n, t, d** are formed by contact of the fore part of the tongue against the upper gum-ridge. For **n** again, the lowering of the uvula allows the nasal emission of breath, while the difference between **t** and **d** is once more only of voice. Thus we have a labial group **m, p, b,** and a dental group **n, t, d** ; the nasal member of each group being characteristic of a state of discomfort.

The connection between these labial and linguo-dental movements and those involved in sucking is obvious at once. It has often been mentioned in a general way, as for instance by Wundt (VP 352) and Jespersen (ND 105). But no attempt has, I think, hitherto been made to analyse the phonetic basis of this similarity.

If we observe the movements made by the lips and tongue

in sucking, we find that it is essential for the lips to be brought together, while simultaneously, or immediately afterwards, the front of the tongue is pressed against the upper gum-ridge. The former of these movements is precisely that involved in saying **m, p** or **b**; the latter in saying **n, t,** or **d.** How then do these consonants become expressive of discomfort or comfort ?

Front Consonants Expressive of Discomfort.—A common observation helps us here ; at a very early age the child is found to be making anticipatory sucking movements when he is hungry or expects to be fed. Darwin (BI 286) noticed it as long ago as 1877 in the case of his own child, 32 days old ; and the fact has been repeatedly corroborated by careful observers such as Bühler and Hetzer (FY 30) who noticed it of children in their second month. Curti also (CP 143) reports some Russian observations which go to show that if the child, in the third or fourth week, is merely held in the normal feeding position, this will be sufficient to evoke sucking movements, in the absence of any other stimulus.

In the case of K, these sucking movements were very marked. From his first days he was accustomed to having a bib tied under his chin before being given his food. After his thirty-fifth day, when the bib was tied at feeding-time he definitely pursed his lips into the sucking position, before he was brought within reach of the food. Nine days later, at the time of his evening feed, this reaction was most definite. " He was crying lustily. His mother put the bib under his chin. His cries gradually lessened, and ceased within about 30 seconds. Then he very definitely began to make sucking movements. His lips were pursed, and the tip of his tongue slightly protruded."

We are here introducing a third factor into our discussion—that of training or conditioning—in addition to our two principles of Darwinian expression and the differentiation of affective states. But it is a factor that is certainly not in dispute. We may take it as a generally accepted principle that when an organism has experienced a pattern of events, the recurrence of any salient item of this pattern will tend to cause the organism to behave as though the rest of the pattern were present. Here the child when hungry has felt the bib being tied under his chin, and this followed by feeding ; sooner or later the touch of the bib when he is hungry, or the mere sight of preparations for food, will evoke sucking movements appropriate to feeding.

It is evident that if the child phonates while making these anticipatory sucking movements, the sounds produced will approximate to the labial and dental consonants. If, further, he is in a state of discomfort such as hunger, and phonates *nasally*—as we have seen he does—then the consonants produced will inevitably be **m** and **n.** Many observers have noticed (Stern KSp 356) that these nasal consonants appear when the child is hungry, but I do not think that they have been shown to arise out of anticipatory sucking movements made during nasal phonation.

The occurrence of these front consonants is so marked— they are indeed the first definite sounds that a casual observer of a child notices—that their origin has sometimes been ascribed to imitation. Wundt, for instance (VP 295), reminds us that mothers commonly make a sound like *mum-mum* when coaxing their infants to take food, and obviously this might have some influence upon the child's own utterance. But it is clear that imitation can at most be only a secondary factor in the production of these front consonants. For neither blindness nor deafness in children seems to prevent their occurrence. Wundt himself cites the case of a deaf-mute aged nineteen who habitually used *mum* to signify food. Jespersen (ND 105), doubting the influence of imitation on the production of the front consonants, suggests that we should find that they regularly occur in blind children also. Since the publication of his work a case has been described by Bean (PL 183) ; the child, who was afflicted with congenital cataract in both eyes, nevertheless uttered *ŭa, ŭa* in states of discomfort soon after birth, and *mmuh* at the age of 0;3,2, when hungry.

There can be little doubt that the origin of the nasals, **m, n,** is that they are expressive of hunger ; that is, they are the audible manifestation of the mouth movements which are bound up with that state. And because the expression of hunger is the most important function of the child's utterance during his earliest months, these nasal sounds become one of the chief means by which the child enters into linguistic communication with those about him—a process which we shall discuss in Section III.

Front Consonants Expressive of Comfort.—The appearance

of front consonants—**p, b, t, d,** sometimes **m** and **n**—in a state of comfort is not so easy to observe as the consonants expressive of discomfort. The child when contented does not articulate with the same definiteness as when moved by the urgency of discomfort. Yet if one listens carefully, one hears sooner or later, emerging from the welter of semi-articulate guttural sounds, consonants which approximate to the labials and dentals.

They occur when the child is contented; chiefly, that is, either after a feed or when he delightedly perceives his food already before him. If we bear in mind this fact of their appearance, their expressive nature is at once evident. They are the vocal manifestation of sucking movements, made usually without nasal urgency, the child uttering them while phonating contentedly on seeing food, or while continuing to make sucking movements after a feed. And, just in the same way as the back consonants expressive of satiety, these front consonants may ultimately become expressive of other states of contentment.

One tendency will clearly bring all the child's early consonants into the stream of contented utterance—the rise of babbling or vocal play. And an important feature of this activity, we shall show, is that even consonants which are primarily expressive of discomfort may become transformed into play, and so appear in a state of contentment (see p. 57). Before, however, we consider babbling and its relation to expression, we must turn to the manner in which the child responds to the speech of others.

Our phonetic analysis of the child's earliest utterance has enabled us to demonstrate its expressive character, in the Darwinian sense. In particular, we have found that the origin of the earlier back consonants and of the later front consonants lies almost entirely in the expression of hunger and of its satisfaction. This is not surprising, for by far the greatest part of the child's life in his earliest months is taken up by food and sleep. And it is inevitable that any utterance made by the child in connection with feeding should become shaped by the movements of feeding; in discussing the nature of language we cannot evade the fact that the organs of utterance are also the organs of sucking.

We have shown also that some order and regularity may be

found in what has often been regarded as the chance and chaotic occurrence of the child's earliest sounds. We have shown that they fall into groups which may be explained by referring to three generally accepted factors—the principle of Darwinian expression, the differentiation of affective states, and the occurrence of behaviour anticipatory of a sequence of events.

CHAPTER IV

EARLY RESPONSE TO SPEECH

THE Child's First Response to Sounds.—Until recently, it was supposed that the child was physiologically deaf for some days after birth. This, for instance, was the view accepted by Stern in 1922 (KSp 144). But already in 1919, Watson (PB 236) had reported definite wrist-movements of a one-day-old child in response to loud noises ; in 1926, Hetzer and Tudor-Hart, in an extended series of observations, found—as Stern records in the last edition of his work (KSp 160)—that a child shows some response to hand-clapping within the first three days. More recently still, in 1927, Löwenfeld, from his own observations and a review of the literature (RS 66) concludes that the child may normally be said to hear on his first day.

The Child's First Response to the Human Voice.—Here we are concerned to trace the development of the child's response to human speech. But again the available records of the earliest stages are very scanty. No doubt the difficulty of observation is considerable ; the child's responses to any sounds at all are at first not overt ; later, when they become more obvious, they are often still so slight as to be passed over by the casual observer. Moreover, the responses at first are often made to the human voice in its context of circumstances—the whole activity in which an adult is engaged when he is concerned with the child, and very few observers have hitherto thought it of sufficient interest to record systematically from the outset all the varied behaviour of a child in response to those about him.

When does the child begin to respond to the human voice ? The older view (as stated, for instance, by Meumann in 1902) was that by the end of the second month the child usually shows a marked response to the voice of one with whom he is familiar—his mother, for example, or his nurse (EK 170). In the third month (O'Shea pointed out in 1907) the child seems to respond more readily to speech than to any other sign of the presence of a human being (LD 18).

Recent systematic work has revealed the difficulty of accepting these statements as they stand. The first question is, when is the earliest moment at which children begin to respond to the human voice ? According to experiments by Bühler and Hetzer (VA 58) we might have to date this event within the first fortnight of a child's life. They tested 27 children, all less than 14 days old, 30 times each by bringing a crying child within the hearing of a silent one, and in 84 per cent. of the cases the silent child responded by crying. We must, however, be careful how we interpret this. Löwenfeld concludes (RS 95) from a series of experiments that children in their first month respond not to the quality of a sound but to its intensity. The more intense the noise, the more likely is the child to cry. And as Bühler and Hetzer did not test the effect of sounds other than children's crying upon their subjects, we cannot at present be sure that these heard cries are more effective than other loud noises in evoking cries from the child. We can in fact only be certain that the child is responding to the human voice as a voice and not merely as a noise when he begins to respond to it in a specific way. The course of this development is well illustrated by Hoyer's observations of his son (LK 373) :

In the 1st week : The child seemed to fix his eyes upon the speaker. (Hoyer is doubtful whether this response was really due to hearing, as it only occurred when the face of the speaker was immediately in front of the child.)
At 3 weeks : The cry of the infant ceased in response to an adult voice.
At the end of 4th week : The child showed pleasure in response to a lullaby when this was accompanied by a caress.
In 6th week : He smiled in response to a heard voice.
In 7th and 8th weeks : He turned at the sound of a voice ; sometimes in the direction from which the voice proceeded.

In brief, the child by the end of his first month responds to an adult voice by ceasing to cry ; in the second month this response takes the form of a smile. These conclusions have been corroborated by systematic observations by Guillaume (IE 185) of his own two children, and by Hetzer and Tudor-Hart, as reported by C. Bühler (KJ 28), observing 126 children of ages ranging from one day to five months.

The question that further arises out of this is whether the response by a smile is a specific one, showing that the child is differentiating the human voice from other sounds. To this the answer now seems fairly definite. The two-months-old child, Löwenfeld (RS 95) found, discriminates by his response between different heard sounds ; the work of Hetzer and Tudor-Hart shows that at this stage the response to a sound by smiling is confined to the hearing of a human voice. Their experiment consisted in submitting their 126 subjects to a series of tests, in which the responses were noted to twelve different sounds, four being forms of human utterance— friendly speech, angry speech, normal conversation and song. Only these four sounds evoked the specific response of smiling, this first occurring at the end of the second month.

The next question is whether we can accept O'Shea's conclusion that the child responded by a smile to the human voice only and not to other human stimuli. The answer to this seems rather doubtful. Thus Valentine—corroborating an observation by Dearborn—found (PA 184) that his son at the beginning of the second month laughed with delight on being placed in position to take food. But C. Bühler (KJ 27) refuses to accept this conclusion as final, maintaining from the extended work of Hetzer and Ripin that at this stage only the human voice or the human glance can evoke a smile ; thus during feeding not the stimulus of the bottle, nor any other of the accompanying stimuli are effective in arousing a smile when the human voice or glance will do this.

It is evident that the problem is complicated by the fact that the human voice (and glance) are inevitably bound up for the child with the situation of being fed. This can be illustrated by gathering together a series of observations by Guillaume of his daughter (IE 185) :

At 2 days : The child smiled after feeding.

From 2nd to 9th day : She smiled on various occasions, but never on seeing or hearing another person.

On 9th day : She smiled on seeing or hearing a familiar person, *but only after feeding.*

On 23rd day : She smiled on being spoken to by a familiar person, *before feeding.*

On 27th day : She smiled regularly at the sight of father, mother or brother.

At 1 month 12 days : She smiled on hearing the voice of any of these familiar persons.

In brief, although it is true that in the child's second month she smiled merely on hearing an adult voice, we must notice that this perhaps occurred only because the child had heard the voice while being fed, a situation in which she was already accustomed to smile.

Finally, we have to take into account this special effect of the adult voice upon the child, that it readily arouses a vocal response from him. Hoyer found that this occurred at the early age of seven weeks ; Guillaume observed it at the end of his son's second month : in Stern's daughter it occurred a fortnight later ; in Bühler's daughter in the eleventh week. And Guernsey, studying 200 children of ages 0;2 to 1;9, concluded that vocal responses to the adult voice begin at the former date.[1]

Can we reduce these varied conclusions to any order ? The main points seem to be as follows :

(i) By the end of his first month the normal child responds by crying to various intense noises, among these being the sound of another child crying.

(ii) At this same time the sound of an adult voice has the effect of soothing him.

(iii) In his second month he responds to an adult voice by smiling, and often by speaking.

What is not yet clear is whether these responses are specifically to the adult voice in itself, or to this simply as a result of its occurrence during feeding.

Divergent Theories of this Response.—The uncertain nature of the evidence is reflected in the divergent views current to-day as to the origin of the child's response to the human voice. There are two alternatives, both strongly maintained at present : one, that this is an instance of the maturation of an innate tendency, the other that it is the result of training.

The former view is Darwin's hypothesis of an " instinct of sympathy " ; the organism, he held, is attuned to respond appropriately to the expressive movements of other members of the same species. Darwin was, however, by no means certain whether this was indeed the functioning of an innate tendency or the result of training, although inclined to favour the former view as more likely.

In one form or another this view is held by the Hormic School (McDougall) and by the Gestalt-theorists (Koffka).

---

[1] Hoyer LK 374 ; Guillaume IE 33 ; Stern KSp 160 ; Bühler KJ 42 ; Guernsey SN 145.

The alternative view is maintained by the Reflexologists and the Behaviorists—that the child's earliest response to speech is the result of training. Thus Bekhterev points out that the primary response of the child to food may rapidly be conditioned so that ultimately it is evoked by the mere movement of an adult ; and it is evident that this explanation might equally well be applied to the child's response to adult speech. Among the Behaviorists, an exactly similar explanation is adopted by Landis.[1]

There is not sufficient evidence to enable us to decide between these two alternatives of maturation and learning. In favour of the latter view we have the fact that some conditioning certainly does take place in the child's behaviour within the first month—for instance, the observation reported by Curti (CP 143) that the mere position of the child when held as in feeding becomes sufficient to evoke sucking-movements. On the other hand, in favour of the hypothesis of maturation as against mere conditioning, we have these facts : that in the child's first months infant cries, and in his second month the expressive acts of smiling and speech, seem to be particularly effective in evoking somewhat similar responses from him.

The question must remain open ; but we may suggest that the alternatives are not mutually exclusive. It seems possible that there is both an innate tendency in the child to respond to speech, and that also within the first month this tendency is reinforced by conditioning. A compromise of this kind is certainly in keeping with Darwin's cautious attitude in stating his theory, and also with the conclusion of Bühler and Hetzer (VA 53) that in this question above all a broad view is desirable. And it is all the more acceptable in that it embraces the two alternative hypotheses of maturation and learning without coming into conflict with either.

The Further Development of Response to Speech.—From the outset, heard adult speech comes to the child steeped in affective quality. In his first month it soothes him ; a month later it makes him smile. We must recognise that heard speech continues to have a strong affective character throughout the child's early development.

This point is of considerable importance. Everyone recognises that the child's own speech is, from the outset, an

[1] Darwin EE 359 ; McDougall OP 156 ; Koffka GM 131, 398 ; Bekhterev ER 280 ; Landis EE 489.

expression of affect ; and in the last chapter we have traced the differentiation of his speech corresponding to the differences in the underlying states of comfort and discomfort. But the fact that the speech which the child hears has also an affective character for him is largely neglected ; yet, as we shall see, it is of the first importance in his linguistic growth. We have to bear in mind that both the speech that he utters and the speech that he hears are from the beginning experiences strongly affective in nature.

The first clear recognition of this seems to have been due to Meumann, who suggested—now more than thirty years ago—that the child's discrimination of intonation in the speech that he hears is an essential feature of his acquirement of language (EK 180). But until quite recently this clue was neglected. Stern, for instance, having said (KSp 160) that the child soon comes to respond discriminatively to differences of intonation and rhythm in the speech that he hears, discusses this no further, taking up the story of the child's discriminative responses only at the time of his comprehension of specific words.

It is not too much to say that a study of the child's responses to intonation provides one of the chief clues to the nature of his later use and comprehension of language. The intonational character of speech is of three kinds, and each has its effect upon the child : first there is its acoustic quality—it is harsh or melodious ; secondly its expressive quality—the features innately linked up with the speaker's affective state ; finally the intonational characters given to it by convention.

Our only evidence, as far as I know, of the development of response to intonation occurs incidentally in the work of Löwenfeld and of Bühler and Hetzer, the former being intended to record the child's reactions to sounds in general, the latter his responses to the various forms of expression. The significance of this work in the study of linguistic growth has not, I think, hitherto been shown.

Löwenfeld (RS 95) summarises his observations of the development of responses to musical tones and noises, as follows :

1st month : The child responds *negatively*[1] to all sounds, but with greater or less force according to their *intensity*.

---

[1] The child is said to respond positively when his movements involve or indicate fuller enjoyment of the stimulus, negatively when he avoids or turns from the stimulus, neutrally when he shows nothing but mere awareness of the stimulus.

0;1 : Different responses according to the *quality* of the sound : response to noises, negative ; to tones, neutral.

0;2 : The child turns his head in the direction of the heard sound.

0;3 : Earliest occurrence of positive expressive response to tones, in the form of a smile.

0;4 : Beginning of definite differentiation of responses according to the *affective* quality of sounds. Thus a pleasant sound (e.g. a bell) arouses a positive response ; an unpleasant sound (e.g. a shrill whistle) a negative response.

0;5 *onwards :* Responses according to affective quality become increasingly uniform ; sounds with less well-marked affective quality evoke fewer and fewer responses.

Thus we find a progressive discrimination in the course of the child's development. In his first month he discriminates only between the *intensities* of the heard sounds ; during his next two months, 0;1 to 0;3, he discriminates between the *musical qualities* of the heard sounds, by responding at first neutrally, later positively, to musical tones, while responding negatively to mere noises. Finally, after 0;4, he discriminates between the *affective qualities* of the heard sounds, and makes few responses to sounds which have little affective quality.

When, therefore, we consider the child's response to speech we must recognise that apart from its expressive functions and conventional meaning it will have an effect upon him merely because of its musical and affective qualities.

The course of these changes in the child's responses to speech has been studied in further detail by Bühler and Hetzer. We have already mentioned their observation that in the first month the child cries on hearing the cry of another child. In this work (VA 60) they were also able to show that there is a progressive diminution in the occurrence of this primary undifferentiated reaction. 80 children of ages ranging from 1 day to 11 months were observed, a crying child being brought near to another one lying peacefully in his cot. The results were as follows :

TABLE II

Age-group.	1–14 days.	1 month.	2 months.	3–12 months.
Proportion of the age-group to respond by crying	84%	60%	32%	24%

How do we account for this diminution of response ? An answer is provided by a further observation made in the course of the same work. When a screen was brought between the crying and silent child so that they could not see each other, this made no difference to the frequency of the crying responses during the first two months ; but by the end of the second month the percentage of children who responded by crying fell from 32 (as shown in the Table) to 10. This goes to show, as the observers point out, that at first the heard cry is merely a " sense-stimulus ", that is, merely a loud sound which evokes a negative response ; but by the second month the cry is being responded to in its context, that is, in relation to the presence of the speaker. In other words because the child is beginning to respond to the situation in which he hears a cry, he is less likely to respond to a cry heard in isolation.

The same change may be seen taking place if we observe the child's responses to an adult voice. In his second month, as we have noticed, he begins to respond uniformly by smiling on hearing adult speech, whatever the tone may be in which this is uttered. Further observations by Bühler and Hetzer (VA 57) give us some indication of the subsequent development. In this work, 10 children of each month of age from 0;3 to 1;0 were observed, the experimenter being hidden behind a screen and the child's responses noted to a friendly and an angry tone of voice. From their results I have drawn up the following table ; the responses are classified according to whether they express a positive or negative affective state, or are " neutral " —that is when the child is attentive but does not respond expressively :

TABLE III

PERCENTAGE OF RESPONSES TO DIFFERENT TONES IN SUCCESSIVE MONTHS
(*from* BÜHLER AND HETZER, VA 57)

Stimulus.	Response.	Age in months.								
		3	4	5	6	7	8	9	10	11
Friendly Tone	Positive .	100	100	100	80	80	80	60	40	80
	Negative .	0	0	0	0	0	0	0	0	0
	Neutral .	0	0	0	20	20	20	40	60	20
Angry Tone	Positive .	90	40	40	0	0	0	0	12	40
	Negative .	10	60	60	100	80	40	60	68	20
	Neutral .	0	0	0	0	20	60	40	20	40

Here the positive response to a friendly tone gradually becomes less frequent, being increasingly replaced after five months by neutral non-affective responses : then at eleven months there is once more an increase of positive responses. This course of events is exactly paralleled in the child's responses to an angry tone, once he has arrived at a full discrimination between the two tones, a point which he reaches at six months, when he invariably responds negatively to an angry tone. From this point onwards his negative response is frequently replaced by a neutral non-affective response, until at ten months we notice an increase once more in the frequency of his positive responses.

It is clear that there are definite points in the child's first year at which we witness the appearance of successive modes of response to speech :

0;2 : Beginning of positive response to adult speech.

0;3 : Growing discrimination of positive response to friendly tone and negative response to angry tone.

0;6 : Beginning of neutral, non-affective response to either affective tone.

0;10 : New increase of positive response to either affective tone.

We have then to consider the significance of these three facts : first, the discrimination between friendly and angry tones ; secondly the appearance of neutral responses to affectively-toned speech : and thirdly the somewhat surprising recrudescence of positive responses towards the end of the year.

Bühler and Hetzer (VA 55) themselves describe the course of events by saying that after the initial period when the child responds alike to all adult speech, he first comes to " reflect " its affective character,[1] and then to " understand " it—that is, to respond to it in relation to the situation ; this last period (from 0;8 onwards) including the occurrence both of neutral responses and of the new positive responses. But their statement cannot be taken to mean that there are these simple successive stages. A consideration of the results shows rather, after the initial period of response, the simultaneous working of both factors of " reflection " of affective character, and of " understanding ". For when the first positive response of the child is differentiated into two " reflective " responses,

[1] That is, to respond positively to a friendly tone, negatively to an unfriendly one.

this already is the beginning of "understanding"; further, this "reflective" differentiation continues at work while new forms of "understanding" show themselves—first in the appearance of the neutral responses at 0;6, and secondly in the appearance of the new positive responses at 0;10.

In brief, during this first year we find the operation of two factors working together in a complex manner—the response to the affective tone of heard speech and the response to the situation in which this speech appears.

As a preliminary to the discussion of these two factors one point must be mentioned: Bühler and Hetzer's own interpretation of the increase in the positive responses towards the end of the year. They point out (VA 55, 57) that in the conditions of the experiment, even the angry tone of voice is not accompanied by any unpleasant circumstances; on the other hand, the child clearly recognises that the situation has the characteristics of play, and it is to these characteristics that he responds positively. This we must accept, and with it the converse conclusion that it implies; that if at this stage a *friendly* tone of voice were constantly introduced in an *unpleasant* situation, the child's response would often be *negative*. In a word, the child now begins to respond to speech according to the immediate situation in which it occurs.

But if we accept this we must also recognise that the same process occurs even earlier. For, as we saw, the child of two months is more strongly affected by the cry of another child, if he can see the latter. Further, even though in Bühler and Hetzer's experiment the adult was hidden from the child, every child is accustomed to hear adult speech in situations of outstanding importance to him. Thus when he comes upon adult speech in the *absence* of such a situation—as in this experiment—his response (as we find after 0;6) will frequently be neutral.

The Two Factors: Affect and Situation.—Apart perhaps from his first month, the child's responses to speech are never exclusively due either to the intrinsic affective character of what he hears or to training by the conditions in which it occurs. Both factors are present in the child's second month and continue to be present for the rest of his life. Unless we recognise this we cannot fully understand his linguistic growth.

The observations are few. The best-known illustration is the experiment of Tappolet's, reported by Meumann (EK 180).

The child had, at an age between 0;6 and 0;8, been trained to turn in the direction of the window on hearing *Wo ist das Fenster ?* One day his father said, *Où est la fenêtre ?* with a similar intonation, and the child responds equally well. To this we may add Pavlovitch's remark (LE 24) that his son responded in a specific manner at 0;3 to each of several words ; Delacroix (LP 297) referring to this observation suggests that it was to the intonation rather than to the phonetic form that the child responded. Further, the work of Schäfer, which we discuss later (p. 113), has shown that when a child does come to respond specifically to given sound-groups, intonational form plays a large part in determining this response.

But when we turn even to such a standard work as Stern's, we find an almost complete neglect of facts of this kind, as important in the child's growth. Stern's view (KSp 166) is that the early responses of the child to heard speech are fundamentally built up on natural gestures (*Gebärde*), whether of the speaker, or of the child himself. For gestures, he tells us, have an internal connection, speech-sounds only an external (*äusserliche*) connection, with their meaning. The child responds first to a gesture, then to the gesture accompanied by words, finally to these words in themselves. How far this account is acceptable we shall discuss later (p. 110) ; but in any case this is clear, that it leaves out of consideration the fact which Stern himself elsewhere (KSp 126–9) emphasises—that all speech, however cultivated, retains some expressive characteristics, and that the child from the outset responds to these.

Now there is no doubt that when a child does begin to " understand " adult *words*, his response to their affective character is modified also by their phonetic pattern—as in the examples given by Meumann, Delacroix and Schäfer—and by accompanying gestures, as Stern points out. But we must go farther back into the child's linguistic history and recognise, from the evidence of Löwenfeld, Bühler and Hetzer, that long before the child responds to the phonetic patterns of adult words or to the accompanying gestures, he is already discriminating between friendly and unfriendly intonation.

On the other hand, it would be a mistake to suppose that here we have a period of pure " reflection " of the expressive characters of speech, followed by a period of response to speech as related to the accompanying situation—as might seem to be implied by the remarks of C. Bühler and Hetzer (VA 56), and also of K. Bühler (MDC 160), that only after the eighth month does the child begin to respond to a given sound in relation to the situation in which it occurs.

For it is clear that when these observers say that responses before this date merely " reflect " expression, they do not mean to exclude the effect of the accompanying situation. In dealing with the child's response to another child's cry, they point out, as we have mentioned, that as early as the second month the heard cry is taken in relation to a situation—in isolation it is not so effective in evoking a cry as when accompanied by the sight of a crying child. And they have also explicitly given it as their opinion (VA 53) that we cannot exclude the possibility of training even at the very beginning of the child's responses to speech.

Thus on the one hand we must recognise that the middle months of the child's first year are certainly marked by an increase in the effect of the accompanying situation upon the child's responses to speech. On the other hand we must also recognise that this is no sudden change in his development : from the outset his responses are due partly to the affective character of heard speech in itself, partly to training by the conditions in which it is heard.

What form does this training take ? It would seem that we can include all the successive stages of development in one statement : the growing apprehension of speech-sounds in relation to accompanying experiences.

At the outset (0;2), it seems probable that the adult voice already carries a pleasant affective quality for the child, and that the accompanying pleasant situations in which it is heard serve to reinforce this affective quality for him. This is the first stage of training.

Out of this there arises (0;3) a discrimination between pleasantly and unpleasantly toned speech. This may in part be due to maturation of an innate tendency to respond to expression ; but it is also likely to be due to training by the conditions in which the speech is heard. These conditions are some of them inherently bound up with the actual utterance—such as the speaker's facial expression : other conditions might be the presence or absence of caresses, or the satisfaction of bodily needs. The details need yet to be investigated.

At the third stage (0;6) the accompanying situation begins to play the dominant part in determining the child's response. In this way, even affectively-toned speech may—as Bühler and Hetzer found—fail to arouse any overt response : here the initial affective quality would appear to be neutralised by the accompanying situation.

At the fourth stage (0;10), the accompanying situation is the dominant factor. Now speech unpleasant in tone may be responded to positively because the conditions are pleasant : the conditions have become more important than the affective tone.

Theories of the Nature of Training.—How does this change come about ? Our problem is the development of a response to situations more and more complex in character, and of this the outstanding theories are three : association, conditioning, and the development of configurations. Our representative of the first view shall be Ward, as giving us the most modern statement of the case ; for the second view we shall take Watson, for the third Koffka.

On one clear point Ward and Koffka agree in differing from Watson ; they emphasise the progressive emergence of " wholes ", while Watson seems to regard conditioning as a piecemeal process in which a stimulus, previously ineffective, becomes capable of arousing a response by being linked up with a stimulus already effective. Yet when we come to examine the doctrines of the three schools, we find that they agree on essentials : the differences seem to lie in the hypothetical physiological activity which is said to characterise the process of training.

Thus Ward tells us (PP 192) that " any presentations whatever, which are in consciousness together or in close succession, cohere in such a way that when one recurs it tends to revive the rest ", but he immediately points out that presentations do not really occur as successive entities but rather as a continuum. The interested attention of the individual fashions a " new whole " out of this continuum ; then when some of the sensory or motor constituents of this new whole recur, they tend to reinstate the rest.

Applying this to our own case we may say that the child's attention is determined by his biological needs ; at first his interest is aroused by the mere affective quality of the heard voice, then increasingly by the nature of the accompanying conditions. The " whole " which these interests fashion out of the continuum of experience, embraces, as time goes on, a wider range within the situation in which the voice is heard.

In very similar fashion Koffka points out (GM 149, 150, 260) that the child's primary experience is undifferentiated : from this there arises a new whole, a mental configuration, which he defines as " a co-existence of phenomena . . . in which each member possesses its peculiarity only by virtue of, and in connection with, all the others ". Now if a particular phenomenon which has been present as a member of a configuration " reappears while still possessed of its ' membership-character ', it will have a tendency to supplement itself . . . with the remainder of the configuration ". Under what circumstances then do phenomena form a configuration for the child ? It is when they possess qualities that will bring about his activity ; in particular when they possess affective character for him. This account corresponds exactly to Ward's description of interested attention fashioning a " new whole ".

It is perhaps more surprising to find no real conflict with these views when we come to Watson. His conclusion is simply this (PB 236) : that " when an emotionally exciting object stimulates the subject simultaneously with one not emotionally exciting, the latter may in time (often after one such joint stimulation) arouse the same emotional reaction as the former ". Now the two important points to notice here are the use of the word " object " and the fact that this must be " emotionally exciting ". Watson, that is, does not speak of mere stimuli or sensations : the child responds not to a sensation of sound but to an " object "—his mother's voice. Further, Watson insists upon the affective character of the original experience, in entire agreement with Ward and Koffka. Finally, his statement in no way precludes the emergence of " wholes " : indeed, when he says that two objects " simultaneously " stimulate the child he is suggesting that they are being taken together as one whole.

The fact of this agreement on fundamentals is implied in the remarks of several recent writers—for instance, Markey (SP 119) ; and it has been explicitly stated by H. E. Jones in dealing with this very question of the " conditioning of emotional responses " in infants. From experimental observations he concludes (ER 496) that the results of Pavlov's work on conditioned reactions are applicable here, but adds : " This much can be stated without the necessity of accepting

Pavlov's neurological corollaries, and without denying that some other statement of the learning process, as in terms of contiguity, combination, redintegration or insight, may possibly equally well fit the facts." He brings together the association, Gestalt and Behaviorist theories.

In brief, where these three schools agree is in insisting upon the affective aspect of the process ; where they disagree is on the question of conditioning or the emergence of wholes, but even on this latter point the disagreement hardly seems fundamental.

It thus becomes possible to make a statement of the development of the child's discrimination in response to the human voice which shall be acceptable to the main divergent schools of thought. We can say that when in his second month, the child begins to smile on hearing adult speech, this is due partly to the affective character of the speech in itself and partly to the presence of the human speaker to whom the child responds by smiling—again either as a primary or as a learnt reaction. The voice at the outset is not a " neutral stimulus " ; it possesses an affective character for the child—in other words, it evokes a response from him. And this affective character persists, so that when at the second stage the child discriminates between pleasant and unpleasant tones, this development is again due partly to a primary response which has now matured and partly also to a training resulting from pleasant or unpleasant concomitants. The whole course of development seems to take this form : an undifferentiated response to the voice as a whole becomes more and more discriminatively differentiated according to circumstances.

So far we have considered only the child's discrimination of intonational form. But towards the end of the first half-year another factor enters ; the influence of phonetic form. Although in Bühler and Hetzer's experiments this factor was excluded, there can be little doubt that it had some influence upon their subjects, for these were normal children who must have undergone the everyday training by the adult speech spoken about them. In the child's linguistic growth intonational forms evoke their typical responses increasingly as a result of their occurrence in conjunction with phonetic forms.

But before we can consider the child's response to phonetic form in the speech of others, we must consider its development in his own. This leads us to the discussion of two characteristic activities : babbling and imitation.

SECTION II

TWO IMPORTANT FEATURES OF THE CHILD'S SPEECH

CHAPTER V

BABBLING

WE have seen that the child's earliest utterance may be divided into two groups : (*a*) characteristic sounds uttered in a state of discomfort, (*b*) characteristic sounds uttered in a state of comfort ; and that in each case the specific sounds may be regarded as expressive of the child's state. We have now to consider a further characteristic of sounds uttered in a state of comfort ; the common observation that the child utters them not only expressively but also apparently for their own sake, for the mere pleasure of producing them.

We may thus distinguish two lines of development of the comfort-sounds ; (*a*) they are expressive, (*b*) they are uttered for their own sake—as " play ". For the purpose of our analysis it is necessary to keep these two functions distinct because of the distinct parts which they play in the child's development. Some obscurity has, as we shall see, been allowed to remain in accounts of this development by failure to make the necessary distinction. Thus Stern at times uses the term " Lallen " to mean play with sounds, at other times to cover all sounds uttered in states of comfort, whether expressively or for the sake of the pleasure they give. In French, the word " babillage " is also used in this double way, as for instance in Delacroix, and this again is true of our English word " babbling ", as used for instance in the translation of K. Bühler and in Lorimer.[1] Here, as an aid to clearness, I propose to speak of one function as " expression ", of the other as " babbling ". I am thus giving a narrower meaning than usual to the term " babbling ", to denote the utterance of sounds only for their own sake.

Development of Babbling in the Child's Early Utterance.— From the records given in Appendix I, supplemented by the summaries of such writers as Stern (KSp 153–6), we can draw up the following account of babbling :

(i) At an early stage—from within the first month onwards

[1] Stern KSp 153, 156 ; Delacroix LP 291 ; Bühler MDC ; Lorimer GR.

—the child utters characteristic isolated sounds in a state of comfort.

(ii) Repetitive chains appear after a time which varies according to the child : Preyer's son, 0;6 ;[1] Hilde Stern, 0;2,2 ; Günther Stern, 0;3 ; Hoyer's son, 0;6 ; K, 0;3,21. Charlotte Bühler (FY 175) says that normally the onset is in the third month.

(iii) The child seems to take delight in some of these sounds for their own sake ; they often seem " meaningless " i.e. to have no expressive function.

(iv) In this respect, as babbling, they are to be regarded as " play " ; thus they have some of the rudimentary characteristics of language as a form of art.

If we are to obtain a clear view of the nature of babbling, several questions arising out of this statement need to be considered. First we have to ask when babbling begins, and what is its relation to sounds expressive of comfort and discomfort ; next we have to consider how it arises, and finally what is to be understood by naming it play and a rudimentary form of art.

I

The Beginning of Babbling.—In Chapter III we characterised the early sounds made by a child in a state of comfort as expressive of that state. But the remarks of some writers seem to suggest that these early comfort-sounds are not expressive, but really babbling. Thus Lorimer characterises even the earliest comfort-sounds as " vocal play " (GR 40). And Bühler makes a contrast between the child's discomfort-cries—" which are built into an instinctive mechanism " to draw attention to his needs—and his babbling, which remains ' " for a considerable time free from any meaning " (MDC 53).

These statements seem to suggest that at a definite moment in his life, the child who has previously expressed only states of discomfort, begins to make new sounds solely for the delight of making them : that the comfort-sounds, at their very first appearance, are not expression but babbling. But a closer consideration of their remarks shows that these writers do not really mean to suggest this. For Lorimer also tells us that the child's comfort-sounds are of a reflex character,

[1] I infer this from Preyer's general remarks.

being an expression of the child's state when discomfort is absent (GR 40) ; while Bühler refers to babbling as " instinctive expression " (MDC 52).

It is clear that they are really in agreement with all other observers on this point ; that the comfort-sounds arise in the first instance as expression, and that only subsequently are they transformed into babbling, that is, sounds uttered for the delight of uttering them. The obscurity is in some measure due to that double use of the term " Lallen " or " babbling " to which we have already referred ; but it also goes deeper than the mere use of a term. It is frequently not recognised that babbling may be not only a transformation of sounds originally expressive of comfort, but also of sounds originally expressive of discomfort.

For if we look at the records in Appendix I we find this : that while on the whole (as we saw in Chapter III) the nasal consonants **m** and **n** are used early to express discomfort, they only occur in states of comfort rather later. Thus in the case of Preyer's son, apart from the isolated instances of *amma* and *ma* at 0;1,15 and 0;2,9 as comfort-sounds, the nasals **m** and **n** are—as he specifically tells us (MC II 104)—characteristic of discomfort during the first five months ; only after that date do we find them regularly in states of comfort. Stern's observations of early discomfort-sounds are unfortunately imperfect ; but in the case of Hilde a nasal (**n**) appears in Lallen for the first time as late as 0;9, while in the case of Günther there is no record of nasals in states of comfort at all. In the careful records of the Hoyers **m** appears only as a discomfort-sound up to 3 months, and only after that date in states of comfort. In my own observations of K, nasals were well established as expressive of discomfort by 0;1,10 ; then—apart from one instance at 0;2,7—they do not appear in states of comfort until 0;5,14. Thus, while one observer after another—Stern (KSp 355), Preyer (MC II 104), and Hoyer (LK 366)—tells us that the nasals are characteristic of discomfort, no attempt is made to reconcile this fact with their appearance in states of comfort, either as expression or babbling.

It would seem that the observations point in this direction : that in states of discomfort the child utters characteristic nasal consonants ; in a state of comfort he not only utters a wide range of sounds expressive of this state, but also transforms into babbling both these comfort-sounds and also those which are expressive of discomfort.

Babbling in Isolated and Repeated Sounds.—When does this transformation of the expressive sounds take place—while the child is still uttering isolated sounds, or only when he begins to utter repetitive chains ? Now, although a common view associates babbling with the repetition of sounds, both Stern (KSp 153) and K. Bühler (MDC 52) imply that babbling may occur while the child is still uttering isolated sounds, the former dating this as early as the first month, while Charlotte Bühler concludes that it normally appears in the second (FY 72).

But so long as the child is uttering isolated sounds, it is certainly very difficult to be sure that he really is babbling. The only criterion is whether he appears to be attending to his own sounds and enjoying making them, and for this we have to rely upon the judgment of the observer. We can begin to be more certain that we are listening to babbling when we hear repetitive chains, but even here the only objective criterion seems to be the occurrence of a rhythm and a " tune " in the course of this repetition. Thus in the case of K, the first repetition of sounds in a state of comfort occurred when he was 0;1,20, but the first fairly certain case of babbling occurred in my opinion at 0;3,21, when he began to utter repetitive chains (see Appendix I, pp. 239-40). Although, therefore, the available evidence is somewhat scanty, we must admit the possibility that babbling occurs both in isolated sounds as well as in repetitive chains. It seems reasonable to accept the statement of so careful an observer as Charlotte Bühler (FY 72, 175) that babbling in isolated sounds occurs in the second month, to be followed by repetitive chains in the third month. The question then immediately arises, is babbling the source of the repetitive chains ? This view is implied by K. Bühler (MDC 52) when he tells us that the child derives so much pleasure from uttering single sounds that he utters them repeatedly. But it is a view which we cannot accept, for it fails to explain how repetition occurs in sounds expressive of *discomfort*. Pleasure in uttering isolated sounds cannot be the main source of repetition : this must arise independently of babbling.

On this point there is considerable agreement : Wundt and Baldwin among the older psychologists, Freud speaking for the psychoanalysts, McDougall for the Hormic school, and

Lorimer for the Behaviorists [1] are at one in this. Where they differ is in their view of the true origin of repetition, and here as in other cases we find the two alternative hypotheses of maturation and training. The former—Wundt's—asserts that one aspect of the primary response to a situation is a recurrence of sounds ; the other—Baldwin's—asserts that in some way the hearing of one's own sound acquires the power of arousing further utterance of a similar sound. It is worth noticing, however, that there is a tendency for some primary repetition to be postulated even by those who, in the main, follow Baldwin. We can in fact trace the growth of a compromise if we compare Baldwin's account with that of one of his strictest disciples, Allport (1924), and this again with that of Lorimer (1928). According to Allport (SP 182) the child hears his own voice uttering sounds, a conditioned reflex is established between the auditory—and kinæsthetic—sense-impressions and the motor mechanism, and thus the hearing of the sound gives rise to utterance. But to this Allport now adds that the most likely explanation is that the " return stimulations are received while the speaking response is still going on (as in a prolonged vowel sound) "—a suggestion which certainly does not exclude the possibility of some primary repetition before the process of establishing a reflex sets in. This implication is clearly brought out by Lorimer (GR 41, 45) who, in following Allport, says plainly that " a situation which evokes a specific type of vocalisation once is apt to evoke its repetition ". In this way he obtains the sequence of utterance . . . hearing . . . utterance that will form the basis of a conditioned reflex.

It would seem therefore that the opposition between the two views is not irreconcilable. Those who insist upon the effect of training need not exclude the possibility of repetition prior to this training. And as both the primary existence of repetition and the subsequent training in it have been well demonstrated by the divergent schools, we should do well to adopt this eclectic view.

In any case, one point stressed both by Allport and Lorimer needs to be noticed : that the child not only hears himself saying sounds but also feels himself doing so—the stimulations are kinæsthetic as well as auditory. This has recently been

[1] Wundt VP 287 ; Baldwin MD 249, 279 ; McDougall OP 174 ; Freud PP 43, 44 ; Lorimer GR 41.

independently corroborated in a most interesting way : Kampik, in a study of babbling in children born deaf, concludes (LT 355) that as a rule this is just as common, though not so definite, among them as among normal children, and adds further that the sense of vibration (*Vibrationssinn*) must take the place of hearing in the circular process that occurs in repetition. The child who cannot hear will nevertheless begin to babble ; what hearing does for the normal child is to make his babbling more definite, and also to render it a means by which he learns to approximate his own sounds to those of the adult language.

Summary.—Our discussion up to this point may be summarised as follows :

(i) *Differentiation :* possibly within a few hours after birth, the child's utterance is differentiated into cries expressive of discomfort and sounds expressive of comfort.

(ii) *Babbling of single sounds :* possibly within the second month, among the sounds uttered in states of comfort, some babbling of isolated sounds may occur.

(iii) *Babbling of repetitive chains :* possibly within the third month, in states of comfort, the child utters repetitive chains apparently for the sake of enjoying them.

(iv) *Babbling and repetition* may arise independently of each other ; but each will foster the development of the other.

II

Babbling as Play.—When we say that babbling is play, what do we mean ? The current view of play, including babbling, is that in a state of comfort, when the child is full of energy, he will make various movements—including sounds—for the mere sake of making them. This view is sponsored by such men as Stern (KSp 156) and McDougall (OP 171) ; in the words of the latter, play arises as " random movements " and is " purposeless, striving towards no goal ". I believe that neither of these statements is truly applicable to play in general or to babbling in particular.

The Source of Play Movements.—The former characteristic of play, that it arises at random, is stated with great emphasis by McDougall (OP 171, SP 400) ; the superabundant " hormic energy " of the child finds an outlet in the " motor mechanisms " with which he is innately endowed ; thus play movements are not in themselves instinctive, they arise by chance, as the manifestation of blind energy.

Casual observation of infants at play seems to bear out this view. Their kicking and stretching movements do seem to be aimless, and strongly contrasted with the movements by which they secure some desired object.

But now it is essential to distinguish between two questions, first, what is the origin of play movements as movements; secondly, how is it that they subsequently arise as play? The answer to the first question can scarcely be in doubt. Careful observation of play of every kind convinced Groos that it arises from movements which are themselves instinctive, and that we call them play when the child pursues them for their own sake; so that play may be regarded as an adaptation of instinctive movements.

Now when we examine McDougall's own treatment more carefully, we find that he too does not really mean to say that play springs from movements which are wholly random in character. For he tells us that these movements are the expression of hormic energy; and in all other places, wherever he speaks of hormic energy, this is always thought of as directed towards some end, it is never merely a blind force : " the fundamental nature of the hormic impulse is to work towards some natural goal " (SP 483). Thus the notion of hormic energy finding vent in merely random movements is self-contradictory. If a movement is a manifestation of hormic energy it is, to use McDougall's phrase, directed towards some natural goal, and thus is not more random than instinctive behaviour in general.

It would seem that McDougall has been led into an extreme presentation of his case by his desire to refute the view that there is a special instinct of play, which, he implies, is maintained by Groos (OP 170). But Groos is really very far from maintaining this : on the contrary, he explicitly asserts : " It seems to me unnecessary to suppose a particular play instinct in addition to all the others " (SM 488, PM 378). Groos's view of the relation between play and instinct is that in play instinctive movements are being practised ; that play movements arise as instinctive movements which then undergo the special adaptations characteristic of play.

This is actually quite in keeping with McDougall's hormic psychology as we can see from Drever, who follows McDougall's treatment almost entirely without however committing himself to the inconsistency which we have pointed out. Drever accepts the principle that in every case of apparently purposeless movement in play, the child is really following an instinctive line of behaviour (IM 223). Play comes in to supplement the working of the specific instincts (IM 167).

This is, in essence, Groos's view restated with the greater definiteness that comes from the work that has been done since he first wrote. We need not therefore accept McDougall's statement that play movements arise at random ; it is much more in keeping with his general system of hormic psychology to recognise that they are, fundamentally, adaptations of instinctive behaviour. And in the case of babbling we certainly find that the sounds which the child is now uttering in play were originally expressive either of comfort or discomfort : that is—to use the term broadly—" instinctive " in origin.

The Goal of Play Movements.—When these instinctive movements have become adapted as play, are they then directed towards any end ? A commonly accepted view of play—to quote McDougall once more—is that " it is a purposeless activity, striving towards no goal " (OP 171). This can hardly be denied, in so far as the child seeks, in play, nothing beyond the activity itself.

But we are then bound to ask, what is it that sustains this activity in the behaviour of the child ? To this again the answer can hardly be in doubt ; he finds satisfaction in the activity itself, and seeks the activity for the sake of this satisfaction. Even McDougall, anxious as he is to rebut the view that the search for satisfaction can be one of the primary springs of conduct, allows that the overflow of vital energy " generates a vague appetite for movement " (OP 172). This can only mean, if we take appetite in the sense in which he generally intends it, that on occasion the desire for movement may arise, independently of any external stimulus ; that the child may seek to make the movement because this has become desirable in itself.

Moreover, while he questions the role of hedonism as a primary motive of action, McDougall is always willing to allow that it may, as a secondary motive, supplement the main hormic impulses (SP 456). This, as he himself points out, is the view of Drever and of Freud ; we may add further that it is also the view of Groos (PM 31).

There seems to be no question then but that play movements —whatever may be the cause of their occurrence—will certainly soon be made by the child for the sake of the pleasure which they bring ; and this surely may be called their goal. At what stage in the child's development this goal becomes clearly envisaged is perhaps open to question ; but even on this point, it may be noticed, some psychologists are in no doubt : C. and K. Bühler maintain (KJ 71) that intention enters into a child's play within his first three months and that this indeed is the first appearance of intention in any of his activities.

It is clear then that the contrast between the " aimless ", " random ", " purposeless " nature of play and the purposiveness of reflex or instinctive behaviour may easily be overstressed ; we have to recognise that purpose certainly is present in play, but that it is of a different kind from that which dominates the specific reflexes or specific instinctive tendencies. The purpose of play is to secure the satisfaction which arises in the course of the activity itself. And if this is true of the child's play in general it is certainly also true of his babbling, even though it may be difficult to determine objectively at which point in his development he begins to make sounds for the sake of the pleasure they bring.

III

The Incentive in Babbling.—We come now to the crucial question : What kind of delight is it that the child finds in uttering either isolated sounds or strings of them ? Although we may say that play movements in general are made for the mere sake of making them, this is inadequate as an explanation of babbling.

For speech, even at the rudimentary level we are considering, is already a very special kind of activity. It is expressive, and expressive both of comfort and discomfort. Our problem then is this, under what conditions is the child likely to engage in the utterance of sounds not as expression, but for the mere pleasure of uttering them ?

If it were only a matter of repeating sounds which have been expressive of comfort, one might be tempted to say that it is their association with a pleasant state which now brings about their repetition. It might be said that something of this pleasantness would tend to be reinstated whenever the sound were uttered ; the back consonant **g,** for instance, or the labial **b,** would carry with it something of the pleasant feeling that follows a good meal. Then we might suppose that the child, " when he had nothing better to do ", that is, when all his primary needs were satisfied, might try in a vague way to make those noises that bring such a pleasant feeling with them. Or alternatively, we might suppose that the child, when quite comfortable, might utter one or other of these sounds " at random ", and then, something of the original pleasant condition being reinstated, he would seek to prolong this by repeating the sound.

But this, although it may cover some cases, is certainly not a complete explanation, for it leaves out of account the fact, mentioned above, that sounds primarily expressive of *discomfort* also become transformed into babbling. No theory of babbling can be regarded as adequate unless it embraces this transformation.

It is therefore worth pointing out that this kind of transformation in other forms of play has recently received some attention, although as far as I know it has not hitherto been demonstrated in the case of babbling. Thus Freud (PP 43) finds great significance in the fact that in play the child often repeats experiences that were unpleasant in the first instance. Guillaume (IE 85), without referring to Freud, records several examples from the behaviour of his year-old son ; the child, having pricked his finger with a pin, repeated the action several times with a tiny shriek ; on another occasion he tried to replace his finger in a door where it had been pinched. Guernsey (SN 161) tells us that a child of 0;11, having accidentally struck his head so hard against a bed that he cried, proceeded then to repeat the experience several times in rapid succession. And Bekhterev (PO 222) mentions the case of a child of 2;0 who, having been hurt in stumbling over a threshold, then amused herself by stepping backwards and forwards over it a dozen times.

Freud's explanation of such facts is well known. The child, he tells us (PP 43), by repeating what was in the first instance an unpleasant experience thereby gains mastery over it ; an unpleasant impression—which, when it occurred, had to be endured—now becomes something that the child freely wills, something under his control. C. and K. Bühler have applied this theory in a thoroughgoing way to the early play of children (KJ 71) ; but nobody has hitherto, I think, shown that it also applies to their babbling.

For there can be no doubt that here we have a hypothesis that provides adequately for all the facts of babbling, especially if we couple with it—as the Bühlers do—some reference to the form or pattern of the activity. The view that pleasure may arise from the mere pattern of an experience is accepted as a hypothesis by divergent schools of psychology, although it has perhaps been stated with most insistence by the Gestalt-theorists. As Koffka says (GM 246, 144), an experience of a sequence of events forms itself into a pattern, which becomes more definite by repetition. Then if an adequate portion of this pattern is experienced, it will tend to arouse an expectation of the complete pattern, and satisfaction will only arrive when completion takes place.

Now there can be no doubt that repetitive play in general, and babbling in particular, is characterised by having a regular pattern. The most obvious feature of babbling is the reduplication of sounds ; but in addition to this phonetic pattern there is frequently a pattern of intonation—a " tune " —which, though it may not be exactly repeated, has certainly a definite form. Further, in any series of babbling there is a marked rhythm ; Guernsey (SN 161) found in her observations of 200 children up to the age of 21 months that the rhythmical character of babbling contrasted most strongly with the formlessness of the child's imitation of adults uttering the same sounds.

We may well say, therefore, that the desire for " mastery " and the delight in a pattern are the two fundamental incentives in babbling as in other kinds of play. We must, however, go further and again point out that babbling is different from all other play by the very fact that it is play with the medium of language. For since language is expressive, when the child utters a cry in the course of any experience, a double pattern is formed for him : the pattern of the experience and the pattern of the accompanying cry. And when in babbling he recalls his earlier cry he not only is mastering this, but at the same time reinstating and also thereby mastering the experience which accompanied it. We might say, in fact, that when a child who has cried *mama* while hungry later says it in babbling, he is both playing at crying and playing at being hungry, and obtaining a " mastery " over both experiences.

The significance of this, both for the understanding of babbling itself and of its place in the development of language appears when we come to our next question : In what sense may babbling be regarded as rudimentary art ?

IV

Babbling as a Form of Art.—As soon as we recognise that babbling is a function of language standing by itself in the child's development we are recognising that he is occupied with a form of art, rudimentary indeed though this may be. To what extent can this view be justified ? Certainly it is a commonplace of æsthetics that there is a close relation between art and play. In the case of babbling this is generally covered by the statement that babbling is a form of art, or that it represents the beginning of the art of language in the life of the child.

But the acceptance of a vague general resemblance is not enough. It is not enough to say that babbling is play, that play gives rise to art, hence babbling is rudimentary art. We need to make a closer comparison, for the importance of recognising the æsthetic character of babbling is twofold. First, it enables us to complete our picture of the child's early linguistic activity, and secondly it gives us further insight into the later æsthetic function of language by enabling us to trace its development from the beginnings.

We are not, of course, called upon to make any analysis of " art " in general, if indeed any such analysis be possible. We need only make a summary of the broad characteristics of the æsthetic use of language, as contrasted with its scientific or practical uses.

Characteristics of Language with an Æsthetic Intention.— Language—whether the intention of the writer be æsthetic, scientific or practical—is used to symbolise experience. Are there any special characteristics in the nature of the experience, and in the nature of the symbolisation, which enable us to distinguish the æsthetic from the other uses of language ?

It will be agreed that the main difference between the artist—as we may call him—and the practical or scientific writer lies in the *intention* of his activity. The practical or scientific use of language is a means to an end, whereas æsthetic activity is self-sufficing : this of course is one of its affinities with play. And this difference between the æsthetic and other uses of language is found to exist both in the nature of the experience symbolised, and in the manner of its symbolisation.

(i) *The Experience Symbolised.*—All instances of utterance with an æsthetic intention involve the reinstatement of experience. So too does the use of language either with a practical or with a scientific intention. But we may contrast these with the æsthetic use in that here the reinstatement of experience is for the sake of the satisfaction which this very reinstatement brings ; whereas in the practical or the scientific use previous experiences are reinstated as a means to an end— the reinstatement is brought to bear upon the situation in hand.

Where the experience—" actual " or " imagined "—is pleasurable, it is easy to understand why it should be reinstated. This covers a large proportion of descriptive and narrative verse and prose, and much of the drama.

It is more difficult to understand why we should seek to reinstate an experience—actual or imagined—which is not pleasurable, which is perhaps even painful in itself. This is the problem of much lyrical poetry and of tragedy. What is the motive that causes Shakespeare to bring up before us the events of *King Lear* ? Here we are not called upon to do more than mention this ancient problem ; we have only to notice that when an experience is symbolised with an æsthetic intention, it is for the satisfaction which the reinstatement brings, a satisfaction which arises irrespective of the pleasant or painful nature of the original experience in itself.

(ii) *The Language that symbolises the Experience.*—Turning now from the experience to the language in which it is symbolised, we may say that this has a twofold function : referential and expressive—the words not only call up a situation, but they also express the writer's emotion. But does this emotion arise from the original situation in itself : is poetry primarily the expression, as Wordsworth says, of emotion recollected in tranquillity ? We may follow Alexander (BV 129) in doubting this, for although in some forms of poetry the emotion aroused in the writer by the original situation may be expressed, in other forms—the drama, for instance— it may be almost entirely absent.

But this does not mean, continues Alexander, that poetry is not born of emotion; there is another source of affect which is not only legitimate in art but indeed its distinguishing feature. Following Clive Bell, he calls this " æsthetic emotion "; the delight engendered by the act of æsthetic symbolisation. There is a joy in the manipulation of the material, and it is this joy—more than the emotion aroused by the original experience—which drives the artist to creation, and which he communicates to some extent in his work of art (CP 310).

Here is to be found one source of our delight in tragedy. The painful qualities of the original experience are not only transformed by the present reinstatement, but also subordinated to the pleasure which arises in the course of the work of symbolisation, so that while we might shun the mere repetition of the actual experience in itself, we find pleasure in the æsthetic symbolisation of it.

Presence of these Characteristics in Babbling.—It may seem ludicrous to attempt to trace the presence of these features of the æsthetic use of language in the babbling of an infant. But their existence is certainly implied in all comparisons made between babbling and art. To what extent, then, are these features actually to be found ?

It is clear from our discussion in the earlier part of this chapter that they certainly exist in a rudimentary form in babbling. Such differences as there are arise necessarily from the immaturity of the child. Thus there is as yet no question of the symbolisation of experience, there is only the expression of affect : but in so far as in babbling the child must partly revive bygone affective states when he repeats the sounds which once expressed them, we have the rudiments both of the reinstatement of an experience and the symbolisation of it—the two aspects of the æsthetic process.

In both respects babbling is rudimentary art. With regard to the experience reinstated we have seen that in babbling the child may come not only to repeat sounds originally expressive of pleasant states—possibly because they were pleasant—but also sounds expressive of an unpleasant state. We find that in order to explain this latter fact we had to invoke the hypothesis of " mastery "; the problem is, at its own primitive level, exactly parallel to that of the nature of tragedy in dramatic art. The poet who makes the tragic verse of *King*

Lear an embodiment of human suffering is, at an immeasurable distance, like the child who in a moment of play repeats his own cry of hunger.

Again, we find a similar parallel when we compare the child's attention to his sounds in babbling with the artist's attitude to the language he uses in symbolising experience. In some measure the sounds uttered in babbling may still express the emotion which they originally expressed : but undoubtedly this is subordinated to the emotion now present—the joy of babbling, the joy of manipulating the material : spoken sounds. In a word, the affective attitude, " æsthetic emotion ", which Alexander finds peculiarly characteristic of the artist, we find present in a rudimentary form in the babbling child.

Thus even in this brief comparison it is evident that babbling presents in a rudimentary form the features of the æsthetic use of language. We must recognise therefore that there is much more than a vague general similarity between the two activities : the child's babbling is actually the beginning of his æsthetic use of words ; so that almost from the very outset the practical and the æsthetic functions of language develop side by side. Thus there are twin impulses in the development of language in the child's life : on the one hand, the satisfaction of his primary needs, and, on the other, the satisfaction of æsthetic tendencies which, arising in the first instance out of his expression of these needs, soon become an independent activity.

CHAPTER VI

IMITATION

IMITATION obviously plays an important part in the development of the child's speech. But when we come to consider the nature of linguistic imitation, we find ourselves confronted with difficulties similar to those which encumber the discussion of babbling. For studies of imitation are usually of a general character, in which hypotheses are formulated to embrace not only the wide range of imitation in human behaviour, but often also its features in animal behaviour.

Here we are concerned only with linguistic imitation, so that while we must take account of the light that is thrown on this particular activity by general studies of imitation, we must also be careful not to allow conceptions derived from them to take us beyond the facts as we find them. In accordance with our general plan, we shall here attempt both to give an outline of the actual course of events, and also to consider their theoretical implications.

One difficulty arises from the form of the available records. Clearly, accounts of observations should necessarily begin at birth, in order to avoid the omission of any possibly relevant facts. But the child's earlier behaviour does not, as we shall see, obviously appear to be imitative, with the result that some observers, such as Preyer, concluding that imitation does not begin until towards the end of the first year, omit any earlier observations.

Evidently much depends upon our criterion of imitation. If we accept as imitation only that fully-fledged activity in which one behaves in a fashion closely resembling a model, it is certainly true that behaviour of this kind rarely occurs in the first eight or nine months of a child's life. But on the other hand, it is equally true that the child, in his earliest months, will engage in behaviour which partly resembles that which he perceives at the moment ; and whatever name we may give to this behaviour it is essential to take account of it in order to see what relation it bears to the undoubted imitation which appears later.

This means that there are two ways in which children's imitation is simpler than imitation in adult life. In the first place the young child imitates only simple activities, the adult more complex ones. But there is another and perhaps more fundamental difference : imitation in infancy is not merely imitation of simple activities, it is in itself rudimentary. That is to say, early imitation is only a primitive form of the conduct to which we give the same name in adult behaviour : imitation itself develops. In our particular study here we have to recognise that linguistic imitation grows and changes while language itself grows, and in order to give an adequate account of its place in the behaviour of the infant, we must begin with the very first behaviour which in any way resembles imitation.

It is also essential, as in the case of babbling, for us to be able to relate the child's imitative behaviour to the rest of his linguistic experience at the same moment. Even if imitation were an isolated phenomenon, this would still be necessary in order that its immediate function might be understood ; but actually, as we shall show, what we mark off as imitation is very closely related at every stage to the general linguistic behaviour of the child. We therefore need records which show the child's imitative responses in their contemporary setting.

The Data.—As in the case of other speech activities, the records may be either statistical or individual. The only statistical work I have come across is Guernsey's study of various kinds of imitative behaviour, including language, in 200 children of ages 0;2 to 1;9. In Appendix II, I have given fully all the individual records which I have been able to find and which are sufficiently complete to be of use—the work of Preyer, Stern, Hoyer, Guillaume and Valentine. To these I have added my own observations of K, giving in all cases any available notes of the other concurrent linguistic behaviour of the child.

Three Stages of Development.—We shall see that these five records, together with the general conclusions of Guernsey's statistical work, enable us to divide the progress of linguistic imitation during the child's first year into three broad stages :

(I) *First three or four months :* the child responds to human utterance by making sounds.

(II) *A period of pause :* at the outset of this period there seems to be a diminution, if not an entire cessation, of the vocal responses to speech typical of the first stage ; then vocal responses gradually reappear.

(III) *After about* 0;9 : the child's behaviour becomes more definitely marked by those features which are to characterise imitation during infancy and childhood.

This is simply a summary of the available observations, but —at first sight at any rate—it does not bear out either of the two main views of early imitation which till recently have held the field. On the one hand many writers, following Darwin, have maintained that imitation does not begin until towards the end of the first year ; on the other hand Stern, until the last issue of his book, held that imitation begins in the third month and continues steadily from that point onwards.

But on closer examination we find that there is really a good deal of general support for the summary we have made. As for our Stage I, it has never been denied that children two or three months old normally make some vocal responses to human speech, but only that these responses are imitation. This doubt, first put forward by Darwin in 1877 (BI 290), has since been repeatedly expressed—by Preyer in 1882 (MC 109), Baldwin in 1894 (MD 124), Ronjat in 1913 (DL 41), and Delacroix in 1924 (LP 275).

But as we have already suggested, this is simply a question of the criterion of imitation. Of course, these early responses are not imitation of exactly the same kind as we find later on. But they are unquestionably the rudimentary beginnings of imitation. There is a continuous development, as we shall show, from the child's behaviour at this first stage right through to those later responses which all observers alike regard as imitation. The importance of considering this early behaviour is recognised in the recent work of Stern, Hoyer, Guillaume and Valentine, who all begin their studies of imitation with the child's first months.

As for our Stage II, we shall later bring forward the evidence which justifies it. But this may be said here : until recently those who agreed with Stern that imitation begins in the child's second or third month also held that it continued from that time onwards, though—to use Stern's own word—only in a " sporadic " fashion (KSp 151).[1] In the last edition of his book (1928) he has, however, altered his statement so that

---

[1] 3rd edition, 1922.

now he stresses the *suspension* of imitation for some time after the earliest months (KSp 162). But in spite of this and the evidence which I have cited in Appendix II, no attention has hitherto been given to the existence of a period of slackening in the development of imitation.

Let us now consider in turn each of the three stages set out above.

I

Stage I (up to about 0;4).—During this, the first stage, the child definitely takes a step in the development of imitation— he responds to human speech by making sounds. We have seen (p. 39) that one form of this kind of response may occur even as early as the first month, when the child cries on hearing another child cry. And if the nature of this behaviour is not yet certain, and we may have to regard it merely as one instance of the child's vocal expression of discomfort on hearing loud noises, there can be no question that in the second and third months children normally respond vocally to speech as speech —that is, as emanating from human beings. At this time, as we saw, the child's vocal response to another child's cry occurs more readily when he can see the crier than when he cannot (p. 45) ; and again—as Guernsey concluded from her survey of a group—the child's vocal response to the adult human voice now becomes a marked feature of his behaviour (p. 41).

Instances of these early vocal responses to adult speech occur in all the observations given in Appendix II, and three of their characteristics are to be noticed : first, they most readily occur when the child is attentive to the speaker ; secondly, they are imitative in this sense, that the child's utterance is specially evoked by hearing adult speech ; and thirdly, that this utterance consists of his own familiar sounds.

(i) *The Importance of Attention to the Speaker.*—It has often been observed that vocal responses to heard speech occur most readily if the adult smiles when speaking to the child. In my own observations I noted repeatedly that unless I smiled and caught the child's eye while speaking, I obtained no response at all from him. Again, Hoyer tells us (Appendix II, p. 244, entry 0;1,24), that his son's vocal response was first aroused by adult speech when this was accompanied by a smile. And Valentine makes the point, throughout his discussion of imitation in infants (PI), that it depends on the child's interest in the person before him. Finally, Guernsey (SN 121), summarising her own observations of vocal and other imitation in 200 children, and reviewing the literature, agrees with Pillsbury that imitative behaviour is to be regarded as one of the characteristic accompaniments of attention ; she points out that the responses of a child to speech in his second or third month are brief, precisely because his attention is rudimentary.

All this suggests that while in his first month the child's vocal responses to crying may be no more than a simple reaction to a loud noise, certainly this is no longer true of his responses either to infants or adults in his second and third months. At this time he responds much more readily when his attention is attracted to the speaker.

(ii) *The Effect of the Human Voice.*—Next we have to notice that even at this early stage the human voice already seems to have a special power of evoking speech from the child. Many varied stimuli, of course, tend to rouse him to vocal expression, but the human voice is more effective than any other. This is accepted as a fundamental fact by Stern (KSp 160).

When does this special effect of heard speech first appear ? We have noticed above that we cannot yet be sure whether in a child's first month the cry of another child is more effective than other harsh noises in evoking a responsive cry. But even on the most cautious view there cannot be any doubt that in the child's second or third month he responds vocally to an adult voice. On page 41 we have already given some instances of this—the observations made by Hoyer, Guillaume, Stern and Bühler between the seventh and the eleventh weeks. It is also strikingly illustrated in another way in the experiment made by Valentine with a child in his fifth week (Appendix II, p. 247, entry 0;1,2). Here, at a moment when the child was already making sounds, the adult intervened and spoke to him, with the result that the child's sounds immediately became more frequent. It so happens that I myself, before the publication of Valentine's work and in ignorance of it, carried out the same experiment with K when he was 10 weeks old (Appendix II, p. 249, entry 0;2,19) ; the results it will be seen are similar.

(iii) *The Form of the Child's Response.*—We next have to

ask how far the child's response resembles the sounds which
he hears ; and on this point again some observers are in no
doubt : they agree with Stern (KSp 15, 161) that if the adult
makes a sound chosen from the child's repertory, the latter
will respond with an exactly similar sound.

Further, this would appear to be true both of intonational
and of phonetic form.   Intonation, as we have said before, is
rarely recorded ; but we do happen to have a few incidental
observations of children's intonation in responding to speech.
Hoyer, for instance, tells us (LK 377) that from the outset
his son's imitative responses were characterised by the correct
intonation and stress ; C. Bühler (KJ 42) that her daughter's
re re at 0;2,18 was spoken with exactly the same intonation
as her own ; and Guillaume also notes particularly of his son
(Appendix II, page 246), that at 0;3,24, and again at 0;3,30
and 0;4,10, the child's intonation was rather like his mother's
as she spoke or sang to him.

For similarity of phonetic form we have the testimony of
Stern (at 0;2½), Valentine (on the 38th and 39th days), Hoyer
(at 0;2), C. Bühler (at 0;2,18), and Guillaume (at 0;2,11, at
0;4 and at 0;5) ; see Appendix II.

But against all this it must be also pointed out that sometimes the child's responses resemble what he hears neither in
intonation nor in phonetic form.   In my own case, being
particularly interested in this point from Stern's account, I
was somewhat disconcerted to find repeatedly that the child K
responded by making a sound only very slightly similar to my
rendering of one of his.   For instance, at 0;3,12, when I said
gu, which he had been saying for some time past, he answered
very definitely **ǔɛ**.   When therefore I came across Guillaume's
work, I was strongly impressed by his remark (IE 43, 44) that
he often failed, in the early months, to obtain from his two
children a sound at all similar to the one which he had borrowed from their repertory.   Further, this was exactly the
experience of Valentine in observing those three of his children
who made some vocal response to speech in their second
month (PI 109).   It would appear, then, that we are able to
accept Stern's statement only in these modified terms : that
the child's vocal response to adult speech in his earliest months
consists of his own familiar sounds ; when he hears a sound
drawn from his own repertory, his response may occasionally
resemble it in intonational and phonetic form.

The Nature of these Responses.—Having described these responses as occurring when the child is attentive to a speaker and consisting of his own familiar sounds, we have next to ask how they arise.

It is evident that they are only to be understood if taken in relation to the rest of the child's linguistic behaviour : that is, his own speech and his response to the speech of others. Looked at in this way these early imitative responses may be regarded as a special case where two kinds of behaviour happen to coincide—the child responds to speech, and his response consists of speaking. But we must not forget that the child's speech at this time is of two kinds—expression and babbling. How is it likely to come about in these two kinds of speech that the child shall speak when he is spoken to, and also that what he says shall sometimes resemble what he hears ?

Three explanations appear to be current : first, that there is an innate tendency for the child to respond to speech by speech ; secondly, that the child responds by expression to expression ; and thirdly, that vocal responses to speech arise from intervention of the adult into the child's activity of babbling. We shall try to show that in the light of the evidence at present available none of these three hypotheses can definitely be rejected ; that all three factors indeed seem to be present to some extent.

(i) *The Innate Tendency to respond Vocally to Speech.*—There is a general belief in the existence of this innate tendency, usually coupled with the qualification that it takes some time to mature. Some writers—for instance, Marichelle and Delacroix—suggest that physiologically the organs of speech and hearing function in a parallel fashion ; others—for instance, Stern—postulate an instinct of imitation ; while a third group —for instance, Guillaume, Koffka and McDougall—reject the notion of a specific instinct in favour of what the last-named calls an impulse to respond to sounds by some vocal utterance.[1]

On the other hand, there are a number of writers—particularly in America, where the influence of Baldwin is still strong —who deny the existence of any innate tendency of this kind. Perhaps the best exponent of this view is Allport. But, as we shall show later (p. 80), the facts of babbling, at any rate,

[1] Le Dantec MI 279 ; Marichelle RA 786 ; Delacroix LP 294 ; Stern KSp 321 ; Koffka GM 330 ; Guillaume IE 33-6 ; McDougall OP 175.

demand that we shall accept the existence both of an innate tendency and of subsequent training.

In adopting the hypothesis that the mere perception of the human voice is naturally a stimulus to the production of sounds, we must however remember that the situation is never isolated in this way. Soon the three main functions of language for the child begin to develop—he responds to the expression of others, he expresses himself, and he babbles. Thus while the tendency persists for him to respond to speech by speech, it is these other factors which determine how far what he says shall resemble what he hears.

(ii) *The Expressive Response to Expression.*—We discussed in Chapter IV, page 41, the fact that the child in his second month will normally be found responding expressively to the expressions of others, although we cannot estimate how far this is the manifestation of an innate tendency, and how far due to training. These expressive responses form one of the main conditions in which imitation arises ; for it is when the child is attending to the speaker that his vocal response most frequently occurs.

We can trace the occurrence of these responses in the records of Hoyer and of Guillaume, part of which have already been cited in Chapter IV (pp. 39-40). In Hoyer's case we noticed that by the seventh week the child had begun to smile in response to an adult voice ; to this we can now add that next day, on hearing a voice he spoke as well as smiled, while a week later he had begun to make sounds similar to those that he heard, if they were drawn from his own repertory (Appendix II, p. 244).

Guillaume's records of his daughter give us a similar series ; though not so detailed as those of his son (Appendix II, p. 245) they show more clearly the relation between the child's vocal responses and his other responses to human beings. To complete the account given in Chapter IV (p. 40) which traced the development of this child as far as the occurrence of smiles in response to a voice, we can now add further incidental observations scattered up and down Guillaume's book (IE 33, 44, 185) :

At 2 days : The child smiled after feeding.

From 2nd to the 9th day : She smiled on various occasions, but never on seeing or hearing another person.

On 9th day : She smiled on seeing, and hearing the voice of, a familiar person, but only *after* feeding.

On 23rd day : She smiled on being spoken to by a familiar person, this time *before* feeding.

On 27th day : She smiled regularly at the sight of father, mother or brother.

At 1 month 12 days : She smiled on hearing the voice of any of these familiar persons.

At 2 months : She responded to the voice of familiar persons by movements as well as by smiling.

At 2 months 13 days : She responded in these ways to a familiar voice, even when she could not see the speaker.

At 2 months 15 days : She *spoke* in response to her father's voice, carrying on a " dialogue " with him.

Now by the time a child reaches the end of such a series, we may reasonably say he is beginning to imitate—he carries on a " dialogue " with an adult. But at what point in this series does his speech cease to be expression, or the response to expression, and become imitation? In Hoyer's case, for instance, the child had been gurgling as expressive of his satisfaction since the age of 0;1,20 ; he had been making some positive response to a heard voice since his fourth week ; at 0;2,0 it happened that the two events coincided—he spoke in response to speech. It is clear that although this may be called the child's expressive vocal response to heard speech, it may also be called rudimentary imitation and is, as we shall show, one source of later complete imitation.

This early vocal response to speech will appear to be imitation, and provide the conditions for the further development of imitation, in so far as the child's own expressive sounds resemble the sounds that he hears. Later, with the entrance of conditions that we shall subsequently describe, this will frequently occur ; it is likely to be less frequent at the stage we are now considering. For the child's response to speech is —as we have seen in Chapter IV—partly a primary response and partly subject to training : thus at the age of three months he will reply positively to a friendly tone, with the appearance of imitation ; but he will also reply positively to many angry tones, and may fail to reply at all to speech which is not affectively toned (see pp. 44 and 45). In these last two cases imitation will appear to be absent.

It is not surprising then that any observer, whose criterion of imitation is a frequent vocal response resembling what is heard, should hesitate—as many since Preyer have done—to regard these early responses as imitation. But just as we cannot draw a clear line between the occurrence of a " dialogue " and the child's earlier vocal response to a smile, so we shall find that later fully-fledged imitation develops directly out of these " dialogues ".

(iii) *The Effect of Babbling.*—We come now to the third condition under which the child's vocal response to speech may occur—the intervention of an adult into the child's babbling. This is the commonest of observations, and the accepted view is that it is due to associations set up in the course of such interventions. It is, in fact, Baldwin's view, based upon his hypothesis of " Circular Reaction " (MD 126, 249), and there are few writers on children's imitation who do not accept this principle in one form or another. We find it in Bekhterev, Stern, McDougall, Koffka, Guillaume and Allport, who is followed by Lorimer and Markey.[1] In the course of repetitive babbling, a pattern of alternating hearing and utterance is set up ; if an adult repeatedly imitates one of a child's own sounds while he is babbling, the heard sound becomes a part of the pattern of alternation, so that ultimately it remains effective in evoking speech which may resemble the stimulus both in phonetic and in intonational form.

But it is important to notice that several writers—Stern, McDougall, Koffka and Guillaume—have found it necessary to supplement Baldwin's principle by accepting at the same time the principle of a general tendency to respond to speech by speech. Of these only Guillaume and Koffka make it clear that they recognise the inadequacy of Baldwin's view to explain the facts. Guillaume (IE 39) tells us that the process cannot be that the mere auditory memory of one of the child's own sounds is of itself automatically effective in evoking a similar sound—there must be an incentive to produce it ; while Koffka (GM 329) urges the importance of the facts which show that there is an innate tendency, prior to any training, to respond to speech by speech.

These two writers base their criticism upon general considerations ; but I do not think that it has been shown before

[1] Bekhterev PO 220 ; Stern KSp 161 ; McDougall OP 175 ; Koffka GM 329 ; Guillaume IE 38 ; Allport SP 183 ; Lorimer GR 42, 45 ; Markey SP 32.

that the actually observed facts of early babbling and imitation demand that Baldwin's principle shall be modified and supplemented. According to him, the child, having uttered a sound such as *ba* repeatedly in babbling, will have formed an associative connection between the sensation of hearing the sound and the movements of saying it. Then an adult says *ba* ; the sensation of hearing this chimes in with the child's auditory memory of his own sound *ba* and he makes this sound. But how does this explain the fact mentioned above (p. 75) and noticed by such observers as Guillaume and Valentine, that the child often responds with a different sound ? When, for instance, I said **gu** very carefully to K (imitating one of his commonest babbling sounds) he replied with **ŭɛ,** certainly one of his familiar sounds, but nothing like the one spoken by me.

To explain this on Baldwin's lines we must assume that the sound of my word **gu** chimed in with the auditory memory of the child's own word **ŭɛ,** and was " confused " with it sufficiently to evoke the utterance **ŭɛ**—which seems very improbable. This is the weak spot in Baldwin's theory. Our only alternative is to recognise that the hearing of the adult word can merely stimulate the child to the utterance of his *own* babbling sounds, and that from this the child may become trained to respond with a particular sound to a particular heard sound. Baldwin's hypothesis is certainly valuable, so long as we couple it with the fundamental assumption that the child tends to reply to speech by speech. On this view we could explain the observed facts as follows : an adult says **gu,** thereby inciting the child to make a sound, which— because it is uttered in a state of comfort—is likely to be one of his babbling sounds, for instance **ŭɛ.** Then it is the hearing of *this* sound—the child's own—which may set in motion a train of babbling, so that the child repeats **ŭɛ** several times. Instances of this stimulation of a train of babbling by an adult word are common enough. I have already cited one from Valentine's record and one from my own (see Appendix II, pp. 247 and 249). Now if an incident such as we have just described were to happen frequently, it is evident that a process of training might take place—as Baldwin suggests— so that the particular adult sound **gu** would become the stimulus to the child's particular sound **ŭɛ.**

But could this ever be called imitation ? It might certainly be called this by an observer who, making guttural crooning noises rather like the child's customary babble, received somewhat similar noises in return. Or, even if a stricter criterion were demanded, there will often be some appearance of imitation because at this stage the child's repertory in babbling is comparatively limited, so that the child's response must sometimes coincide with the sound which the adult has chosen from the child's own repertory. And, a coincidence of this kind having occurred, any adult who set himself to make it the beginning of training might well succeed in establishing a regular response by the child of a particular sound on hearing this sound uttered.

Thus it is extremely doubtful whether a view which relies entirely upon Baldwin's theory as an explanation of the effect of the adult's intervention into the child's babbling is tenable ; and this is a criticism which may be made of Allport (SP 183) and those, such as Lorimer (GR 42, 45) and Markey (SP 32), who follow him closely. Allport does, indeed, say that the process as he describes it is hypothetical, and—although he presents it in physiological terms—even adds that " precise physiological data are wanting ".

All the observations go to show that the child is very far from behaving with machine-like regularity. Once again then it is not surprising that careful observers such as Preyer have refused to admit the existence of imitation at this stage. And once again we are bound to say that if fully-fledged imitation is certainly absent, the beginnings of imitation, and the conditions out of which its later developments spring, are certainly present.

From what has been said in the present section, it would seem that at the stage we are now considering three factors may combine to determine the child's vocal response to speech : the primary stimulus-effect of a heard voice, the expressive response to expressive speech, and the effect of an adult's intervention into the child's activity of babbling. But it is important to notice that as the child develops, probably none of these factors alone remains powerful enough to bring about a vocal response. This is illustrated by an observation of my own, given in Appendix II, pp. 249–50. Stern (KSp 133) and Guillaume (IE 57) mention that the sight of a speaker's lips moving silently as in speech may evoke a vocal response from the child. What happened in the case of K was this :

at 0;2,20 I noticed that he would not respond vocally either to my smile or my voice alone, but only to a combination of both. And again at 0;3,12 when I said **gu** without smiling, he did not respond ; nor did he when I smiled without speaking or making any lip-movement. But when I both moved my lips and smiled he said **ŭɛ.** This suggests that the child's vocal response was aroused not by facial expression (the smile) alone, nor by vocal expression alone, nor by my voice as a primary sense-stimulus alone, but to a combination of facial expression and vocal expression, even if this were presented merely as a movement of the lips.

In addition to these two factors, the intervention of the adult into the child's activity of babbling would also play its part in this way : it would help to maintain the identity of his response through training. Together then the three factors would tend ultimately to bring about vocal imitation.

Summary of Stage I.—From this discussion the following statement may be made of the probable character of the beginning of vocal imitation :

1. During his first three or four months the child responds positively to adult speech, making one of his own familiar sounds. The factors present seem to be :

(i) The primary stimulus-effect of heard speech.

(ii) Expression : heard speech, as uttered by a smiling friendly person, arouses a state of pleasure, which is expressed by characteristic expressive sounds.

(iii) Babbling : heard speech becomes, as a result of training, effective in evoking the child's own familiar babbling sounds.

2. There will probably not be at this stage any but a broad similarity between what the child hears and what he says in response.

3. The three factors above mentioned together determine the nature of the response at this stage, as well as the subsequent development of closer imitation.

II

Stage II.—This is a period during which there seems to be a diminution, if not an entire cessation, of the vocal responses characteristic of the first stage.

This period of pause is clearly illustrated in the records

given in Appendix II of the five children observed throughout their first year. In the case of Hilde Stern the period lasted from the age of $2\frac{3}{4}$ months to $7\frac{1}{2}$ months : in Hoyer's son from the age of 2 months until 8 months $1\frac{1}{2}$ weeks ; in Guillaume's son from 0;2,23 until some time towards the end of the year : in Valentine's son apparently from 0;1,9 until 0;6,0 ; and in K from 0;3,12 until 1;0. There are, it would seem, individual differences in the rate of development, but in all five cases the characteristic behaviour of the earliest months is followed by a period during which vocal response to speech ceases altogether or occurs only rarely. We shall show later that the marked recurrence of imitation usually appears some time after the ninth month.

It is only recently that any attention has been given to this period of slackening, although observations showing its existence have long been known. Darwin, as we should expect, missed nothing ; in his observations made in 1840 and published in 1877 he tells us (BI 290) that after some doubtfully imitative responses in his son's fourth month, no further imitation occurred until the tenth. This observation was exactly corroborated by Preyer in 1882 (MC 109) ; but Stern, writing in 1907 (KSp 151), speaks of the sporadic occurrence of imitative responses from the third month right through the first year. It is not until the revised fourth edition of his work, 1928 (KSp 162), that he stresses the lapse of imitation during a period extending from the third until the eighth month. In the meantime Guillaume (IE 36) had drawn attention to the fact that vocal imitation after the fifth month is rare, appearing in force only towards the end of the year. But the value of his discussion is diminished by his refusal to recognise that the child's frequent vocal responses to speech before the fifth month are imitative in nature, so that our second stage appears in his account not so much a pause as the rare rudimentary beginnings of imitation.

But this will not do, because in accordance with such observers as Stern, Hoyer and Guernsey, we must take into account imitation in those earlier vocal responses which Guillaume himself has observed, but dismissed as " exceptional ".

Imitation and the Growth of Meaning.—Our problem, in fact, is to explain how it is that these earlier responses lapse, and this seems inexplicable, so long as we take imitation as an isolated activity, apart from the rest of the child's linguistic behaviour. But if, as before, we continue to observe his vocal responses to speech in relation to his general development, we certainly do not find that these responses merely cease; what happens is that they are mostly replaced by behaviour of a different kind. The child, in fact, begins to respond to the meaning of what he hears; there is a corresponding inhibition of simple vocal responses to heard speech.[1]

We have already seen that a development of this kind takes place, within the child's first two months, in his responses to other children's cries; a similar change accounts for the inhibition of simple vocal responses to adult speech.

Let us notice, for instance, what occurred in the case of K during a couple of months, as given in Appendix II, pages 249–51.

At 0;2,16–24 : Considerable vocal response to the voice of his father, when the latter attracts the child's attention by smiling while speaking.
No response to voice of his father out of sight.
At 0;3,12 : Observation similar to above.
At 0;3,22 : For the first time the crying child responds positively to the voice of his father out of sight, by *ceasing* to cry.
At 0;4,2 : Very infrequent vocal response to voice of his father, even when the latter attracts the child's attention by smiling while speaking.
Marked vocal response to presence of his mother, mainly when he is in *a state of need*. But no vocal response to mere presence of his father.
At 0;4,4–26 : As in previous two entries.
At 0;5,4 : No vocal response to voice of his mother when he is in a state of comfort, and she attracts his attention by smiling.

In two months, then, this child's vocal responses to the mere hearing of speech have become extremely rare instead of frequent; while at the same time both his own articulate utterance and his responses to speech have become more meaningful. They have become meaningful in a special way : by being linked up with the presence of particular persons. As we see in the entry at 0;4,2, the appearance of the child's

---

[1] After coming to this conclusion from my own observations and the other sources I have mentioned, I found that the clue had probably been given to me in a remark added by Stern to the 4th edition of KSp (p. 135). He points out that the child's interest in meaning may sometimes directly inhibit imitation.

mother now evokes a specific utterance ε ε ε, at a time when he is in need ; it is therefore less likely that her words, when he is not in a state of need, will arouse any merely " imitative " response (0;5,4). In the same way, the entry at 0;3,22 shows the child responding for the first time to his father's voice in the absence of the speaker ; soon after this (0;4,2) the child tends to respond less frequently to his father's words when these are spoken for the mere purpose of securing imitation.

This change in the child's response to speech is seen very clearly if we compare the entry at 0;3,12 with that at 0;4,2 or any that follow (see Appendix II, p. 250). In the first case, the child usually responded to a smile by smiling, and to speech uttered with a smile by speaking. By 0;4,2 the picture had changed ; the child responded to smiling in one of two ways, either by smiling or neutrally, that is, although his attention was held, he made neither a positive nor a negative response. My note runs, " Sometimes he remains stolidly looking at the speaker without any other response." In the same way, his response to speech accompanied by a smile was now either a smile or neutral ; very rarely did he respond vocally. At 0;4,18, I noted, " When he makes a vocal response, there is not much resemblance to the word spoken to him ; and then it is not certain that it has merely been aroused by the stimulus, for repetition often fails to bring forth the response." In other words, the child's response had no longer the character of the simple arousal of speech by the hearing of speech ; it was becoming much more definitely an expression of the effect of this speech upon him ; he was beginning to respond more certainly to its meaning—mainly, its affective quality.

In considering vocal imitation, we must in fact constantly bear in mind that it is peculiarly different from all other imitation in that it is imitation of speech : an activity, that is, which has a symbolical function in the life of the adult speaker, and already possesses some rudiments of this function, in the life of the listening child. And although the child may find a meaning in what he hears very different from the meaning intended by the speaker, nevertheless it is a meaning ; and it is the increasing preoccupation with this meaning which brings with it a lapse of the purely imitative responses which we are able to observe in the earliest months.

The course of progress of vocal imitation is, indeed, an exact reflection of the development of the child's responses to the meaning of adult language, as shown for instance in the work of Bühler and Hetzer to which we have already referred (p. 45). We have seen that after about the fourth month imitative responses become rare ; while Bühler and Hetzer show that it is about this very same time that the child begins to respond to speech no longer in a uniform positive fashion, but in relation to its affective quality. Thus we cannot resist the conclusion that the lapse of imitative responses is only another way of looking at the fact that the child is coming to respond to the meaning of the speech that he hears.

It is evident that the development of discrimination will inevitably diminish the possible scope for the occurrence of the simple primary response to speech by speech. The mere growth of neutral responses will in itself of course lessen the possible number of imitative responses. On the other hand, the discrimination, by a positive or negative response, between positively and negatively toned speech, might at first sight appear to increase the semblance of imitation, were it not for the fact that at the same time the child's utterance is becoming more defined in its articulation. In this way the difference between what he utters and what he has heard becomes more apparent. So long as he responds to all that he hears by somewhat inarticulate positive noises, we may be ready to take them as imitation ; but this identification becomes less possible as both his comfort-sounds develop their own distinctive features, and as his discomfort-cries, already well-developed, enter as a response to negatively-toned speech.

Effects of the Growth of Meaning.—The growth of meaning in heard speech will have its effect upon each of the three tendencies mentioned in our discussion of Stage I : first, the innate dependence of utterance upon hearing ; secondly, the child's expressive response to utterance ; and thirdly, the entrance of adult speech as a stimulus within the course of a repetitive chain of babbling.

The mere dependence of uttered speech upon heard speech will obviously be greatly affected by the growth of meaning in the latter. We might even say that this dependence dies out after Stage I, were it not that it reappears in the subsequent period, Stage III, particularly in the form of " delayed imitation " (see p. 95). It seems more reasonable to say then that in Stage II the dependence of speech upon hearing falls into abeyance, or at least is obscured ; for while the child will still tend to respond to speech by speech, what he says will be determined more and more by the meaning of what he hears, by its accompanying circumstances. The child's utterance, as I have said above in my observation of K at 0;4,18 (p. 85), will no longer appear to be automatically stimulated by the mere occurrence of an adult word, but will begin to be a reply or meaningful response to it.

The child's expressive response to utterance will also evidently be affected by the growth of meaning in both what he says and what he hears. The result is a diminution of apparent imitation both when we speak expressively to the child and when we address ourselves to secure his imitation. In the former case, the tendency does, of course, persist ; if the child's mother speaks to him in a caressing tone of voice, he will continue to respond by making comfort-sounds. But this response becomes less inevitable as he learns to respond not simply to the affective character of speech, but to speech in a context of circumstances ; thus his response may be inhibited where his own state or the context is unfavourable. Further, his response, when it does occur, is now less likely to be vocal, for his own utterance is also becoming more definitely linked up with specific situations. As a result he will certainly appear to be less imitative, on the whole, when he is simply being spoken to.

In the same way, he will respond less frequently when we address ourselves to secure imitation from him. For as heard speech comes to acquire meaning from its context, it will become progressively meaningless in the absence of such a context. When we speak to him in order that he may imitate, the situation is a peculiar one both in intonation and in gesture, and the child's response—which might be forth-coming in a " meaningful " context—is inhibited. Thus again he seems to be less imitative.

Finally, the effect of the adult voice upon a repetitive chain of babbling will also be influenced by the growth of meaning in heard speech. For if an adult happens to speak in a manner that has begun to be meaningful for the child, the latter will respond to this either expressively or neutrally, according to circumstances. If, on the other hand, the adult deliberately utters a sound from the child's own repertory in order to arouse a chain of babbling, there may be no result, simply because the child by now tends to inhibit responses to meaningless speech. Nevertheless, as Guillaume found (IE 45), throughout this period of Stage II, the adult voice does occasionally set going a chain of babbling. This will occur either when the child is actually babbling or, we must suppose, is in a state conducive to play. For in babbling the child is not concerned with the meaning of what he says—the stream flows on in an automatic self-maintained fashion. If now, while the child's attention is withdrawn from concern with meaning, a sound from without drops into the stream of his utterance, the effect may still be seen in an increased flow of babbling. And even if he is not actually babbling, but yet in the right mood, the hearing of one of his familiar babbled words may cause him to speak it.

Thus, while the growth of meaning in both heard and uttered speech operates now in an inhibitory fashion upon all three factors which have tended to produce imitative responses, it does not entirely abolish these responses. They occur sporadically, though to a diminished extent, throughout this period, which we have named Stage II. It is only when the child becomes aware of the activity of imitation in itself that this activity becomes frequent once more ; this is the next stage.

III

Stage III (from about 0;9 onwards).—We have placed the beginning of the third stage during the tenth month, as an intermediate point among the varying estimates of the different observers. Their records show that about this time certain marked changes occur in the frequency and the nature of the child's imitative responses. These changes are :

(i) A readier imitation of sounds drawn from the child's own vocabulary.

(ii) The more certain imitation of intonational form.

(iii) The appearance of delayed imitation.

(iv) The more definite imitation—perhaps the first imitation—of sound-groups new to the child.

(v) The development of " echolalia ".

The earliest time for the beginning of this third stage of quickened imitation is that given by Guernsey, who tells us (SN 146) that imitation of unfamiliar words begins at 0;7, while delayed imitation occurs not before 0;8½ (SN 165). Stern's observations of his daughter, as given in Appendix II (p. 243), show the period of quickened imitation as beginning with the eighth month, and he records (KSp 82) a similar observation of his son.   In the case of Hoyer's son (Appendix II, p. 244) the third period does not begin until the ninth month; while in the case of K, I did not observe the recurrence of frequent imitation until 1;0, an observation which agrees with Guillaume's general statement (IE 36) that imitation appears in force towards the end of the child's first year.

Clearly it is not possible to fix the beginning of this third stage with any certainty ; something perhaps depends on individual differences among children, something also upon the judgment of the observer.   It is interesting to notice that the result of systematic experiment, such as that of Guernsey, tends to put the date a good deal earlier than it is found to be by non-experimental observation ; this suggests that while normally the child does not manifest a quickening of linguistic imitation until towards the end of his first year, the development may be hastened if he is stimulated by an adult.

Of the five characteristics we have mentioned above, three —the readier imitation of sounds drawn from the child's own repertory, of intonational form, and of new sounds—are illustrated in Appendix II in the records of Stern, Hoyer and myself.   In none of these three cases, however, do we find any special mention of delayed imitation or of echolalia. The former is recorded by Guernsey (SN 165) as generally appearing at 0;8½ and by Valentine (PI 115) as occurring in the case of his child Y after 1;0.   But apart from any special observation, it is clear that delayed imitation enters whenever a child first uses a conventional word some time after having heard it ; so that we can include here Stern's observation (KSp 18) of Hilde saying *didda* at 0;10½ on hearing the clock tick, as well as my own observation of K saying **nana** at 1;1,8 on seeing the maid (see Appendix IV, p. 302).

As for the fifth characteristic—echolalia—this is mentioned by Preyer (MC 113) as occurring in his son's thirteenth month, and by Stern (KSp 163) and Guillaume (IE 37) as generally appearing towards the end of the first year.

How is it that these five characteristics appear together in a marked form at about this same time ?

The Growth of Awareness.—A simple answer would be that,

as the months pass by, the child's auditory perception becomes increasingly refined : he learns to distinguish more effectively between one sound and another, and—under the incentives which we have noticed as present at the first stage—he comes to imitate more accurately. But this, though true, is only one part of the story. As we have seen in Chapter IV, the child's main advance in the auditory perception of speech is that he learns to apprehend it in relation to its accompanying conditions, that is, he comes to respond to its meaning.

Once more, then, we must look for the explanation of changes in imitation in the general development of the child's linguistic behaviour, as well as in the special development of imitation itself. And the point that strikes the observer at once is that this very period, the last quarter of the child's first year, is precisely the time when he makes his first real advance in the use of conventional language ; that is, he begins to utter and respond to specific adult words as referring to specific circumstances. Postponing our survey of this important change until the next section, we have here to notice how it is reflected in the special behaviour which we call imitation.

The child begins to be aware that specific words, whether spoken or heard, are followed by specific sequels, so that he can secure satisfaction by speaking a given word in given circumstances, or, on the other hand, by behaving in a given way in response to a given word. This growth of the instrumental use of words brings with it two important effects on the child's imitative behaviour : he pays closer attention to the forms of words because they are used instrumentally for him and by him, and he becomes aware of imitation as an activity in itself.

In the first place, it is clear that the attempt to use and understand conventional words will bring about a closer imitation of them. The child, as we show in the chapters which follow, tends at first to use his own primitive forms and to advance from these to the forms used by the adults around him. As he begins his attempts upon conventional language, the influence of this adult environment will be exercised very powerfully upon him. Sometimes the difference between the child's own form and the adult word which he intends to use will be so great that he is simply not understood ; then he must either give up his attempt or imitate the model more accurately. At other times, when he is inaccurate but yet

intelligible, an adult will help him by supplying the correct
form at the moment of responding to the child's demands.
Throughout his development, the influence of society will be
continually at work selecting the correct forms from out of
the welter of baby-talk that pours from his lips.   Even the
busiest of mothers can spare time for an occasional smile of
approval at her child's successes, and not even the most sympa-
thetic of mothers can always repress a smile of amusement at
the quaint turns of speech that mark her child's failures.   In
these ways, social selection will be at work, resulting in closer
imitation of conventional words by the child as he pays more
attention to their phonetic and intonational patterns.   Thus
the tendency to respond to speech by speech, which we noticed
as characteristic of the first stage and which fell into abeyance
during the second, now receives a fresh impetus from the rapidly
growing use and comprehension of adult language.

This connection between imitative attention to words and
interest in their meaning is implied in a remark of Stern's
(KSp 163) that imitation by his three children of *isolated*
sound-groups (that is, speech heard in the absence of a context)
greatly diminished during the last quarter of their first year
and did not become frequent again until some months later,
when they were already understanding and using conventional
words.   A similar conclusion was arrived at by Guernsey in
her work with 200 children ;   she found that while from 0;7
children imitate single tones, they gradually cease to do so
after about 1;3, while their imitation of a series of two tones
begins at 0;10 and of three tones at 1;0, in both cases continuing to increase throughout the second year.   This change,
she suggests, is connected with their growing interest in words
(SN 146).   And both Guillaume (IE 45, 200) and Valentine
(PI 111) conclude, from observation, that an interest in heard
sounds will foster more accurate imitation of them.

A second effect of the growth of the instrumental function
of language is a new attention to the activity of imitation in
itself.   At the same time as the child is becoming aware of the
instrumental sequels of words he also becomes aware, by contrast, of another kind of sequence ;   the pattern of events
which is made up by hearing a word and imitating it.   He
may come across this kind of pattern in two different ways ;
either when he quite spontaneously imitates a word or when
he is called upon to do so by some adult.   He will find in both

cases a satisfaction in the mere business of imitation, the satisfaction which comes from completing a pattern previously
experienced when now one element of this pattern recurs.
And in both cases this satisfaction may be enhanced by the
approval which his performance brings him from adult on-
lookers.

Thus, as a result of the growth of the instrumental functions
of language, conditions at this third stage are particularly
favourable when an adult addresses himself to secure imitation
from a child. For some time past, during Stage II, such
attempts will frequently have been met by a neutral response
on the part of the child, for the word which has become
meaningful in one context of circumstances will be correspondingly meaningless in other contexts, including this context
of imitation. But now, as the child becomes increasingly
aware of the close instrumental linkage that exists between
certain heard words and their contexts, he also becomes aware,
in the course of this development, that certain other words
have peculiar contexts of their own ; they demand imitation.
He realises that when, for instance, an adult says *papa* in a
certain manner and with a certain intonation, the " correct "
response consists in replying *papa* ; or—to put it another
way—that this response is a means of obtaining satisfaction
in the shape of approval from the adult. In brief, the child
is being trained to imitate, he learns how to play this game.

An interesting example of this occurs in my record of K.
At 1;2 I heard him one morning saying **bæ** . . . **baba,** the
bæ being low-pitched and held for three or four seconds, and
the **baba** following suddenly in a loud voice. I imitated this
sequence, and after a few repetitions by me, he chuckled and
proceeded to say **bæ** . . . **baba** in great apparent glee. Then,
by way of variation, I said **bæ** . . . and stopped short ; he
came in immediately with **baba** in the correct way. He
enjoyed this game on several successive days.

Of course, this increase of imitation as a game is only a symp-
tom of a more general tendency for imitation to take place.
Much more important than this demanded imitation is the
spontaneous appearance of the five features we have mentioned above as characteristic of this third stage—the readier
imitation of familiar sounds, of new sounds and of intonational
form ; delayed imitation and echolalia. In one way or
another these all hasten the child's acquisition of the adult

language. It is therefore worth while to show briefly how they arise partly from the tendencies already present in the two earlier stages and partly as a result of the rapid development of the instrumental functions of language during the latter part of the child's first year.

(i) *The Imitation of Familiar Sounds.*—Little need be said about the child's tendency to imitate sounds drawn from his own repertory. We have noticed its beginnings at the first stage and its subsequent weakening at the second when the child's attention begins to be taken up with the meaning of the words that he hears. Now, at the third stage, it reappears with growing force ; both when an adult takes the trouble to make one of the child's own sounds, or when in the course of everyday conversation the child hears sounds that resemble his own.

In both cases imitation will become readier with the growth of the child's awareness of the relation between words and the situations in which they occur. For when on occasion he imitates the adult utterance of one of his own familiar sounds he finds that this brings the approval of adults as well as a satisfaction in itself—the satisfaction of completing a pattern. Now as he becomes conscious of these sequels he may set himself to secure them when he hears his own familiar sounds. In this way the child's involuntary response to heard sounds may be reinforced by voluntary imitation.

In two respects this imitation of familiar sounds is important in the child's linguistic development. In the first place, the child's approach to conventional speech occurs—as we shall see in the next chapter—by adults adopting sound-groups from his own repertory and stabilising their meaning. On the whole the adult will tend to choose from the child's repertory just those groups of sounds which have a currency as nursery-language. Thus the child obtains exercise in the production of those sounds which will constitute his entrance into conventional speech by way of the semi-conventional speech of the nursery. Reference is often made to Groos's view that babbling is a preparation for the acquisition of speech. But, clearly, not all babbling is of equal value for this purpose. By the process we have just described the most valuable part of the child's repertory of babbling is given a predominance over the rest. The child develops a habit of responding to these particular sounds when he hears them.

Secondly, and this is perhaps even more important, the child's response to adult speech by making his own sounds is a step on the way to the imitation of unfamiliar sound-groups. But before we can describe this achievement we must consider two other features of the child's behaviour at this third stage ; his response to intonational form, and the rise of " delayed " imitation.

(ii) *The Response to Intonational Form.*—Response to intonational patterns occurs, as we have indicated, in the earlier two stages ; markedly in Stage I and whenever the child is stimulated to babble during Stage II. Now in Stage III it shows itself more frequently and more definitely. The number of syllables, the stress pattern and the pitch pattern are all imitated. As for the number of syllables and the stress pattern, Stern tells us (Appendix II, p. 243) that at 0;7½ his daughter Hilde replied correctly to *hä*, to *hähä* or to *hähähähä* ; and that his son Günther at 0;8 responded equally well to *ä* or to *ää*. Hoyer's son at 0;8 repeated *ä ä ä* sung to him, while Preyer's son at 0;9 said *ätä* on hearing *tatta*. Lorimer reports that a child Diane responded correctly at 0;10 either to *hahaha* or to *hahahaha*. In the case of K, I have no record of such an exact response as early as this, but at 1;0,6, when his mother several times said **bububu** he replied **bø bø** on each occasion. By 1;1,8 he was saying **ɛbɔ** in response to *Peep-bo* and three days later **iːkibɔ** in response to *Peeky-bo* (Appendix II, p. 252). For a general statement we may recall here Guernsey's summary of her observations of 200 children that imitation of a series of two tones begins at 0;10 and of three at 1;0.[1]

As for the response to pitch, we have to distinguish here between the imitation of pitch in itself and the imitation of a pitch pattern. Stern tells us (Appendix II, p. 243) that when Hilde was 0;9 she would reply to her father's high-pitched whistle with a similar high-pitched shriek. This is the only instance that I have come across of the imitation of pitch itself before the end of the first year ; and it would seem that Guernsey is right in maintaining (SN 148) that this is very rare even throughout the second year. But we are here more concerned with imitation of the *pattern* of pitch, an achievement of much greater importance in the development of

[1] Stern KSp 83 ; Hoyer LK 375 ; Preyer MC 109 ; Lorimer GR 47 ; Guernsey SN 146.

language : and although observations are very few we cannot doubt that this must persist from the first stage (see p. 75) and now develop further. Hoyer's remark (LK 375) that his son at 0;8 repeated $\bar{a}$ $\bar{a}$ $\bar{a}$ sung to him, Stern's (KSp 163) that all his three children at about 0;9 imitated intonation (Tonfall), and Preyer's observation (MC 129) that at 1;5 his son imitated sung tones, all point in this direction.

The whole question of intonation in children's speech is, as we have already noticed, extremely obscure. In the absence of detailed observations one may hazard the suggestion that what happens at the stage we are now discussing is that first the adult's speech evokes from the child intonational patterns of which he is already capable, and that he advances from these to the imitation of unfamiliar patterns. The increased attention to the forms of adult speech, arising out of its growing instrumental function for the child, provides a fresh impetus for the working of that tendency to respond to speech by speech, which has been present from the outset of the child's development. And the closer imitation of intonational patterns fosters, of course, the instrumental use of conventional language.

(iii) *Metalalia or Delayed Imitation.*—This process, as we have said, now appears for the first time in the child's development. He hears a word in a specific situation and does not respond imitatively at this moment. Later, in the absence of the auditory stimulus, he utters the previously heard sound.

As we have pointed out above, delayed imitation occurs whenever the child first uses a conventional word some time after having heard it. Is this imitation ever perfectly " meaningless " ? Stern's definition of metalalia (KSp 135) provides no answer ; it is simply this : " imitation in which there is a period of latency between the stimulus and the reaction ". From his incidental remarks, however, it is clear that he regards the stimulus-word as normally having been understood ; this is certainly the case in all the examples that he cites. The point is important—it illustrates once more the difficulty of attempting to isolate " imitation " from the rest of linguistic behaviour.

I think we must accept Stern's implied view that delayed imitation is never really meaningless. For even if the external conditions when the word is repeated are unlike those in which it was heard, the child will still tend to reinstate (or " remember") these earlier conditions.   In brief, this context of recalled conditions—which gives the word its meaning—will also aid the child's repetition of it.

What is the nature of this persistent effect of an earlier heard word ?   Unfortunately a good deal of difficulty has been imported into the discussion of the subject by the use of the term " emmagasinement ", which since its introduction by Le Dantec in 1899 (MI 354) has been repeatedly adopted, for instance by Delacroix (LP 290) and those whom he cites, and by Lorimer (GR 43, 49).   But it seems no more justifiable to speak of " storing-up " in this than in any other case of reinstatement of a past experience.   What is it that is stored, and where ?

A more helpful analysis is made by Guernsey (SN 164), who suggests that delayed imitation is most probably a combination of " memory " and of " physiological perseveration ".   Some form of " memory " there certainly is : both in the case where the external conditions recur and the child supplies the sound, and in the case where the child apparently reinstates both the conditions and the sound.

The former case is the more obvious.   To take, for instance, an observation of Stern's (KSp 135) ;   his daughter Hilde at 1;10, having often heard *Gute Nacht* at bedtime without imitating it, now on the occasion in question said *Nacht!* unprompted just as she was about to be taken to bed.   Here the experience of the incomplete pattern of events was sufficient to evoke from the child a completing response.

Of the second kind of case we must be less certain—that in which the child utters a previously heard sound in the apparent absence of any of the accompanying conditions.   Thus Stern (KSp 136) cites an instance in which a French child of 1;3, a month after losing his Italian nurse, began to speak with something of an Italian pronunciation.   Clearly, in a case like this, one can never entirely exclude the possibility that some external circumstance served to evoke the sound from the child.

However, allowing that cases of the second kind as well as of the first may occur, we now have to ask, how is it that the child, who in the original situation merely heard the sound without speaking, now speaks it ?   This is the gap that Guernsey's second factor, " physiological perseveration ", is no doubt meant to fill.   It suggests that in some way the original auditory stimulus leaves a persistent physiological effect, so that—since there is a tendency to respond to heard sounds by speaking—what was heard yesterday issues in speech to-day.

But if we examine the case more closely we find it quite unnecessary to invoke this new factor: it is enough to accept the hypothesis that we tend to respond to hearing by speech. It comes to this: that whenever a child hears a spoken sound, there is a tendency for him to speak,[1] although frequently his utterance may be inhibited—as we have seen in discussing the facts of Stage II. Now, on a subsequent occasion, he either experiences a similar pattern of events or reinstates the original pattern: in both cases this reinstatement including a revival of the implicit utterance which accompanied the original experience. If the present incentive is strong enough, this implicit utterance finds expression and the child breaks into speech. In a word, it is not that the child remembers hearing a sound which he now reproduces, but rather that he reinstates his *total perception* of the sound, this perception including both the hearing of the sound and the implicit utterance of it.

How is it that delayed imitation does not appear until the present stage of the child's development? The answer is that it depends upon two features of the child's growth which only appear in force towards the end of his first year: his memory of spoken sounds, and the power to respond to human speech in its context of a pattern of events.

With regard to the former point, there are two ways of judging the child's power of remembering words—his utterance of them and his response to them. The evidence is not very plentiful: but as summarised by C. Bühler (KJ 103) from the work of Scupin, Stern and Valentine, it certainly shows that (in children of the class we are here considering) the last part of the first year is the normal period in which any delayed recall of the utterance of sounds or response to them appears.

With regard to the second point—the growth of the child's power to respond to a word in relation to its setting—it is evident that metalalia may be regarded as a process exactly

---

[1] Guernsey notices (SN 164) that frequently when a child heard a sound which he did not immediately imitate, he did not remain passive, but made " rudimentary movements ".

complementary to " understanding " a word heard apart from its usual context of circumstances. When a child " comprehends " a word, he responds to it as though the rest of the usual context were present ; the word alone arouses his previous response to the whole situation. In metalalia the reverse happens : the situation is supplied (or remembered), and the accompanying word is absent ; then the child responds to the situation as though the word alone were ·present : he imitates the word. Sometimes, of course, this word at the moment of imitation will be used instrumentally ; but this is a question which we must leave for later discussion (see Chapter VII, p. 136).

Now, since, as we have said above, it is only in the latter part of his first year that the normal child shows a regular awareness of the place of heard speech in an experienced situation, it is only then that metalalia appears. This form of imitation may therefore be considered as arising from that attention to heard speech in its pattern of events which is characteristic of the present stage, together with the growth of memory of heard sounds, a new impetus thus being given to the persistent tendency to respond by speech to speech.

(iv) *The Imitation of New Sound-Groups.*—With this we come to an achievement which is obviously of the greatest importance in the child's linguistic development ; he begins to acquire the forms of adult conventional language. Every observer has of course recorded this event—nothing could be more striking than a child's earliest imitation of an adult word. But it was not until Stern's account of his daughter Hilde that we were given a series of observations sufficiently detailed to enable us to analyse the process.

This child's earliest imitation of a word not in her own repertory occurred, he tells us (KSp 16), when she was o;8. During the past week she had often made the sound *p* while babbling, and when her father said *papa* to her with the intention of getting her to imitate she always answered with this same sound *p*. On this particular day when the same thing had repeatedly occurred, he gave up the attempt, but coming back a few minutes later heard her in her cradle babbling *pa pa pa* again and again to herself. Now when he said *papa* to her she answered him with the right word.

There are three phases in this process : first the child responds to the new sound-group by uttering her own familiar sounds ;

then when she is left alone she says the new sound-group in the course of her babbling ; finally, when she again hears this combination spoken by the adult she comes out with it correctly. In these three phases we see the various factors at work which we have described as characteristic of the child at the present stage of development. The first phase consists simply of the stimulation of the child's own familiar sounds, for she is already capable of saying *p* and *a* ; then follows a period in which metalalia occurs—the persistent effect of a close attention to the form of what has been heard, with the result that the child babbles the new combination of sounds: *papa*. Finally, when the adult again says *papa*, this acts once more as a stimulus to the child's own babbling, and she produces *papa*, a chain of sounds which has now become part of her babbling repertory.

In this case of Stern's, the whole process fortunately took place slowly and overtly, but in the ordinary life of a child it no doubt often occurs more rapidly and without any period of practice being observed. A child hears a new word, and subsequently when a similar situation occurs accurately imitates what he has heard.

It is important to notice that in this instance the child's imitation consisted in a combination of sounds already familiar to her : all that Stern demanded was that the child should bring together two sounds which had frequently appeared in her babbling. Allport maintains (SP 186) that this is characteristic of every kind of imitation of unfamiliar activities within the child's first eighteen months ; the records of children certainly show that it is true of early vocal imitation. For, as we shall point out in detail later (Chapter X), for a very long time the forms used by the child in imitation of adult language consist of his own familiar sounds spoken as approximations to those that he hears. Only gradually, as he attends more closely, are the movements of his vocal organs subordinated to his auditory perceptions. At first he is satisfied to make broad, crude attempts : as time passes his vocal movements become more and more refined. Slowly he comes to pronounce his mother tongue in the accepted fashion, under the stress of social selection, that is, the responses made to his attempts by others.

In the course of the everyday instrumental use of words and—where adults take the trouble to play it—the game of imitation, the adult's concern with the child's responses must prove to be the very strongest possible incentive to the correct production of new forms. If Stern, for instance, had been content to accept his daughter's *p* . . . *p* . . . when he said *papa*, and had shown his approval of her attempt, we cannot doubt that she too would have been satisfied with this approximation—for the time being at any rate. And where the intercourse between child and adult brings the word into use as an instrument, the incentive to conform to adult patterns must be stronger still.

There remains one point of great difficulty : how does the child pass from his familiar sounds to unfamiliar ones ? Even in the case before us, it is obvious that *papa* is something more than a combination of *p*'s and *a*'s—it is a new act. This is a difficulty which has impressed one psychologist after another, so that Claparède (EP 142), in the absence of any satisfactory hypothesis, has been led to postulate an " instinct to conform ". This, however, is itself so unsatisfactory that we must be content to leave the question open for further evidence.

It is clear that what at first sight might seem to be a simple activity—the imitation by the child of a sound-group which he has never himself said—turns out to be a complicated process. Here, as at the earlier stages, we are far from the notion of a simple tendency to imitate : instead of this, a number of factors combine to produce in the child behaviour more or less similar to that which he perceives. And these factors appear to be largely, if not entirely, the persistence of tendencies which have existed in a rudimentary fashion far back in his history.

(v) *Echolalia*.—This is the name usually given to a marked tendency in a child to imitate immediately what he hears, in an apparently meaningless way, and even though the sounds may have been said without any intention of securing imitation from him.

Preyer (MC 113) was perhaps the first to draw attention to the fact : he noticed his son in his thirteenth month imitating the word *papa* that he had just heard, quite correctly but " almost as in a dream ". This kind of apparently involuntary imitation persisted throughout the child's second year, in sharp contrast with his voluntary imitation, which as a rule was by no means so accurate. An interesting example occurred when the child was 1;8 (MC 135) ; in the garden he watched a redstart attentively for a couple of minutes, then began to imitate its piping very closely. Turning round he caught sight of his father. " It was when he saw me that the child first seemed to be aware that he had made attempts at imitation at all. For his countenance was like that of one awakening from sleep, and he could not now be induced to imitate sounds."

There has been some difference of opinion as to the regularity and importance of this kind of imitation in children generally. Guillaume (IE 200) wishing to stress the rôle of awareness in imitation, is inclined to minimise the significance of echolalia; Stern (KSp 135) and Jespersen (ND 115) on the other hand, maintain that it is both of regular occurrence and of considerable importance in the child's linguistic development. In the case of K, I can say this, that it was by no means a persistent tendency, but occurred only occasionally. Lorimer (GR 46) is probably right in his suggestion that individual children differ in this respect ; the degree and nature of the differences are questions open to further investigation.

What is quite certain is that we cannot regard echolalia either as the source of all meaningful imitation or always as the result of it. To take the first point : echolalia cannot be the source of all meaningful imitation, for as both Stern (KSp 163) and Guillaume (IE 37) show, the beginning of echolalia as a persistent activity occurs when the meaningful use of adult words is already well established. On the other hand it would be equally false to go to the other extreme, as Koffka (GM 338) is inclined to do, and maintain that attention to the meaning of what is perceived is the main source of imitation. For echolalia certainly does not appear for the first time at the stage we are now considering. It already occurs in children before they are four months old, at our first stage (see p. 74) ; the only difference between this and the typical echolalia of the third stage being that the latter occurs in response to unfamiliar as well as familiar sounds, and is more accurate and more frequent.

On the contrary, as we have attempted to show (p. 84), if a child from one cause or another is constantly taken up with the meaning of the sounds that he hears, this may inhibit his imitation of them. It is only when a child accepts a sound independently of its meaning that echolalia is likely to take place. Thus this kind of imitation is characteristic of feeble-minded children. As we have seen throughout the present chapter, there are two kinds of response which a word may arouse in a child : on the one hand a response to its meaning, on the other a response to the form of the word in itself. When the latter kind of response occurs in its purity, unmixed with any attention to meaning, we have echolalia.

It is evident that echolalia may play an important part in giving the child practice in speaking the forms of adult speech, both phonetic and intonational. For in so far as the child's attention is absorbed by the mere pattern of a word, to the neglect of its meaning, his close perception of it will find expression in a faithful reproduction of its form. On the other hand, it need hardly be said that persistent echolalia might well prove a hindrance to the acquisition of language as an instrument.

We have now briefly outlined the main features present at this third stage of imitation, and have attempted to show how the factors which were present in the child's early linguistic behaviour—his expressive response to speech, the subordination of his utterance to hearing, and the arousal of his own babbling by appropriate heard sounds—combine, as he becomes more aware of the place of speech in his experiences, to bring about advances of the utmost importance in his acquisition of the mother tongue. He learns to utter forms previously unfamiliar to him, and to utter them some time after he has heard them spoken, in an increasingly accurate fashion. We have now to see how this power of reproducing the forms of words is related to the growth of their instrumental use.

SECTION III

THE FIRST ACQUISITION OF CONVENTIONAL SPEECH

CHAPTER VII

THE BEGINNING OF COMPREHENSION OF CONVENTIONAL SPEECH

WE come now to the point at which the child begins to " understand " and " use " conventional language. On the one hand he begins to respond in specific ways to conventional words, on the other hand to utter conventional words as a means of dealing with specific situations.

These two lines of development are of course closely intertwined ; here, for the sake of clearness, we shall deal first with the growth of comprehension (in the present chapter) ; next with the growth of the use of words (in Chapter VIII) ; finally (in Chapter IX) we shall consider the place of each of these two factors in the development of the child's symbolical use of language.

The Onset of Comprehension.—When does the child first begin to understand conventional words ? If we put the question in this way it can hardly be answered. For, as we shall show, there is no clear line marking off the child's responses to particular conventional words from his earlier responses to the adult voice. But so much may be said : that in the course of the child's first year there comes a time when his responses to particular words become more specific, more regular and more frequent. This point—in normal children of educated parents—would appear to fall towards the end of the third quarter of the year.

At first sight it might appear strange that exact statistical evidence of this date should be lacking. But the fact is that it is not at all easy to mark the point when a child's response to a particular word first becomes stabilised. It is, however, generally accepted [1] that on the whole the first comprehension of conventional language slightly precedes its first meaningful use, and as this later event—which is comparatively easy to observe—is generally put in the last quarter of the first

---

[1] Delacroix LP 297 ; Schäfer RS 319 ; Stern KSp 164.

year (see p. 125), it would seem reasonable to put the marked beginning of comprehension at the end of the third quarter.

The Nature of this Comprehension.—How do we judge that the child comprehends conventional language ? Let us begin by considering some actual cases of children's responses to specific adult words. Here it is not sufficient merely to say that at a given moment the child " understood " a given word ; we need a record of the word, of the circumstances in which it was uttered and of the manner in which the child responded ; and in order to trace the child's development we need a series of such instances noted of a particular child.

Records of this kind, where they exist, are usually incomplete. Stern's list, for instance, of the words first " understood " by his daughter (KSp 17), though of the greatest value in other ways, is not as helpful to us here as it might have been, because he has confined himself to the briefest possible statement of the *act* which the word evoked, and has omitted mention of the circumstances or of other responses.

Perhaps the most helpful record for our purpose comes from Deville (DL) although it was made as long ago as 1890 and in the now despised "anecdotal" fashion; from a very early stage in his daughter's life he noted regularly her behaviour in response to words spoken to her. For comparison with this, I venture to give some of my own observations of K ; my fuller records will be found in Appendix IV, p. 300.

RESPONSES TO SPECIFIC WORDS :

(i) *Deville's daughter*

0;4,5   *Kins.* The nurse for some weeks past had said *kins* (*tiens*) on offering the child food. On and after 0;4,5 if the nurse said this to the *satiated* child without making any other movement, the child would whimper and express displeasure as though being offered food.

0;5,6   *Dodo.* The nurse was accustomed to say this word to the child on putting her to bed ; sometimes the child would cry. After 0;5,6 when this word was uttered without any accompanying movement, the child often showed signs of being about to cry, and would cease to make them only when the nurse ceased to say the word.

0;6   *Bravo!* For some time past the child had imitated her mother clapping hands, and had been rewarded with *Bravo!* On and after 0;6,23 the child responded to *Bravo!* even if this were unaccompanied by movement, by clapping her hands.

eu. Her father was accustomed to say *eu* to her in a severe manner and with a frown. On 0;6,15 the word alone was sufficient to cause the child to draw down the corners of her mouth, as though about to cry.

0;7   *Chut!* When *Chut!* was said to her, she would refrain from touching an article she was about to touch.

0;8,8 *Chauve-souris.* The child had for some time past been interested in bats seen through the window; at such times the word *chauve-souris* was said to her. On 0;8,8 she was sitting with her back to the window when someone said, *Tiens, les chauves-souris!* She turned round and looked out of the window. This was repeated on successive evenings.

0;8,13 *Bonjour.* Waves hands in response to this.

0;8,16 *Les marionettes.* Child makes appropriate movements of hands.

0;8,25 *Lisbonne.* Child turns towards the dog so named.
       La grimace. Child makes a grimace.

0;9,14 *Eh bien!* Child refrains when about to throw some object to the ground.

0;9,22 *Donne.* Gives what she is holding.

0;10,2 *Touche la main.* Touches hand held out to her.

0;10,14 *Voyons les mains.* Looks at her own hands.

0;10,21 *Soupe.* Smacks her lips, as when seeing food.

After this, her advance was steady; by 1;1, Deville reports, she understood 20 words.

Responses to Specific Words:

(ii) K

0;8,20 *Cuckoo!* The child smiled in response to this uttered in a special tone of voice. (Repeatedly observed.)

0;8,24 *Nan-nan.* Turned in direction of maid when this word was uttered by his mother. (Doubtful.)

0;9,5 *No!* He refrained from the movement that he was about to make. (Repeatedly observed.)

0;9,6 *Say Good-bye.* He waved his hand in response to the word alone, while being held at the window to watch his parents leave the house.

0;9,14   *Where is the ballie?*   Many of his playthings were lying about him, his ball being out of sight ; he turned round and touched it. (Repeatedly observed on successive days.)

0;10,12   The following responses were definitely established : *Where's daddy?* Turns in direction of his father when this word is spoken by his mother.

         Where's nan-nan? Turns in direction of maid.

         Where's the ballie? As under 0;9,14.

0;10,27   *Where's doggie?* Many of his playthings about him ; in response to this phrase he reached out and held up his toy dog.

1;0,1   *Give mummy teddy.* Ceased crying, searched in his carriage, found his toy bear and held it out to his mother.

1;0,6   *Give mummy crustie.* He was gnawing at a crust ; on hearing the word, held up the crust and whimpered a little.

1;0,6   *All the way to Paris.* When feeding him his mother sometimes sang, " All the way, all the way, all the way to Paris ", bringing the spoon to his mouth at the last word. On this occasion, he had refused further food, and had thrown himself backward on her lap. She now said, *All the way to Paris*, and at the last word, although he could not see the spoon, he cried out excitedly and waved his hands as if waving away food.

1;0,6   *Give mummy tinkle-box.* For the past week he had had a musical box with which he often played. His mother had often uttered the above phrase, but without effect. On this occasion he handed the toy to her.

1;0,10   *Give daddy crustie.* No response to this when uttered by his mother ; repeatedly observed ; but responded correctly each time to *Give mummy crustie*.

1;0,12   *Give auntie teddy.* His mother and " auntie " both present. No response to phrase uttered by his mother, three times in succession. On fourth occasion he handed the toy bear to his *mother*.

1;0,12   *Come out, Baby!* When he was lying in his bath—of which he was very fond—and his mother uttered this phrase, without any accompanying movement, he immediately crawled away as far as he could get from her.

1;0,26   *Baby, where's shoe-shoe?* He had one shoe on, the other being at some distance out of his reach. On hearing the phrase, he crawled towards the shoe and endeavoured to reach it.

The responses of these two children may be classified in the following way :

	Expression.		Action.	
	The child smiles. e.g. :		*Action is initiated.* e.g. :	
Positive	Deville's daugh-ter. [No example]	K. *Cuckoo* (0;8,20)	Deville's daugh-ter. *Bravo !* (0;6,23) *Chauve-souris* (0;8,8) *Bonjour* (0;8,13)	K. *Say Good-bye* (0;9,6) *Where's doggie ?* (0;10,27) *Give mummy crustie* (1;0,6)
	The child cries (or makes other negative reactions) e.g. :		*Action is inhibited.* e.g.	
Negative	Deville's daugh-ter. *kins* (0;4,5) *dodo* (0;5,6) *eu* (0;6,15)	K. *Paris* (1;0,6) *Come out, Baby!* (1;0,12)	Deville's daugh-ter. *Chut !* (0;7) *Eh bien !* (0;9,14)	K. *No !* (0;9,5)

In brief, the child responds to the heard words either positively or negatively, and in each case by expression or more actively. We have already, in Chapter IV, considered the child's expressive responses to heard speech ; now we have to notice the change from these expressive responses to the performance of overt acts—a change which, I think, has hitherto not been commented upon.

Usually the discussion of the child's first comprehension of language is confined to the consideration of his overt acts in response to words ; but no attention has been paid to the *inhibition* of his acts, or to the relation between the present initiation or inhibition of acts and his earlier positive and negative responses. The reason why emphasis is placed only on the initiation of action is evident enough ; this is certainly the more frequent mode of response and the one which develops with the greatest rapidity in the last quarter of the first year. Further, this mode of response is often the result of specific training, a process which can be closely observed and described in detail. But since the inhibition of action plays a most important part in the child's education, and since also his positive and negative expressive responses to what he hears persist throughout his life, all these must be taken into account in considering the progress of his comprehension of conventional words.

Now there is no doubt that frequently this process of comprehension of conventional words is described far too narrowly as a matter of training. Emphasis is laid on the part played by the adult ; he leads and the child follows. The child is trained, we are told, to perform certain movements on hearing certain patterns of sound. Too little account is taken of the persistence and further development of tendencies already present in his earlier history.

Take, for instance, the summary made by Stern (KSp 166–7). A child, he tells us, is trained to link a word with its accompanying situation, so that he comes at length to respond to the word alone. The chief aid to this linkage is furnished by movements or gestures (*Gebärde*) ; either those of the adult, or those of the child. In the former case, the child responds first to the adult's gestures—for instance, his mother's outstretched arms—and then he is trained to respond to the accompanying words, so that ultimately these alone acquire the power of evoking the appropriate movement. In the second case, the process of training begins from one of the child's own gestures. These may be of three kinds : (*a*) spontaneous—for instance, dancing a doll or looking at a clock ; (*b*) imitative ; or (*c*) induced (*geleitete*)—for instance, the child is induced to touch his nose. The adult constantly introduces a word when the child is making a gesture, and ultimately the word acquires the power of evoking the gesture.

How does this come about ? Stern's explanation (KSp 166) is in general physiological terms; sensori-motor connections are set up. In the first case—beginning with the adult's gesture—the child's movement is linked up first with the sight of this gesture, then with this and the sound of the accompanying word, finally with the sound of this word alone. In the second case—beginning with the child's gesture—the adult merely accompanies this gesture by speaking a word, and ultimately the sound of the word becomes linked to the child's movement and capable of evoking it.

This account, though fruitful, is open to this criticism : that too much stress is laid upon the factor of training and too little attention given to the persistence of tendencies already present both in the acts that the child performs and in the words that he hears. The child's development cannot be fully understood unless we consider these tendencies in relation to whatever appears to be new in his comprehension. The persistent features are these : the child has at an earlier date already begun to perform specific acts, and to respond to sounds by expression. The new features are these : he now performs specific acts (or inhibits them) in response to specific phonetic patterns. These features, the old and the new, must be briefly considered.

The Persistence of Tendencies already observed.—(i) *The Maturation of Purposive Movements.*—The first point on which we must insist is that the active movements, with which the child replaces his earlier expressive responses, are only partly due to training. They are also due to maturation—the child comes to take an increasingly active hold upon his environment. Woolley [1] found that at 0;7 the child's response to coloured objects changed from passivity to activity. Similarly, Schäfer (BV 270) records of his son that at 0;9 the child's passive observation of a clock changed to active manipulation of it— touching it, moving it, and opening the door. C. Bühler (KJ 95) mentions the same date as that at which there is a remarkable increase in the child's handling of objects and in interest in the objective world; and in another publication, (FY 52), she gives in detail observations of this development, made by herself and other workers. These may be summarised as follows :

Newborn child : Closes hands on object brought within his reach.
At 0;2 : His hand explores the object.
At 0;4 : Grasping is directed by sight.
At 0;5 : Grasping with single hand, using thumb opposition.
At 0;6 : Reaching out, and moving body, in direction of remote objects.
At 0;9 : Locomotion towards remote objects.

A similar development takes place in the case of negative reactions in situations unpleasant to the child, for instance, the insertion of a cotton swab into his nostrils (FY 22) :

Newborn child : Cries and makes aimless restless movements. Turns head away from strong stimulus only.

[1] Cited by Schäfer (BV 270), but I cannot trace the reference.

At 0;1 : Turns head away from milder stimulus.

0;2–0;4 : Aversion of head accompanied by " flight movements " of limbs.

At 0;4 : Rearing defence movement of body.

At 0;5 : Child pushes away unpleasant object.

At 0;6 : Child holds adult's hand and prevents action.

The child's response towards other people likewise becomes more purposive and more definitely directed (FY 180, 181, 184). Up to 0;6 the child responds only expressively to the presence of an adult ; from that time onwards he reaches out towards him, and from 0;9 he will seek to attract the adult's attention by touching or grasping.

In this way, apart from any training in reaching or manipulation given to the child, purposive activity develops in him ; moreover, it is activity increasingly directed towards a given object. Thus the movement that the child comes to make in response to a word need not be a trained movement ; what often happens is that the word which previously evoked an expressive response now evokes a directed act.

Stern recognises this to the extent of saying that some of the movements which become linked with words are " spontaneous ", adding that other movements may be " imitated " or " induced ". But there is no question but that the first group plays a larger part in the early comprehension of language than the other two : thus Schäfer found (BV 283) that where the child's movement is spontaneous the response to language based upon it is more stable, and less subject to his varying moods, than when the movement has first to be trained.

It would appear then that the normal process of development is not that the adult first causes the child to perform an act and then causes him to perform it in response to a word. This may happen occasionally, but the direct line of development is this : the heard word arouses an act which has become definite as the child has grown up. When, for instance, K at 0;9,14 reached out and touched the ball in response to *Where's the ballie ?*, all that the adult did was to set this act in motion. It was not that the word *ballie* for the first time caused the child to direct his attention to the ball ; there is not the slightest doubt that this narrowing of attention had developed a very long way in the absence of anything said by any adult.

(ii) *Response to the Intonational Patterns of Speech.*—Next we have to point out that the effectiveness of the heard word is only partly due to training. In the main, adult language is, of course, conventional in character; that is, there is no inherent connection between a specific sound-group and its meaning. Nevertheless, there are certain features of speech which, in themselves, arouse response in the child before he is trained to respond to them in given situations, and which therefore to some extent determine the nature of this training. These features we now have briefly to consider.

We have seen, in Chapter IV, that throughout the child's first year there is a growing differentiation of his responses to the intonational features of adult speech. These features persist in the specific sound-groups to which the child, towards the end of the year, comes to respond by specific activities : all speech is, of course, a complex of phonetic and intonational patterns.

The importance of these intonational patterns in determining the child's responses to specific sound-groups has hitherto been insufficiently stressed. We have in Chapter IV (p. 48) already mentioned the isolated cases discussed by Meumann and Delacroix ; but for a systematic treatment we have had to wait for the recent experimental work of Schäfer (RS and BV). For instance, he trained his son at 0;9 to respond to the phrase *Wo ist die Tick-tack ?* by looking at the clock—a movement which the child had been in the habit of performing spontaneously for some months past. Schäfer found, he tells us (BV 285), that the response was facilitated when the phrase was spoken with the emphasised and exaggerated intonation often used in the nursery (Ammensprache) ; so that when *Wo ist die lala ?* was said to the child with the same rhythm and intonation, he responded as to the original phrase (BV 279).

Stern (KSp 168) mentions this observation in the last edition of his work, but does not discuss the place of the intonational pattern in the growth of response to a word. But this development at once becomes more intelligible if we recognise that the response to intonational form has its roots deep in the child's earliest experiences, and that it continues to operate even in his ultimate comprehension of language.

The part played by intonational form is well illustrated in Schäfer's record of training his child to respond to *Mache bitte bitte* by hand-clapping (BV 276).[1]

[1] For full record see Appendix V, p. 322.

I

At 0;9,7 the training was begun : the father brought the child's hands together saying *Mache bitte bitte* in " *Ammenton*", *and in a definite rhythm* ($\backslash \times / \times \backslash \times$) corresponding to the rhythm of the clapping.

Very soon the child would imitate the movement, on seeing it performed, but not in response to the phrase alone.

At 0;9,19 he responded correctly to the phrase unaccompanied by any movement of the speaker.

In the next few days the response appeared in various degrees of strength, according to circumstances, in particular the condition of the child.

During this time the child did not respond to the phrase *when uttered in an ordinary tone of voice.*

At 0;10, he did respond correctly to the phrase uttered in an ordinary tone.

At this time he also responded with the " *bitte*-movement " to the phrase *kippe kippe* uttered in " *Ammenton* " and correct rhythm ; but not to *lala lala* although this was uttered in the same way.

Here we see the importance of the intonational pattern in determining response at the outset, and—although the point is not discussed by Schäfer—it is evident that we can relate this fact to the earlier stages of development already considered in Chapter IV. There we saw the refinement of the child's earlier crude response to the expressive characters of heard speech, by way of the progressive differentiation of his responses to intonational patterns : and here we see that these patterns continue to be significant to him at this stage when, as a result of training, he begins to respond also to phonetic patterns.

Schäfer's record indicates in a striking fashion the phases of this development. The first stage, when the child's response is largely determined by intonational form, is followed by a period in which this factor plays a less important part than phonetic form. For instance, at 0;9,19 the child would respond to *Mache bitte bitte* only when it was uttered with a specific intonational pattern, whereas by 0;10 he responded correctly when the phrase was uttered in an " ordinary " tone of voice, that is, with an intonational pattern partially different, for while the tone was changed, the original rhythm was retained. But now the importance of phonetic form showed itself ; the child responded correctly to *kippe kippe* (phonetically similar to *bitte bitte*), when uttered with the original intonational features, but not to *lala lala*, a different phonetic pattern, even though this was spoken with the same intonational features.

At this point, then, the phonetic form of the phrase probably begins to be the dominant feature in determining response ; but this does not mean that intonational form no longer operates—as we have said, the meaning of speech even for adults is always partly determined by this factor.

Further, it is very important to recognise that the effect of an intonational pattern may be of two kinds : expressive and representational. In the former case, intonational form— rhythm, stress and pitch—is expressive of the speaker's affective state. In the latter case, intonational form is representational when by rhythm, stress or pitch it pictures the situation. This is a kind of onomatopœia : for instance, *tick-tack* spoken in time with a clock.

Now it is clear that the child's response to conventional words is determined by both of these effects of intonational form. He responds, as he has done for months previously, to the expression of the speaker's affective state : and he responds also to those features of intonational form which picture the situation. Neither of these kinds of response is the result of specific training at this moment ; on the contrary, they supply the basis for further training. The child responds to expression as he has long done, and he responds to the onomatopoetic features of stress and rhythm because they have an immediate connection with the situation in which they are spoken. Thus Schäfer found (BV 285) that saying *tick-tack* in time with the clock or *bitte bitte* in time with clapping greatly facilitated the training of the child's response to these phrases.

The next important step is this : that soon the *phonetic* pattern of the spoken word acquires a dominance over the intonational pattern : *kippe kippe* remained as effective as the phonetically similar form *bitte bitte*, when the intonationally similar form *lala lala* had become ineffective.

It would seem then that we can distinguish these stages in the development of a child's response to a specific sound-group :

(1) At an early stage, the child shows discrimination, in a broad way, between different patterns of expression in intonation.

(2) When the total pattern—the phonetic form together

with intonational form—is made effective by training, at first the intonational rather than the phonetic form dominates the child's response.

(3) Then the phonetic pattern becomes the dominant feature in evoking the specific response; but while the function of the intonational pattern may be considerably subordinated, it certainly does not vanish.

If we bear in mind both the expressive and the representational features of heard speech, it is clear that the specific word to which the child is trained to respond is not a neutral situation. Its expressive intonational pattern is already able to arouse an affective response in him, while its representational features facilitate its linkage with an appropriate situation. We have now to consider how, on this basis, the actual training takes place.

Adult Speech as a Stimulus.—From what has been said we cannot possibly accept the simple view that a conventional fragment of speech, being introduced by an adult into a situation, becomes thereby capable of evoking the same response as the situation did. It is indeed doubtful whether anyone seriously holds this view, although we do find Watson saying (PB 341) that a conventional word such as *box* may become, by simple conditioning, a stimulus which evokes the same reaction from the child as a desirable box had evoked.

For as soon as we get down to close observation this statement turns out to be what Watson himself calls it : a rough hypothetical description. Quite apart from the effect of the adult's voice, the situation—as Stern points out—is frequently made attractive for the child by the intermediary of the adult's gesture, to which he has long been responding. But we are compelled to go further than this, and point out that even the adult's voice itself is far from being a neutral stimulus for the child. We have to reject the suggestion implied in some accounts—that the voice of a child's mother has no more significance for him before special training begins than the metronome had for Pavlov's dogs when they first heard it. It is essential for us to deal explicitly with this point.

Let us take first Stern's remark that the child begins by responding to the adult's gesture, and then from this comes to respond to the accompanying words; it being, as he says, simpler to respond to gestures than to words. But actual observations show that it is really very questionable whether the gesture of an adult is really more potent in evoking a response than his speech. Bühler and Hetzer found (VA 58) that before 0;6 no child observed by them responded to a coaxing or threatening gesture, a further two months elapsing before most of them responded appropriately; whereas as we saw in Chapter IV (p. 45) specific responses to differences of intonation were well established at 0;6.

It is even less clear from Stern's account how it is that the child's own movements come to be aroused by an adult's words; all that Stern tells us is that sensori-motor bonds are established (KSp 167); but we must add that this can only happen because the adult's words are far from being neutral for the child—their intonational patterns have long before this evoked expressive responses from him.

The problem before us, then, is really this: how does the child who has been responding to intonational patterns come to respond to specific phonetic patterns? What is the transition from the time when a child such as K smiles on hearing an adult voice to the time when he seizes a ball on hearing the phrase *Where is the ballie?*

The answer lies in recognising two facts: first, that the phonetic pattern is presented to the child intermingled with an intonational pattern to which he already responds; and secondly that even phonetic patterns are themselves often far from neutral. They may be of three kinds, according to their relation to the given situation: expressive, or onomatopoetic, or conventional.

(i) The expressive patterns are those which the adult takes over from the child's own utterance, in the manner which we describe in detail in the following chapter. For instance, the child has long said **mama** expressively while in a state of hunger; his mother has repeatedly uttered this same word when bringing him food. Ultimately the time comes when the hungry child, on hearing the word **mama** will turn and reach out towards his mother, or even in the direction from which she normally approaches; and we say that he understands the word. Here it is evident that the expressive nature of the sound-group **mama,** as uttered by the child, has already caused it to be linked to the specific situation of the satisfaction of his hunger; the work of the adult consists in stabilising this connection. Now it is a very significant fact that, as we shall show in Chapter X, the great majority of the child's earliest words—both those which he uses and those to which he responds—are of this expressive kind, either originally or by adult adaptation of his own forms.

(ii) The onomatopoetic patterns—using this phrase in a wide sense—represent the sounds of the situations in which they are spoken, while often at the same time the intonational patterns represent the rhythms. Into this group fall the common onomatopoetic words of the nursery—*puff-puff*, *tick-tack* and the rest ; the latter, for instance, representing both the sound and the rhythm of the clock. Further it is not improbable that a phonetic pattern may represent in a subtle way the actual pictorial form of a situation—for instance, in *zig-zag* the tongue makes something of a zigzag movement ; while when *tiny* is pronounced *teeny* in the nursery the closed vowel (and the high-pitched voice) are an attempt to represent smallness. This last kind of onomatopœia must not perhaps be overstressed, although it has been the subject of study by such writers as Paget (HS, Chapter VIII), Grammont (PP 585–90) and Werner (EP 186), and has been attributed to the speech of children by Stern (KSp 184) and Schäfer (BV 285), among others.

(iii) The conventional patterns have neither an expressive nor an onomatopoetic connection with their situations. But although these are the vast majority of sound-patterns in adult speech, they are a small proportion of the forms to which the child first learns to respond. The adult—as we shall show in Chapter X—aids the child by adapting his words to the child's own patterns : conventional words are given expressive or onomatopoetic features.

Bearing in mind then that even the phonetic pattern of a word may help to link it immediately with a situation in which it is spoken, we are now in a position to summarise the actual process by which a child is first trained to respond to adult speech.

The Process of Training.—At the end of Chapter IV we saw that the process of training whereby a child comes to respond expressively to speech in relation to accompanying conditions is generally described in these terms : the child's attention, permeated by affect, fashions a new whole out of his experiences. The heard speech and the accompanying circumstances together form a unity for him, a pattern of events ; and one element in this pattern—the heard speech—

acquires a certain dominance, in that it plays an increasingly important part in arousing the child's response.

In the present chapter we have been considering a further development of this same process, the new features being that now the child comes to respond by active movements rather than by expression, and that the phonetic form of the heard speech acquires dominance over its intonational form. And once more we can point out that it is the affective character of the process which goes far to determine its development.

To begin with the child's movements : these, as we have seen, may arise quite independently of any speech-training as the child's acts become more manipulative, directed more definitely to obtaining a hold upon his environment. In addition to these spontaneous movements there will be, as Stern says, some imitated or induced movements, due to adult intervention. But in all three cases alike—and this is a point on which it is important to insist—the child's movement will have a markedly affective basis. In the case of spontaneous movement this is doubly so ; the child dances a doll or looks at the clock both because it pleases him to, and also because he is encouraged to proceed by the gestures, expression and intonation of an adult, and encouraged to repeat his movements by their facial and vocal expressions of approval. But affective factors determine imitated and induced movements also. With regard to the former—for instance, handwaving in response to an adult's similar movements—we have already seen in our discussion of imitation that this takes place mainly when the child is interested in the behaviour of the adult. And the child is encouraged to repeat his imitation by the approving expression and intonation of the adult. Finally, in the case of induced movements, the child —to take Stern's instance—will certainly not repeat the action of putting his hand up to his nose merely because some one has moved his hand for him in this way a few times. Again he must be encouraged to proceed by gestures, expression and intonation, and encouraged to continue by expressions of approval.

Confirmation of this importance of affect is given by the observation of Schäfer's which we have already mentioned (p. 112) : that where training in comprehension is based upon the child's spontaneous movements the effect is more stable than when the movement itself has first to be trained.

For, we can point out, in the former case there is a strongly-established foundation of affect, whereas in trained movements this is likely to be much more sporadic and fleeting. From Schäfer's remark we may in fact infer that the three classes of trained response mentioned by Stern are decreasingly stable in the following order : when the basic movement is spontaneous, imitated or induced.

It is clear that under normal conditions—where adults are not concerned to cause a child to perform tricks—it is the first of these three kinds of movement which will the most frequently become the basis of a trained response. What is trained in such cases is not the movement itself, but only the initiation of a movement in response to the adult's words. These spontaneous movements arise in the course of the child's attempts to satisfy his needs—ranging from his most vital primary needs to his mere desire for play—and thus are permeated with affect. But even imitated and induced movements are also in some measure affectively toned.

When we turn to the second factor—the intonational patterns of adult speech—we are again confronted with the importance of affect in determining the child's response. For, as we have seen in Chapter IV, the child's responses throughout the earlier part of his first year are positive or negative according to the pleasant or unpleasant character of what he hears. As time goes on, the situation plays an increasingly important part, but the primary affective character of heard speech is by no means lost even when the child begins to respond to specific words.

What the intonational pattern does is this : it encourages the child to proceed with his act, or discourages him from proceeding. Where at an earlier stage he would respond by a positive or negative expression, he now responds by engaging in some movement or desisting from one which he had intended, as the instances which we have cited above from Deville's daughter and K clearly illustrate (p. 109).

Indeed, it is only by recognising the part played by the affective character of heard speech that we can understand one very important class of responses, those in which a proposed movement by the child is inhibited, as for instance Deville's daughter's response to *Chut !* or K's response to *No !* This kind of trained response to a sound-group is not often discussed—Stern, for instance, does not mention it ; although obviously it is an important feature of the child's education, both linguistic and general.

In these cases we find that it is not the situation which brings about the negative response to the word, but rather that the affective tone of the word dominates the whole situation. The situation may primarily be pleasant enough, the child is about to perform some desired action ; but the adult intervenes with his prohibition, and the child refrains from his intended movement. Take, for instance, K's response to *No !* at 0;9,5.

> He had seized a piece of newspaper which he was about to put into his mouth. I said *No !* in a loud voice. Immediately he stopped the movement of his hand and looked towards me. He kept his eyes steadily on me for a minute or so, then turned back to continue the movement of the paper towards his mouth. I said *No !* again. Again he turned towards me, and stopped the movement of his hand. This time he looked at me for quite two minutes. I looked steadily back at him. He began to cry and continued for some minutes.

In this case it is clear that the child's initial response has not been brought about only by training consisting of the experience of the word in relation to a particular context of circumstances. The child is already responding to the intonational pattern of the word *No !*, which in itself startles him, resulting in the suspension of his movement ; ultimately the phonetic pattern of the word acquires this power.

In saying this we do not mean to deny that the adult's gestures and expression may also play some part in determining the child's response. What we cannot accept is Stern's suggestion that the response to gestures is prior to the response to the intonational patterns of speech. The child responds to both : each indeed may facilitate the effect of the other. Together they evoke an affective response from the child, initiating or inhibiting his acts.

We turn now to the third factor—the phonetic pattern— which ultimately comes to dominate the intonational pattern. For whereas a pleasant tone can only encourage the child and an unpleasant tone discourage him, it is ultimately by means of a specific phonetic pattern that he is brought to perform or desist from a specific act. Thus he is trained now to respond by a movement, previously performed spontaneously, to such phrases as *Where is Nan-nan ? Wo ist die Tick-tack ?* or *Chauves-souris !* ; or he performs a movement, acquired imitatively, in response to *Bitte !* or *Bravo !* ; or he makes an induced movement, in response to *Wo ist die Nase ?* ; or he inhibits a movement which he is about to perform, on hearing *Chut !*

This process is commonly spoken of as though a fragment of speech, until this moment entirely foreign to the child's experience, is brought into association with a given situation. Described in this way, the process is decidedly mysterious ; so that those writers who are not satisfied with a " mechanical " account are even driven to invoke a special instinct or innate " power, that of turning more or less spontaneously to an object when its name is mentioned " (Fox, MB 106).

There is no need to postulate this innate capacity ; instead we need only recognise that on the one hand a phonetic pattern is intimately bound up with the intonational pattern in the same word or phrase, and that on the other hand—particularly in the language of the nursery—it may often have an intimate connection with the situation into which it is brought.

Training then proceeds in this way : the child responds affectively both to the intonational pattern of what he hears and to the situation in which he hears it. And at this very same time he hears a phonetic pattern, inextricably intertwined with the intonational pattern and—in many cases—linked expressively or onomatopoetically with the situation. Then his affective response fashions a new whole out of these experiences, this new whole including the intonational pattern, the situation, and the phonetic pattern. When at last the phonetic pattern acquires dominance so that irrespective of the intonational pattern it evokes the appropriate response from the child, we say that he has understood the conventional word. Finally, there comes a time when the child on hearing the particular word refers to a particular object.

So far we have studied only the beginning of this process—the initiation or inhibition of particular actions. We have still to enquire how it is that the phonetic pattern as it acquires dominance also acquires the power of arousing reference to an object. There is no doubt that this development is in some measure due to the fact that the child himself utters the same word—with its phonetic pattern—in the particular situation ; he imitates the adult, or the adult imitates him, or both.

In the next chapter we turn therefore to the question of the child's meaningful utterance of his first conventional words.

The child's response to adult words, and his use of them are sometimes described as though they constituted a sudden new step in his life ; but if we take into account the factors just described and those which are discussed in the following chapters, we find that we are able to trace the growth of symbolisation in him, without a break, from his earliest cries and his earliest perception of the adult human voice.

CHAPTER VIII

THE BEGINNING OF MEANINGFUL USE OF CONVENTIONAL SPEECH

WE come now to the child's first meaningful utterance of conventional words. When we say that the child has begun to use words in a meaningful way, we are describing this behaviour : that now in a specific situation he consistently utters a specific sound-group whose phonetic pattern is either borrowed from the adult language or influenced by its forms.

We have to consider first the occurrence and form of these earliest words, secondly what meanings they appear to have for the child, thirdly the manner in which these meanings seem to arise. (And in the chapter which follows we shall discuss the development of these meanings both in the words that the child understands, and in those that he utters, in relation to his earlier linguistic behaviour.)

The Occurrence of the Child's Earliest Conventional Words. —When does the child first speak words drawn from the adult language, with meaning ? It is certainly easier to mark the point when a child appears to use an adult word meaningfully for the first time than to notice when his response to a word becomes stabilised. Stern (KSp 171) comes to the conclusion that in children of educated parents the former event takes place in the first quarter of the second year ; but in the list he gives (KSp 172) of the first meaningfully uttered words of 26 children, of English, French, German, Danish and Slavonic parentage, the average age at this point is $11\frac{1}{2}$ months, while in 18 (69 per cent.) of the cases it is less than 12 months. Bateman (LD 392), gathering up the records made by 28 observers of 35 children (some of whom are also included in Stern's list) finds that in 43 per cent. of the cases the first word occurred at about $10\frac{1}{2}$ months, while in 75 per cent. of the cases it occurred before the end of the first year. In Bühler and Hetzer's inventory of the observed behaviour of 69 children, of whom 35 were boys, " words expressive of desire " normally occur at 0;10 (Bühler FY 184).

Here we are not in any way concerned with this figure as a standard, for as Descoeudres (DE 102) and Hetzer and Reindorf (SM 455) have shown, children in less favoured circumstances may be retarded in this development by as much as 6 months—as a result, perhaps, both of hereditary and environmental factors. The point of importance for us here is that in children of similar social status, there is a concurrence in the period of the first meaningfully uttered words ; so that we are able to compare it with other equally well-established events in the linguistic behaviour of children of this same status.

In any case, too much stress must not be laid upon any particular date as marking a sudden new development in the child's life ; for, as we shall show, the child's first conventional words, both in form and in meaning, owe much to his earlier expressive speech.

The Form of these Earliest Words.—The great majority of the earliest words are of a definite phonetic form : they consist of single or duplicated syllables in which the consonants are either labials (**p, b, m, w**) or labio-dentals (**f, v**) or tip-dentals (**t, d, n**) : they are made with both lips, or lip against teeth, or tongue-tip against teeth (or gum-ridge).[1] All these may be called front-consonants, the typical words in which they occur being **papa, baba, tata, dada, mama, nana, wawa.** Now if we analyse in Appendix III, pages 253-6, the list given by Stern (KSp 172) of the earliest words of 26 children, together with those from my own observation of K, we find —taking for convenience the first half-dozen words where more are given—that no less than 83 out of 110 (or 75 per cent.) contain only front-consonants, while another 12 per cent. contain one front-consonant. Further, 85 per cent. of the total are either monosyllabic or reduplicated (39 per cent. of the former and 46 per cent. of the latter).

These examples are from the children of parents speaking different European languages : but it has long been recognised, as Wundt points out (VP 324) that similar forms may be paralleled from the great majority of children, of whatever stock, throughout the world.

The Meanings of these Words.—Not only are the earliest words alike in form, but—as has again often been pointed out —they also seem to be alike in meaning wherever they are

[1] The full classification is given in Appendix III, p. 259.

found. And although, as we shall show, it is long before the child utters words with reference to particular objects, at the present stage it is already possible to classify them broadly according to the situations in which they are used.

In the table which follows I have classified in this way the most typical front-consonant words spoken by children of different nationalities. A fuller list, together with the sources, is given in Appendix III, pages 257–8.

TABLE IV

TYPICAL EARLY FRONT-CONSONANT WORDS [1]

Meaning.	Form.						
	m	n	p	b	t	d	w
1. Mother . .	mama			babab			
2. Nurse . . . Aunt . . . Grandmother	amme muhme amma	nana		bäbe baba	tété	dedda deda	
3. Food . . .	mum	nana	pap	bap			wawa
4. Bed, sleep .		nana		bye-bye	teitei	dodo	
5. Child himself .				baby			
6. Father . .			papa	baba	tata	dada	
7. Play : ball . . . clock . . dog . . . pointing . giving . . thanking . going out .			pa	ba ba	titta tatta ta tata	didda da da da ada	wauwau

[1] In the notation of the various observers.

The situations in which these front-consonant words appear are naturally those of primary interest to the child : the people immediately about him, his food, his bed and his play. But the question that immediately arises and has been frequently debated is this : How is it that these situations are universally named alike ?

Some confusion has arisen in the discussion of this question, because two problems, which should be considered separately, have often been treated as one :

(i) How do words such as *mama* come to have their meaning in the nursery ?

(ii) How have these words been adopted into conventional adult language, either as they stand, or as the basis of further developments such as *mater* ?

Linguists have often tried to show that the processes which account for the appearance of nursery-words also account for the appearance of the adult forms. But the factors in the latter process must remain conjectural because inevitably we lack the historical, to say nothing of the prehistorical, data ; there is no reason, however, why we should not observe what goes on in the nursery and deal with the appearance and development of front-consonant words there. And if we confine ourselves in this way, we shall not be tempted to import explanations which, while they may serve to fill gaps in the history of language, only obscure our view of what happens to the child.

On the whole, there is general agreement on two points : first that these front-consonant forms are connected with the child's sucking-movements, secondly that there is some significance in the fact that the mother is usually named with an **m**-form, the father with a **p, b, t** or **d**-form. It is on the question as to how these meanings occur that disagreement exists. We find two types of explanation :

(1) The view that the phonetic characteristics of these words suggest, of themselves, specific meanings to all human beings alike (Wundt, Stern).

(2) The view that these words, which occur universally because of their origin, have been given a series of arbitrary meanings which are traditionally maintained (Jespersen).

Wundt (VP 253) begins with the assumption that the connection between the front-consonant words and sucking-sounds is merely one of association of similar things ; the sounds survive in the child's repertory because they recall sucking-movements to him. He repeats **m** and **p** words with pleasure because they remind him of feeding. Adults aid this survival ; noticing the frequency of these words in the child's speech, they imitate him and he in turn imitates them, and so a strong habit is developed. As for the meaning which these words acquire, this is also suggested by their form. Wundt points out, in particular, that the **p**-forms generally denote the child's father and the **m**-forms his mother ; these attributions, he suggests, are made by adults, who feel that **p** is a " strong " consonant, suited to name a man, **m** a " weak " consonant suited to name a woman. The child then adopts these meanings imitatively.

Wundt's view is open to at least two objections : he neglects the expressive functions which these sounds have long had for the child, and he postulates a sense in us of the relative " strength " of **p** and **m,** for there is no other evidence than these very cases in question.

Stern (KSp 363) is violently sceptical of this theory of Wundt's. Sucking-movements, he agrees, are certainly elements out of which the front-consonant combinations develop into the *ma*-words and *pa*-words of the nursery. But this development depends not on any fancied contrast between " strong " and " weak " ; it is due to the fact that the **m, n** sounds have a " centripetal ", the **p, b, t, d** sounds a " centrifugal " meaning.[1] He does not make it clear whether he intends these meanings to exist only for the adult, or whether the child also is to be regarded as having some inkling of them. In any case, I must confess that I am unable to understand the nature of this somewhat mystical contrast—which, it may be added, is markedly out of keeping with the strong empiricism of Stern's general treatment.

Jespersen (ND 160) rejects the views both of Wundt and of Stern. He is prepared to go so far as to accept the connection between the earliest front-consonant combinations and sucking-movements or vocal play. But the further development into " mother-words " and " father-words " occurs, he asserts, mainly through the adult's " arbitrary interpretation " of the child's " meaningless " syllables. It seems to me that Jespersen's account falls short just in this insistence upon the arbitrary and the meaningless.

All these three views appear to make unnecessarily complicated and questionable assumptions because they endeavour, I think, to find the same explanations for two quite distinct processes—the origin of the nursery-words and the origin of the adult words. Further, they fail to lay sufficient stress on

---

[1] Stern seems to have borrowed this notion from the philologists, for Whitney (SL 430) refers to it as a theory concerning the primitive roots *ma* and *ta* ; a theory for which, he adds, there is very little evidence.

one important fact—that the two classes of front-consonant forms (the nasal and the oral) are phonetically, that is physiologically, bound up with the primary contrasting bodily states of the child. If we ignore this fact, a gap remains in the chain of events from the expressive cries to the fully-formed nursery words, a gap which has to be filled up by invoking some extraneous hypothesis.

But as we have said, it is generally agreed that the form of these words is connected with the child's sucking-movements. In Chapter III we have shown the phonetic basis of this connection : that the front-consonants are indeed the forms taken by the child's expressions of discomfort and comfort, aroused by his need for food and by the satisfaction of this need. It is clear therefore that his earliest words, being reduplicated or monosyllabic front-consonant forms, are fundamentally the child's own expressive utterance, which has begun almost with his earliest cry. These forms become stabilised by the influence of adults, making use of the traditional words already existing in their language. Thus if we confine ourselves to the front-consonant forms of the nursery, and make no speculations concerning the origin of the related words in adult language, we are able to limit the process of development to these three factors :

(i) The front-consonant words arise directly out of the child's expressive nasal and oral front-consonant utterance.

(ii) Their meanings are stabilised in the nursery by adult interpretation of the child's expressive use of them.

(iii) This stabilisation is also determined by the existence of traditional nursery forms.

The Process of Stabilisation.—When we say that the child's earliest words are fundamentally expressive, this does not mean that he always plays the leading part in establishing a given word. Stern—apparently following Meumann (SK 25) —finds that there are three routes by which this may take place (KSp 170) : in the first case the initiative appears to come from the child, in the others from the adult.

(1) In expressive utterance [1] ; for instance, the child's *mamam* comes not only to express his state of discomfort but to refer to a specific situation—e.g. his mother, or the feeling of hunger.

[1] Stern uses the word *Lallen* ; but from the rest of his statement as given above it is clear that he means to describe expressive utterance. This is an instance of that ambiguity to which we have referred on page 55.

(2) Imitation : meaning is given to words which have been meaninglessly imitated ; e.g. having long said *dedda* (Berta) imitatively, one day the child turns to the nursemaid while saying it.

(3) Words which evoke a trained reaction ; the child has been trained—as described in the last chapter—to respond by specific activity to a specific word ; one day he also says the word in the appropriate situation : e.g. *tick-tack* on seeing the clock.

Taking this analysis as a guide, let us consider in each case the actual course of development, as far as it can be observed.

(i) *Expression as a Factor.*—At an early stage, as we have seen, the child's states of discomfort are expressed by nasal sounds, his states of comfort mainly by oral sounds. When the child begins to utter labial and dental consonants, which are phonated sucking-movements, states of discomfort are expressed by **m** and **n** forms, states of comfort by **p, b, t** and **d** forms. Does this distinction, we may now ask, show itself in any difference of meaning at the stage when these early forms become stable " words " ? Only in one respect, although a very important one : on the whole the mother is represented by nasal forms (usually **m,** occasionally **n**) and rarely by oral forms ; while the father, on the other hand, is usually represented by oral forms (**p, b, t, d**)—very rarely (perhaps never among European children), by nasal forms. How is this ?

For the association between the **m**-forms and the child's mother, at any rate, there would appear to be no need to seek beyond the simplest explanation. The child in discomfort makes urgent nasal sounds, he cries **mama** ; to his mother this means that he is " calling her ", the more so when she finds, of course, that her attention to him results in the cessation of the cry.

So much, indeed, is accepted by Stern. But this interpretation demands no feeling, either in mother or child, of the " centripetal " nature of the sounds, or of their " weakness ", as suggested by Wundt. It demands only that the child shall utter expressive nasalised cries, and that he shall make anticipatory sucking-movements in the course of this utterance, with the result that forms such as **mama** appear.

Nor can we regard the mother's appropriation of the name **mama** to herself as in any way an " arbitrary " application of " meaningless " sounds, as Jespersen maintains. No one would assert that the ordinary expression of fear or rage is meaningless—each has an intimate connection with its specific state ; the expression **mama** is similarly a meaningful expression of the child's hunger. To his mother it means that he is hungry and needs her ; but even to the child himself his utterance, once this has occurred, cannot be entirely meaningless : his expression of hunger must carry with it some reinstatement of the pattern of events in which it has repeatedly occurred, including his experience of his mother. And to this extent the mother's appropriation of **mama** to herself is certainly not an " arbitrary " act.

The process, then, by which the expressive sound-group **mama** ultimately takes on a referential meaning for the child has this very important characteristic : it is a progressive development and differentiation of a meaning which this sound-group already possesses for him and which has a long history in his life. At a very early stage indeed this sound-group must already carry with it—whenever the child utters it and hears himself uttering it—some reinstatement of the feeling by which it has regularly been accompanied. To this extent it means to him the state of discomfort. Further it must soon come to mean for him also the whole situation of the appeasement of discomfort, including the person who ministers to him ; so that all that the mother does in this case, by repeating the word **mama** when she presents herself to him, is to bring into higher relief and closer relationship two features which are already in existence in the pattern of events—the child's experience of her and his experience of the sound-group.

This does not leave out of account the fact of the existence of **mama** as a traditional name, which also contributes to the mother's appropriation of the name to herself. And this traditional usage depends in its turn partly on the occurrence of the word in infantile utterance, and partly also, of course, upon other historical factors which we are not attempting to consider here.

The existence of a traditional name plays its part in this way : it helps to stabilise the child's present use of the word. By imitation he comes to approximate his own utterance to it, and tends also to confine its meaning to that which it has in the community about him. But there is no doubt that the expressive origin of the word is at least as effective in determining its meaning as this traditional use in the community. Even if the traditional form **mama** did not exist, it seems likely that most children would still say **ma-ma** (or something of the kind) expressively in hunger, and mothers hastening to feed them would inevitably feel that their children were " calling " them, naming them.

It is also evident why **mama** rather than **nana** should become the usual name for mother.   The labial is much more obviously a consonant than the dental; when the child brings his lips firmly together we can see that he is speaking : he has begun to speak !   But **nana** is not very different from nasalised **a a**— sounds that the child has been uttering from birth.   To the majority of mothers, therefore, **mama** naturally seems to be their child's first word.

This also explains, without any further assumptions, the appropriation of **nana,** on the whole, to the child's nurse. When the child is in a state of discomfort, the **n**-forms are just as likely to appear as the **m**-forms ; but as **mama** is the child's first obvious " word ", and appropriated to the mother, **nana** and such forms are left over for the nurse, or for any other woman in attendance upon the child.

The appropriation of the **p, b, t, d** forms to the child's father can obviously be explained in the same way.   These, as we have seen, are generally uttered in states of comfort.   Any adult who approaches the child while he is vocally expressing his satisfaction will tend to regard the sounds he is making as a way of showing recognition ; the adult will tend to repeat the particular sound-group and so bring this experience into closer relationship with himself, in the manner adopted by the mother when she is appropriating **mama** to herself ; further, the child will tend to imitate the sound-group on hearing it uttered, and this will fix it in his speech.   Finally, its traditional meaning in the adult conventional language will influence the meaning it comes to have for the child.

In one respect the appropriation of these oral forms as names for the child's father may be regarded as " arbitrary ", as Jespersen maintains.   If their meaning grows up as we have described, then certainly we should expect them to embrace any adult whose presence has formed part of a pleasant experience for the child.   And our list does show this, that there is no universal appropriation of these forms to the father alone ; a sound-group such as **baba** may mean, in one nursery or another—or even in the same nursery—father, mother, nurse, aunt, or grandmother. Again, as Stern mentions (KSp 19), a child may be found, for some time, using a form such as **papa** for his mother or father indifferently. It is only through the influence of adult usage that the meaning of the form **papa** becomes confined to a single person, and it is only this limited appropriation which can be regarded as somewhat " arbitrary ". But the fundamental use of these oral forms, to embrace any adult who appears when the child is in no urgent need, is certainly very far from arbitrary. Even though adult usage does ultimately determine the appropriation of a particular form to a particular person, this only occurs by the progressive differentiation of a wider meaning already present in the child's expressive utterance of the form.

We are left now with two situations—" food " and " bed " —which seem to be represented just as frequently by a nasal as by an oral form. Both Wundt with his contrast of " strong " and " weak ", and Stern with his contrast of " centrifugal " and " centripetal " find it difficult to explain instances of this kind, and have to regard them as exceptional. Stern indeed has to go so far as to admit that in **p**-forms meaning food, the consonant ceases to have a centrifugal meaning (KSp 372).

Without pretending that our own explanation covers every possible case without exception—since the factor of tradition is throughout somewhat indeterminate—we may at least point out that it does without difficulty extend to these instances also. For hunger and fatigue are undoubtedly two of the chief states of discomfort in the young child, and also the only two in which a specific *object*—food or bed—as distinct from a specific person, is perceived by the child as a source of relief. Thus in food and bed we have the two principal objects with regard to which the child may definitely experience either discomfort or comfort. It is evident that the urgent anticipation of food might be manifested by a nasal cry of discomfort such as **mama,**[1] while the same child's pleasant anticipation of food, especially when this is already before him, might be manifested by the oral form **papa,**[1] a sound-group expressive of satisfaction. Similarly the tired child might utter the nasal cry **nana** [1] as an expression of fatigue—" longing to go to sleep "—and murmur **baba** [1] or some such oral sound-group on actually seeing his cot or on settling down to sleep. Thus

[1] See Appendix III, p. 257.

two forms, nasal and oral, might both become attached to each of these situations.

Which form, the nasal or the oral, in each case remains the triumphant surviving "word", depends no doubt upon special circumstances; often, we may suppose, upon traditional usage. In these cases, just as in those previously described, the social determination of meaning amounts to this : it helps to link up the word closely with one feature of the situation instead of its being loosely linked up with the whole.

To sum up, we may say that essentially we have here but two fundamental forms, the nasal and the oral sucking-sounds, refined, as they are, into nasal or oral front-consonants. Two primary factors converge to bring about a differentiation of meaning ; on the one hand the expressive utterance of the child, on the other, social response to him and pressure upon him. One great primary differentiation of meaning is potentially present in the difference between nasal discomfort-sounds and oral comfort-sounds ; this differentiation is stabilised by adult response, carrying with it both universal nursery tradition and local linguistic tradition. Further differentiation on the basis of this primary grouping occurs as the child's social environment provides specific sequels, and hence specific meanings, in the form of particular persons or objects. In this way each of the two fundamental modes of expression, the nasal and the oral, each with its own wide undifferentiated meaning, comes to have its specific differentiated meanings.

What we have endeavoured to stress here is that both nasal and oral forms owe their specific meanings in some measure to the fact that they arise directly out of the child's early expressive utterance. The meanings of his first "words" are therefore fundamentally expressive as well as socially determined. These meanings are not casually attached by adults to sound-groups casually chosen by them ; nor even casually attached to those sounds which the child happens to utter spontaneously. They are the social stabilisation of meanings which already exist in the child's utterance.

But in passing from these words which are used in connection with the child's more immediate needs and the people immediately about him to the words used in less intimate situations —such as his games—we certainly find ourselves confronted more definitely with the effects of adult intervention. Before we discuss this, however, a word must be said about the place of babbling.

(ii) *Babbling as a Factor.*—Stern does not give any example of children's words which have clearly begun as babbling. The fact is, that although it is frequently maintained that— as Lorimer puts it (GR 61)—" bits of babble " become transformed into meaningful words, this is not easy to demonstrate. For in babbling the child is attentive to the sounds he is making, he is playing with them, they are meaningless in relation to the situation in which they are uttered. Clearly, sounds which have no expressive, or onomatopoetic or even conventional connection with a situation, must provide the very least suitable material out of which to fashion a medium of intercourse between adult and child.

Once more, in fact, we are confronted with the notion that the adult arbitrarily chooses a fragment of the child's speech and attaches it to an object or situation by a process of training. We have suggested that this view is due to an imperfect analysis of what happens. In the first place one must distinguish between babbling and expression as two different functions which the same sounds may have for the child. Then, as we have shown, it is the sounds uttered expressively by the child which—because they are evoked by particular situations—may readily become stabilised in relation to these situations. Finally, we find—and this is a point which must be stressed—that many words which are clearly of onomatopoetic or conventional origin become transformed by the child and adapted to his own forms of speech. Stern's *didda* for *tik-tak* and *dedda* for *Berta* are clear cases, which might, on a superficial view, appear to be " bits of babble ", when without question they are the child's own expressive adaptations of forms used and stabilised by the adult.

To come now to this process of stabilisation : Stern's view— as seen in the second and third groups of cases which we have cited from him on page 130—is that the adult sometimes provides a model for imitation, and sometimes links the word with a specific situation by training. We shall find that this statement needs some modification, and that instead of there being three independent processes—arising from expression, imitation or training—all three may be present in the development of a single word.

(iii) *Imitation as a Factor.*—Stern describes the course of events in his second group of cases in these terms : " the child may have said *dedda* (Berta) in mechanical imitation, on hearing it spoken ; until one day, while uttering the word, he turns in the direction of the girl whose name it is " (KSp 170). It is important to notice the details of this description of Stern's, for in it he envisages the rise of meaning in a previously meaningless sound-group, by chance. If by chance, he suggests, the child says a certain word at a time when he is experiencing a certain situation, the word will come to have a meaning from that situation. This is just the kind of process which is frequently described in support of the view that meaning develops in the child's meaningless utterance by virtue of chance association with a given situation.

Let us consider the actual course of events in a case of this kind. First of all, Stern tells us, the child has imitated the sound in a mechanical fashion (*mechanisch nachgesprochen*). As the whole point of this account lies in Stern's insistence that meaning is absent from the preliminary imitation, it is essential to notice that this is by no means the only possible, or even the most likely, state of affairs. For, as we have had to conclude (p. 101), pure meaningless echolalia is far from occurring universally among children ; usually when the child imitates, whether immediately or after delay, this in itself is the outcome of interest in the situation of which the word, when heard, has formed a part. For instance, in this case of Stern's, the child would presumably have heard the name *Berta* spoken in the presence of its owner, probably often by the girl herself, and the affective basis of the child's primary response to this person would constitute a strong factor in bringing about an imitation of her name. And even in cases which begin as pure echolalia—for instance, when Stern trained his daughter to say *papa* (see p. 98)—a change must very soon take place if the incident recurs : the child hears the word uttered by a speaker, in a given situation ; and thus almost from the very outset his imitation is something more than meaningless echolalia—the word comes to him with a fringe of meaning.

Further, if we consider the next event in this process, we find that the continued growth of meaning is again not the mere result of chance. Usually training will take place, through which adults foster the connection between the imitated word and one specific element of the situation in which it was first experienced. For instance, in Stern's case, the child might possibly sometimes say *dedda* (in imitation of *Berta*) in the presence of the person so named, without however showing any overt direction of his activity towards that person. But all through this time the direction of his attention would certainly be trained by two processes. Adults saying *Berta* (perhaps even *dedda*) in the presence of the person so named would often undoubtedly turn in her direction, and this alone would serve to restrict the attention of the child at the moment when he imitated the word. In many cases, much more than this involuntary gesture would occur ; there would be pointing and other ways of causing the child to turn in the required direction—as we have described in the last chapter. Moreover, as soon as the child uttered the name, its owner would naturally respond with a smile or some other sign of approval ; this too would help to direct the child's activity at the moment of saying the word. Thus two processes would be going on side by side. The child on hearing the word *Berta* or *dedda* would respond by making some movement towards the nursemaid, and again whenever he said *dedda* in her presence would be rewarded by a smile from her. In the end there would come a moment when he would say *dedda* and turn towards her as he did so.

This is far from being a process in which meaning creeps into a word meaninglessly imitated : training plays a very important part.

Further, in the course of our discussion an interesting point has obtruded itself : that, as Stern mentions, the child, instead of saying *Berta*, says *dedda*. This, as we shall show in Chapter X, is in the highest degree typical of children's imitation at this stage ; it is also very significant of the process of development we are now considering. For *dedda* is a characteristic front-consonant word, either occurring in the course of babbling, or expressive of a state of comfort : both of these factors may play some part in the process.

The former factor would appear to be the one implied by Stern. An adult says *Berta*, which—through its effect upon a train of babbling—becomes the beginning of the circular process of training such as we have described in Chapter VI, p. 99 ; and ultimately comes to evoke the word *dedda* regularly, this meanwhile acquiring meaning in the manner we have described above.

On the whole the second factor—that the word *dedda* arises as an expressive word—here seems likely to be the stronger. What more natural than that the child, seeing a familiar friendly face, should express his satisfaction by saying—among other front-consonant words perhaps—something like *dedda* ? When this was caught by an adult and interpreted as an imitation of *Berta*, the process of stabilisation would begin, based—as we have just described—partly upon imitation and partly upon training.

Our conclusion must therefore be that—instead of meaning entering by chance into the utterance of a meaningless imitation—three factors may really be present at this first stage : expression, imitation (working upon a basis of babbling), and training by the conditions of the situation and the intervention of the adult. The child expresses his satisfaction by uttering some front-consonant word such as **dada** or **deda** ; this is stabilised in form by his being given the model *Berta*, and becomes *dedda* ; and is stabilised in meaning by the conditions under which it is spoken and by a course of training.

The process as we have described it is certainly more complicated than in Stern's account ; but all the evidence leads us to the view that at every stage the growth of language is rarely simple but due to the effect of a number of concurrent factors.

(iv) *Training as a Factor.*—Stern describes the first utterance of words, which have already acquired meaning through training, as follows :

> The child has perhaps for a long time past shown an understanding of *tick-tack*—without uttering it—in that he turns towards the clock on hearing this word. Then when the word is at last spoken by the child, it is straightway spoken with meaning (KSp 170).

In brief, there is trained response to a word, followed by utterance of the word. There seems no good reason, therefore, to restrict our discussion to one only of the three kinds of trained response described in the last chapter (p. 110), and no doubt Stern means his example to be typical of all three. Meaningful utterance of a word might supervene upon trained response to it, whatever its origin ; and we have seen that the original action upon which the response is based may be of three kinds :

(i) "*Spontaneous*" action : e.g. first the child turns to the clock ; later he turns to it on hearing the word *tick-tack* ; finally he says *tick-tack* on seeing the clock.

(ii) "*Imitative*" action : e.g. first the child imitates hand-clapping ; then he performs this action on hearing *bravo!* ; finally he says *bravo!* while performing it.

(iii) "*Induced*" action : e.g. first the child is made to point to his nose ; then he performs the action on hearing *Wo ist die Nase?* ; finally he says *Nase!* while performing it.

Although Stern sharply distinguishes this group of cases —words given a meaning through training—from that described in the last section (words which originate as "meaningless" imitation), the distinction cannot be so clearly maintained when we come to consider the actual course of events. In both instances we have these two determining factors : the child's imitation of a word, and his trained response to the word in its situation. The only difference would appear to be this, that in such cases as that of *Berta* the imitation came first and the training followed ; in the case of *tick-tack* the training came first, and the imitation followed.

But even this distinction is probably slighter than appears at first sight. For when a child listens attentively to a word, he has already begun to imitate it. As we saw in Chapter VI, page 97, hearing is incipient utterance. When the child hears *Tick-tack* or *Bravo!*, in so far as he is sufficiently attentive to it to respond at all, there is a tendency already present for him to say it aloud ; as Delacroix puts it (LP 293) : "percevoir un mouvement c'est savoir le répéter". We have seen (p. 86) how such incipient imitative utterance may sometimes be inhibited when the heard word has a meaning ; the child has been trained to make a certain movement on hearing a word, and this movement is his adequate response to the heard word and may thus exclude imitation. We have seen also (p. 90) that at the present stage the inhibition will often be broken down : we encourage the child to say the word while making the movement, and when he does so we feel that he has spoken it with meaning. Thus, throughout the whole period that the child is being trained to respond to the word, he also has a strong tendency to imitate it.

We may regard this instance of training as a simple case of the completion of a pattern of experience. The chief constituents of this pattern have been three ; seeing the clock, hearing a word, and making a movement ; when one day only two of these constituents are present—seeing the clock and making the movement—the child himself supplies the missing constituent, the heard word, by saying the word himself.   Thus it is reasonable to point out that the imitation of the word and its meaning for the child have been growing up together : while he has been learning to respond to it by a movement he has been learning to imitate it.

In both groups of cases, then, described by Stern (the instance of *Berta* and that of *tick-tack*) the factors of imitation and of training are both present ; the only difference being that imitation seems to operate more rapidly in the former case, training in the latter.

But we can go further.   It would seem that the third factor, that of expression, which we noticed in the case of *Berta*, may also be present in the case of *tick-tack*.   This is not obvious in Stern's statement : he does not tell us what the child would say in imitation of *tick-tack*.   But when we go back to his own careful observations (KSp 18) we find that what his daughter Hilde said at 0;10, under precisely these conditions was *didda* ! Surely nothing could be more significant ; once more we are faced by a front-consonant word.   And this is by no means an isolated case, as we shall show in Chapter X ; thus the child cited by Sander said *dida* under these conditions, and the one cited by Major *titit* (Appendix III, p. 255) ; while K's characteristic forms were **tittit** and **titta** (Appendix IV, p. 312) —all front-consonant forms.

Thus to the two factors of imitation and training we can add either expression or babbling—or both.   When the child at last says *didda* or *tit-tit* on seeing the clock, this is not merely a sound-group mechanically forced from him as an effect of imitation and of training.   He says the word in satisfaction, even in glee ; it is expressive and therefore likely to be made up of front-consonants.   At the same time imitation is certainly also working here upon the basis of his own babbled sounds ; the previously heard *tick-tack* or *tick-tick* will evoke from the child a form somewhat like it from among his repertory of babbling—just as Stern's *papa* drew forth an imitation, after delay, from his daughter (p. 98).

The Concurrence of these Factors.—Our conclusion then, from considering Stern's analysis must be this : that certainly the three factors he mentions—expression, imitation, and training—are present in developing the child's first meaningful utterance of conventional words. So much we owe to him and to Meumann. But we have to add, that so far from these three factors working independently and giving rise to three different groups of forms, actually they are likely to be present, all of them, in the development of any one of the child's earliest words. In each case, no doubt, one of the three factors may be dominant ; and, obviously, the child's earlier words must owe more to expression, his later ones more to imitation and training.

The importance of recognising the presence of these three factors is that it reveals the development of meaning in the child's earliest spoken words as an unbroken continuous process from the time of his first expressive utterance. We see that although his early spoken words may be regarded as expressive, onomatopoetic and conventional in origin, it would be false to conclude that either the form or the meaning of an expressive word such as **mama** is due simply to expression, or of an onomatopoetic word such as **wauwau** simply to its resemblance to the animal's bark, or of a word such as **puppe** simply to imitation and training. In all three cases all the three factors—expression, imitation, and training—may be present.

We have shown that this is true in the case of the expressive forms—**papa, mama** and the rest. It holds good of the other forms also. In the case of the onomatopoetic words, Stern concludes from observation that these are due almost entirely to the influence of adults, both in form and meaning (KSp 379) ; in all the large onomatopoetic vocabulary of his three children —50 per cent. of the total in the case of Hilde at 1;6 (KSp 376) —only five words seemed independent of this influence. What, however, he has not emphasised is this : that the first onomatopoetic words, at any rate, are partly assimilated to the child's own utterance : their forms owe something to expression and babbling, and their meaning is certainly largely expressive. It is surely no mere coincidence that of the eleven onomatopoetic words given in the list derived from Stern in Appendix III (pp. 253–5), six are *wauwau* (or *oua-oua*), three are *didda* (or *tit-tit*) for *tick-tack*, one is another front-consonant form, *m m* for the noise of a cart (Lindner's son), while only one—*ssi-ssi* (Strümpell)—is not front-consonantal. What happens, then, is this, that the child—whether he directly imitates the animal or sonorous object, or whether he only imitates an adult model —uses the word expressively, and that this tends to show itself in the expressive front-consonantal form of the word. In fact, what Lindner observed of his son must often be true of the other cases : that when the child at 1;0 said *m m* on hearing the sound of a cart he did this expressively, and not in a purely imitative way (Stern, KSp 380).

Something similar may be said of those words which arise primarily from a conventional form in the adult language : for instance, Meringer's case of *awa* (*Wasser*), Major's case of *baw* (ball), or Ament's of *deda* (*Tante*) (Appendix III, pp. 253–5). While the child acquires such words by imitation and training, they are also at the same time expressive, and this function shows itself in their front-consonantal form.

All these words, then, owe something to the child's primary activities of expression and babbling as well as something to the influence of the language spoken about him. In the present chapter we have discussed the effect of these individual and social factors upon the entrance of conventional words into his speech ; in the last chapter we observed their influence on his first understanding of conventional speech. We next have to discuss the further development of the functions of these words, a problem which can only be considered by comparing the child's response to language with his use of it, at this stage. This is the topic of our next chapter.

CHAPTER IX

THE NATURE OF THIS PROGRESS

WHAT are the changes in the functions of language which mark the child's advance in the comprehension and utterance of his " first words " ?

The Growth of Objective Reference.—The main development was formulated thirty years ago by Meumann (EK 156). Language, he maintained, is at the outset exclusively affective-volitional in function, becoming as time goes on increasingly objective. This statement has been generally accepted, with slight modifications ; in the first place, the evidence compels us to agree with Stern (KSp 181), Delacroix (LP 295) and Lorimer (GR 64) that even at the outset language is not wholly devoid of objective function—a qualification which Meumann himself hinted at (EK 192). Secondly, to-day we should substitute the word " conational " for " volitional ", for the latter term suggests that the infant is consciously directing his own use of language. In terms current to-day we should say that the function of objective reference grows in language which previously was mainly expressive of affect and conation.

What does this change amount to in the child's actual use and comprehension of words ? In general, we say that a word has the function of objective reference when it serves as a means of directing behaviour towards a specific portion of an experience. Take, for instance, the case of A desiring B to hand him a ball. By means of A's remarks the attention of the listener (or of the speaker) may be drawn to one or other of these elements in the situation : the speaker A, the listener B, A's desire, the action of handing, or the ball. Then Meumann's view, in its modified form, is this : that when a very young child who desires food first says *mama*, this is mainly an expression of his affective state in hunger, and of his striving to satisfy his appetite, and only very slightly expresses the direction of his attention either towards this state, or this striving, or towards the food, or towards the bringer of food ; and further that only gradually does the utterance of the word bring with it this direction of attention towards one portion of the whole experience.

We have now to see how far this formulation is justified by a survey of the facts.

Our Judgment of the Change.—How can we judge that an advance in the function of reference is taking place ? Obviously by noticing the progressive changes in the meaning that language has for the child. But this plan, so easy to formulate in principle, is precisely our chief difficulty in practice. How are we to know what meaning a particular sound-group has for the child, when he utters it or responds to it ? To say that a word means an object, refers to it, because the child utters the word or responds to it in the presence of that object, is an assumption that needs to be tested.

If, for instance, we assert that when a child says **mama** on seeing his mother, the word now means mother to him ; or that when he looks towards the clock on hearing someone say *tick-tick*, this word now means the clock to him, we are making an assumption that might be misleading in two ways. It would suggest, first of all, that until the child utters the word in the presence of a particular object, no referential function has existed in the word for him ; and further, that as soon as this utterance occurs, the word has acquired a referential function exactly of the same kind as it might have for an adult. On this view, throughout the period when the child says **mama** irrespective of the presence of his mother, it is merely an expressive cry, without a vestige of referential function ; and when he does at last say it regularly on seeing her, he is using the word as a name for her.

Now these assumptions might quite possibly prove to be well founded in fact. But until we have actually tested their truth, it would be misleading to regard them as anything but assumptions, arising out of the superficial view that the function of reference enters the use of a word at the moment when a child appears to connect the word with a particular object.

To discover how reference develops, we have to notice, by considering the child's behaviour at times when he is speaking or responding to words, what is the function of a given sound-group both before and after he first appears to attach it to a given object. In other words, we have to judge of the meaning of a word by noticing its place in the child's activity. In this we find ourselves following a trend which recently has become strongly marked in discussions of the nature of language in general; the work, for instance, of Dewey, Malinowski, De Laguna, Markey and Gardiner.

The Data.—Thus we need detailed observations of a child's behaviour when he is using or responding to words. Observations of this kind are, however, extremely scanty, most observers having confined themselves to recording the changes in a child's utterance only, and this by the mere statement in each case of the word's " meaning ". Even when, as in the case of Deville's record, we have successive observations of responses, we are frequently told only that the child " understood " a word on a certain occasion, but are given little indication of the essential fact—what it was in the child's actual behaviour which led the observer to this conclusion.

In order therefore to test Meumann's formulation by noticing the function of language as the child develops, I propose to consider here my own observations of K, in which I recorded his actual behaviour at times when he was uttering or responding to a word.

First of all, by taking cross-sections at intervals in his history, we shall notice the general course of development, and then study in detail the successive changes that occur in the functions of a particular word.

The General Course of Development. (a) *Instances of Response.*—In Appendix IV (1), p. 300, I give three sample cross-sections of K's responses. The first consists of the earliest five entries, as they occur in my record, of his definite overt behaviour in response to words; then allowing three months to elapse I give the record of his next five responses, and again of the next five after a similar interval.

To summarise these observations, we notice that in the first group of entries (9th and 10th months) K's responses—where they are not neutral—consist of the initiation or the inhibition of a given act, and that in one entry (0;9,14) the act consists in touching a given object, one of many present. In the second cross-section (13th month), we find that the direction of the child's activity towards a specific object has become more definite : his movement of giving in response to the word *Give*, learnt since the first group of entries, may be regarded as an advance upon his earlier response of merely touching, for it is more closely concerned with the particular object— the child's crust or his toy bear. In the third cross-section (16th month) we find a further advance in this direction of activity towards a specific object, in one important respect : that now the child will respond to a word in the absence of the object by moving in the direction of the place where this has customarily appeared. In the instructive case of *Where's apple ?* (1;3,5) he goes a step further still ; he directs his activity towards the spot, not where the apple has customarily been, but where he happens to have seen it a short time since.

In brief, we may say that in the earlier entries the child's response to a word is largely affective and conational—consisting of the initiation or inhibition of an act as the result of the affective state aroused by the word ; while in the later entries his response is increasingly directed to and concerned with one particular element in his experience—an " object ".

(b) *Instances of Utterance.*—Turning now to the changes of behaviour accompanying utterance, I have given in Appendix IV (2), page 302, three cross-sections similar to those just studied, except that as, on the whole, the use of words develops after comprehension, it is necessary to begin our selection a month later. As before, the entries are given just as they occur in my record. To summarise them, we notice in the first group (11th month) that there is as yet no certain use of a word of adult form with any objective reference, although the child's own sounds **a a a** at 0;10,28 would appear to be directed in some degree towards the toy dog. Nor is there any considerable advance in the second group of entries (14th month) ; possibly there is some direction towards a specific person in the cases of **nana** and **mama** (both at 1;1,8), and towards a specific object in the case of **a a a** at 1;1,15, but there is more than an element of doubt in all these instances. At the most, there appears to be an increase in the definiteness of the act which accompanies speech : a word like **ɛbɔ** (1;1,9) or **iːpba** (1;1,20) occurs in the course of a specific movement. But by the third group of entries (17th month), the picture has certainly altered. Here there are at least three clear cases of objective reference : **bɑ** (at 1;4,6) is definitely directed towards the bath, **ba** (at 1;4,17) towards the buttons on the mother's jacket, and **ba** (at 1;4,18) towards those on the child's own coat. Further, there is even a case of direction towards an absent object : **ha** (at 1;4,17) when the child at breakfast-time turns towards the cupboard from which the honey has customarily appeared.

From these two series of entries it is clear that the changes in the child's responses to words parallel the changes in behaviour accompanying his own speech, the latter development following, stage for stage, some months after the former. Along both lines we see a progressive increase in the reference to specific objects within the situation, and ultimately reference even to objects which are not actually present. To this extent we certainly find a justification of Meumann's view : the child's linguistic behaviour, both in utterance and in response, seems to have more and more an objective reference.

The Process of Development.—Having illustrated the growth of objective reference, we now have to consider at closer quarters the nature of this development. When language begins to have the function of objective reference for the child, is this equivalent to saying that a particular word has now become the name of an object for him ? This question can only be answered by noticing the changes of his *behaviour* in using and responding to the same word. For the main clue to our understanding of the growth of objective reference lies in recognising that in the early stages language is not something set apart from the rest of the child's activity, but a form of activity in itself. Everything that we can observe leads us to the conclusion that, at least during his first two years, language is only one feature of the child's total behaviour at any given moment, and that only through a process of development does it become a relatively distinct form of his behaviour.

Take first his response to words. As we have seen in Chapter VII, the effect of heard conventional words upon the child is to cause him to engage in or desist from certain acts. These words gradually take more and more the place of the adult's physical activity. At first, when we want the child to do something or cease from doing something, we physically help him or prevent him ; making, perhaps, encouraging or discouraging noises the while. For instance, we put a ball within his reach or we remove him from the hot fireguard towards which he has crawled. Later, to achieve the same results, we say, *Baby, ballie !* encouragingly, or *No !* or *Hot !* in a menacing tone.

Now it is important to notice that the behaviour that our

words set going is on the whole of two kinds. Either we make him turn his attention in this direction or that, or we make him perform (or desist from) a definite act, which may include the manipulation of some object. For instance, we say *Chauve-souris !* to him or *tick-tack !*, so that he turns his attention towards the window through which bats have been seen, or towards the clock. Or we say *Bravo !* or *Give mummy crustie !* so that he claps his hands or holds out the crust to us. Both in causing him to attend and in causing him to act (or desist from acting) our words increasingly replace our deeds.

The same replacement occurs, but of course very slowly, in the child's own instrumental use of language. When the child is not just babbling, playing with words, he is using them with an effect on the behaviour of others. We can reasonably say that he is using language instrumentally, always with the reservation that the *intention* to use speech in this instrumental fashion may only be partially present. And if we look at the child's first spoken conventional words, we find that he uses them instrumentally in two ways, which we may call the *declarative* and the *manipulative*. In the former use he is drawing our attention to some object—as when K, for instance, said **tita** pointing to a picture of a watch—Appendix IV (6), page 312, entry 1;6,11. In the latter use he is not only drawing our attention to an object, but at the same time demanding that we shall satisfy his needs in relation to that object, for instance, when K said **goga,** wanting chocolate—Appendix IV (7), page 313, entry 1;6,15. In both uses, the declarative and the manipulative, there is expression of the child's affect and conation as well as the rudiments of reference to an object.

When used instrumentally, the child's language has the effect of bringing others within his circle of activity. In the declarative use he attracts another's attention and so assures himself of company. If he is delighted, the presence of another person enhances his delight ; if he is afraid, the presence of another person alleviates his fear. The word becomes for the child a means of securing this enhancement or alleviation. In the manipulative use the child is again using the word as a social instrument ; this time as a means of securing the help of others in satisfying his practical needs. Sometimes, of course, both declarative and manipulative uses will be present.

Now there is no doubt that the use and acceptance of the

instrumental functions of words play an important part in hastening the growth of objective reference in the child's language. Thus, to trace the growth of the meaning of a particular word for a child we need to trace the changes of his behaviour both in responding to and using the same word. The matter is simplified a little for us by the fact that comprehension generally precedes use, so that for a time we can often watch a child's responses to a word without the complication of the child's uses of it.

(a) *Response to a Word.*—In Appendix IV (3), page 304, I have given my observations of K's responses to the word *ballie*, a word to which the child responded in a number of definite ways before he himself uttered it with meaning, in the form of **bo:**. During this period that he was responding to *ballie*, if he wanted the object in question he would say **a a a a**—a sound-group also used by him for the expression of many other desires.

The child was given his first ball about a fortnight before the date of the first entry here. In the course of this period, he must often have heard the word *ballie* while seeing the ball. At 0;9,14 he shows himself capable, for the first time, of turning towards and touching the ball on hearing the phrase, *Where is the ballie?*, and does this repeatedly during the next six weeks, usually without any attempt to touch the other things that may be present ; excluding even another ball (0;10,21). Some definite progress seems to be recorded at 0;10,27, when the child learns to hold up one object in response to *Where's doggie?* and another in response to *Where's ballie?* A further development also appears on this same day, when in response to this latter phrase the child holds up a large coloured ball instead of the original small white one ; the application of the word seems to have become extended—partly, at least, on a basis of objective similarity.[1] At 0;10,29 we have an instance of the kind of experience which helps to bring about fuller objective reference. Here, as it happens, the word *Ballie!* does not evoke the touching or pointing movement ; but direction of attention towards the object nevertheless occurs, an experience which we may regard as of some importance. For up to this moment only two kinds of behaviour have been linked up for the child with the specific word : either he

[1] This question of the extended application of a word we discuss in Chapter XI.

performs the total act of handling the ball, or he fails to respond entirely. Now a third kind of behaviour has appeared : the child's attention is directed towards this single portion of the whole situation, without the rest of the be-haviour—the handling—taking place. It would be reasonable to describe this by saying that the child now responds to the phrase by directing his attention to the object, ball ; we could say that the heard phrase causes the child merely to refer to the ball.

Two months later, at 1;1,5, a further advance is recorded. Now the word has come to arouse, not simply direction towards a specific object which is present as part of a total situation, but behaviour directed by the reinstatement of a previous experience of the object. It would be reasonable to say that now the word helps the child to *recall* the object. There are two factors in the process : the child's previous experience of the ball while playing with it, and his present hearing of the phrase. The effect of the previous experience persists and is able to direct the child's activity at this present moment ; and this present activity is initiated by the hearing of the phrase *Where's ballie ?* We may therefore say that the phrase causes the child to refer to an absent ball ; the behaviour that was previously aroused by the presence of the ball, is now aroused by the hearing of certain sounds.

Thus a series of observations of this kind makes it possible for us to interpret the phrase " the growth of objective refer-ence " in terms of the child's behaviour. We see how the adult using a word such as *ballie* both declaratively and manipu-latively, causes the child sometimes to attend to an object, sometimes to deal actively with it, and that all the time the object itself is becoming clearly lifted out of the whole situa-tion, and given a closer linkage with the particular phonetic pattern of the heard word.

But this is only a very small part of the story. To say that the child, while learning to understand the word *ballie* adopts it and then uses it as the adult does, would be to give an extremely one-sided account of what happens. A very im-portant part of the process is the simultaneous development, in an instrumental direction, of the child's own cries, and their replacement by conventional words—a development which has rarely been considered in any detail. To this we must now turn.

(b) The Growth of Utterance. (i) *The Child's Primitive Cries.*—
As early as his first month, a child—as we have seen in Chapter
III, page 23—will normally be using differences of intonation
as expressive of different affective states. Although he may,
for instance, use the same vowel-sound **a** both when he is
unhappy and when he is pleased, we have no difficulty in
distinguishing his contentment from his dissatisfaction even
though we cannot see him. In the course of the next few
months further differentiation of intonation takes place, these
varieties of intonation being the chief vocal means by which
the child makes us aware of his different moods.

In Appendix IV (4), page 305, I give my records of K's later
uses of these varieties of intonation. It will be seen that in
his tenth and eleventh months he was using the sound **a** with
at least three different patterns of intonation, expressing
these distinct affective states :

(*a*) Delight in obtaining or seeing some desirable thing (0;9,16).

(*b*) Dissatisfaction at inability to obtain such a thing (0;10,28).

(*c*) Rage at being reprimanded (0;10,28).

He expressed delight, dissatisfaction and rage.

But although these three intonation-patterns express the
child's moods they also do something more : they draw our
attention to the object or situation with which he is concerned. The child in fact is beginning to use sounds in declarative and manipulative ways, calling upon us either to share
his feelings about things, or do something for him. In the
case of K again this was seen in rather an interesting way in
his different uses of the sound **ɛ**, a form which seems to have
been a variant of **a,** but used in a more urgent manner, with
more definite direction towards the situation.[1] He used this
sound **ɛ** in the course of his second year in the following ways
(Appendix IV (4)) :

(i) In reaching for an object—a form of " I want this ! "
(1;0,15).

(ii) Demonstratively—" Look at this ! " (1;4,8—1;6,26—
1;8,10).

(iii) Interrogatively, asking for a name to be given to a
thing—" What is this ? " (1;6,3).

[1] See Chapter III, p. 28.

(iv) Again interrogatively, asking for approval of some act; " May I do this ? " (1;9,12).

In each of these cases the sound clearly has a double function ; not only does it express the affective state of the child, his attitude towards something, but it also serves to direct the attention of others to the particular thing with which he is concerned. The child is using a word in a declarative or a manipulative way, with definite reference to the situation before him.

Now it is important to notice that this increase of definite reference to a situation may occur before the child learns the conventional adult word for it. Because the child has an urgent need to direct attention to a situation, he will use his own primitive sounds instrumentally for this purpose.

But of course, while he is still using his own sounds in some situations, in other cases he will certainly be influenced by adult words. To refer to K again, while his use of ε was being differentiated as I have just described, his use of a was being affected by various adult words that he heard. In the early part of his second year he was using ɑ or a in the following ways (Appendix IV (4)) :

(i) With reference to an apple (1;1,24—1;6,24—1;6,25).
(ii) Expressing satisfaction in certain pleasant smells, flowers, for instance (1;4,12).
(iii) Caressingly (1;5,30).
(iv) With reference to his eiderdown, a beloved bedfellow (1;7,1).

In at least two of these cases we can be quite certain that the child's use of a was influenced by a word of the conventional adult language. a in the first case is the child's form of the word *apple*, and in the fourth case his form of the word **aidi** (used by his mother for *eiderdown*). In the second and third instances we probably have something in the nature of a reinforcement of the child's own primary sounds. He said, we may suppose, a or **aha** when smelling a flower, or a when caressing someone. These sounds taken up and imitated by an adult would thus be given a closer connection with the situation. Now in all these four cases it is clear that the child's use of his original sound a has been given a more definite objective reference by becoming assimilated to a somewhat similar sound used by the adults around him.

All these cases, in fact, are examples of the process described in Chapter VIII. The child—using his own or an acquired sound—expresses his affective response towards an object ; where the conventional name has some resemblance to the child's own uttered sound, this tends to become stabilised with closer reference to the particular object which has evoked it.

The next stage in the process is a further conventionalisation of the child's speech, when he adopts a conventional adult word in place of his own sounds. K, for instance, having responded regularly to the word *flowers* for a couple of months, during which time he himself only said **a a** on seeing or smelling flowers, suddenly at 1;6,14 said **fa fa** on catching sight of some hyacinths (Appendix V, p. 318).

A similar development can be found in his use of the sound **ε** (Appendix IV, p. 307). At 1;8,10, for instance, seeing one of his shoes, he said **ε ε,** his own urgent sound signifying that he wanted the object. But on this occasion he also added **ʃ ʃ,** his attempt at the adult word *shoe*. Six days later again we find him replacing his customary sounds **ε ε,** when wanting butter at table, by the word **bʌti** ; while at 1;9,27 he said **pei** on seeing an aeroplane, having during the previous week frequently said **ε ε** on similar occasions.

To reach this point the child has had to pass through these stages :

(i) Varied intonations of the sound **a** to express different affective states.

(ii) The use of the same sound (or a more urgent variant of it) with increasing reference to the situation.

(iii) The conventionalisation of the sound or the adoption of a conventional substitute (such as **fa** or **pεi**) for it.

A record of this kind clearly brings out the following points. First that there is a regular development, without any sudden break, from the child's expressive use of his own primitive sounds right up to his instrumental use of conventional words. Further, that the child's need to bring others within his circle of activity will lead to the growth of reference to a situation in the sounds he is using, before his adoption of conventional words. Finally, that the adoption of conventional words, linked closely as they are with particular situations, helps to develop further the growth of reference to these situations.

(ii) *The Utterance of Conventional Words.*—We next need a similar series of observations to show what changes of behaviour take place when the child has adopted a specific conventional word. But, as we have said above, it is not easy to find a series of this kind where behaviour in utterance of a word is not influenced by experiences of response to the same word. For even when a child does not obviously respond to a word, as soon as he is heard to be using it with any degree of regularity, it is taken up by the adults around him, and inevitably he responds to them. In giving, therefore, one example (**mama**) of expressive origin, one of onomatopoetic origin (**tik tik**) and one of conventional origin (**goga**), we shall have to place observations of utterance and response side by side.

Appendix IV (5), pp. 308–11, summarises the development of **mama** ; as the complete series of entries is rather formidable, I give here only those which record some new form of behaviour.

The earlier uses of this sound-group have, as we should expect, an affective-conational function : they express both the child's affective state and also his impulse to secure an alleviation of his distress or a continuance of his satisfaction. But some traces of direction towards an object soon begin to appear, and this before there is any overt response to the same word heard ; for instance at 0;8,20 K says **mammam** while reaching for a plaything ; at 0;9,6 while looking up at his mother, and at 0;9,29 while reaching out for his ball. It is not until 1;0,6 that he makes his first overt response on hearing *mama*. Thus it would seem that the beginning of objective reference in speaking a word may occur independently of the training which a child may undergo in responding to that word.

On the other hand, the child's first responses to a given sound-group may show few traces of direction towards any specific object : this is illustrated in K's earliest responses to such phrases as *Give mama crustie* or *Give mummy tinkle-box*. The effect of these—as we saw in Chapter VII, page 109, is merely to initiate action. It is true that on each occasion the action involves a particular person, and to that extent is directed ; but quite clearly the word *mummy* does not arouse objective reference to the child's mother only. The entries at 1;1,6 and at 1;1,15 show that it is really the phrase as a whole which arouses the action as a whole ; for when the child's mother says *Give daddy crustie*, he may offer the crust to her, and when she says *Give mummy crustie* he may offer it to his father. There is not yet any clear direction towards a specific person in response to the word *mummy*.

Meanwhile the growth of objective reference seems to proceed in the child's own utterance, as we may see from the entry at 1;2,1. At 1;4,2 and at 1;5,8 this reference also begins to appear more clearly in his responses. The second entry on the latter date is particularly interesting. *Where's baby?* evokes the specific movement of pointing at the mirror, but *Where's mummy?* arouses no response at all, although the child has had a much longer experience of response to *mummy* than to *baby*. We seem to be confronted here (and again in the entry at 1;6,13) with something in the nature of an inhibition. The word *mummy*, both as spoken and heard by the child, will have gathered around it a very special significance. When he says **mama** the word expresses affect and conation; it expresses his discomfort or delight, and the desire for the discomfort to be removed or the delight to be maintained. And when he hears the word—in such a phrase as *Give mummy crustie*—he responds to it by a specific movement, one which he has been trained to perform and which gives him pleasure. Because the word has come to have for the child this special affective and conational significance both in speech and response, it is difficult for its use to be extended to any further new situation, even though his mother may appear in it; for instance, he cannot easily be brought to respond to the word by pointing to her reflection in the mirror.

But unless some extension of this kind occurs, objective reference cannot develop in the use of the word. The child's behaviour both in speech and response, must be directed to this one abiding feature—his mother—in many different situations. This process we shall study in detail in Chapters XI and XII; here we may observe a particular instance of it in the entries at 1;6,2 and 1;6,15. On the former date when the child hears the phrase *Where's the newspaper?* he makes the movement of lifting the object; when he hears *Give mummy newspaper* he makes this same movement and an additional one—lifting the paper and giving it to his mother. In this latter phrase, it would seem, the first two words evoke the customary response towards the mother, and the last word the customary response involving the newspaper. In this way the hearing of the word *mummy* has the effect of directing the behaviour of the child towards this particular person, in a new situation. And it is interesting to find that two weeks later, at 1;6,15, the child shows the first certain instance of objective reference in speaking this same word.

The whole series illustrates the gradual emergence of objective reference, in the utterance of a word of expressive origin. To complete the picture, we also give instances of its development in a word of representational (onomatopoetic) origin (**tik-tik**) and in one of conventional origin (**goga**).

Appendix IV (6), page 312, shows K's use of **tik tik,** to which he was trained to respond in the usual way. Here the very first utterance of the word, at 1;5,22, might already be said to have the function of objective reference : the child is directing his father's attention to the watch. But there can be no doubt that when he first says **tik tik** in this way, pulling at his father's coat, the word is also, perhaps mainly, expressive of affect and conation : it expresses the child's longing to secure a particular satisfaction—the pleasant ticking sound and the bright shining thing that sometimes emerges from his father's pocket. The entry at 1;5,24 illustrates how objective reference in such a case may grow : the child points to a picture of a watch on hearing the woru **tik tik.** This is a form of training : the word incites the child to find similarity between the picture and the watch [1] ; later, at 1;5,30, the sight of the picture evokes the word from the child, and by this time is becoming closely bound up with the visual impression of the object. It is no longer merely a stimulus that sets going a whole train of behaviour in the child : it is much more a means by which he is caused to refer to an object within the situation.

The next three entries show the persistence both of the affective-conational and objective functions of the uttered word. The entry at 1;7,18 is interesting as illustrating the extension of the word to include a situation objectively similar to that in which it was first acquired (the little clock was much further in resemblance from the original watch than the picture in the book had been) ; while the final entry, at 1;8,28, illustrates a further extension due to objective similarity. We are not, however, justified in supposing that these two last cases are wholly without affective colouring ; the child's cry of **titta** presumably expresses his delight in recognising the

[1] This is discussed in Chapter XI.

object. Thus, as we shall show more fully in Chapter XI, page 196, the child's application of the word to a new situation may be regarded as having not only an objective, but also an affective basis.

Turning now to the case of a word of conventional origin, we show in Appendix IV (7), page 313, the changes in K's behaviour accompanying his use of **goga** (chocolate). When he first says it, at 1;6,9, its function is clearly both expressive of affect and conation as well as referential—there is an expression of longing, together with some reference, if not to the chocolate itself, at least to the desirable experience of eating it. We cannot, indeed, be sure that the child's attention is directed towards the chocolate itself, as an object, even though we have such cases as that at 1;6,13, where there is certainly a sharp discrimination between the experience of eating the banana and the experience of eating chocolate. At 1;6,23, however, the objective reference to the chocolate itself appears with more certainty ; while the amusing instance at 1;7,28 shows to what extent the word is now bound up with a particular visual pattern. The final entry, at 1;8,18, reminds us that even when considerable objective reference has developed, a word may still be used to embrace a comparatively wide situation, which may include, together with objective direction, both affective and conational features.[1]

(c) *Mutual Effect of Utterance and Response.*—In these cases, we see, an important factor in bringing about the growth of reference is that the child both hears and speaks the same conventional word in the particular situation. For instance, he responds to *tick-tick* by looking at the clock, and says **tit tit** (or something of the kind) when he sees the clock. Every time that he says **tit tit** he tends to respond to it in the same way as when he has heard it : that is, his own use of the word causes him to turn to or refer to the clock. Thus, although the child begins by using a word instrumentally in either a declarative or manipulative way—it is directed mainly towards bringing other people into touch with him, and is perhaps only slightly directed towards the situation—yet it is clear that the function of reference in the word must rapidly develop. When the child hears the word he turns to the clock ; when he speaks it he turns to the clock (either actually or incipiently), while at the same time the person addressed also turns to the clock.

[1] We consider this case in detail in Chapter XI, p. 207.

Everything combines to develop the function of reference in the child's use of the word.

This process of the child's self-stimulation has been studied in great detail by Markey (SP 126), who perhaps tends to over-emphasise its importance in the growth of the referential function of the child's language, at the expense of the other factors which we have found to be present. On the other hand, there can be no doubt that Markey is right in maintaining that the growth of reference only becomes intelligible when we pay attention to the parts played both by the child and the adults around him : it is a social process. As we have seen, language becomes referential for the child because it is a form of behaviour by which he calls upon others and in which he responds to their calls upon him.

(d) *The Child's Resistance to Change.*—It is, however, important to lay stress on what is already, indeed, partly recognised : that the process is not merely one in which the child straightway adopts a conventional word, with its instrumental use. Even though a child has imitated the word in its appropriate situation, some time will often elapse before he shows signs of using this word instrumentally. And this, we suggest, is not because the child "forgets" the new word, but rather that in the stress of a declarative or manipulative need, he tends to make use of his own familiar means—reaching out and uttering expressive cries.

This may be illustrated by two entries from my record of K, showing the beginning of his acquisition of the word *cake* (see Appendix IV, p. 303) :

1;4,0 : At tea there was swiss roll. K held out his hand for some. His mother said *Cakie, Baby ?* and gave him a piece. He repeated **kæke** softly and with a smile. Every time he was offered a small piece of cake he said **kæke** ; and while eating it he repeated in a whisper, **kæke, kæke.**

1;4,1 : There was swiss roll for tea again. He saw it and stretched out his hand for it. His mother offered him some but withdrew it before he could reach it, in the hope that he would remember the word, but he only signified his desire for the cake by saying **ε ε ε**, with growing impatience. Then she said *Cakie*, and immediately he said firmly and loudly **ka ka.** Later, while eating the cake, he said **kæke, kæke.**

On the first occasion the child imitates the word ; but next day an exactly similar situation does not immediately evoke this word ; the child's attention, in fact, is so much taken up with the cake and the need to secure it, that he begins by reaching out for it, and when he finds this unavailing, says urgently ɛ ɛ ɛ. It is reasonable to say that the stress of the situation *prevents* rather than fosters the imitation of the conventional word.

In the same way, Schäfer found (BV 280) that when he had trained his son to make a conventional clapping-movement on hearing *mache bitte bitte* (see Appendix V, p. 322), and then frequently gave him a piece of cake as a reward, it was some time before the child used this movement on seeing the cake. Instead, he used his own primitive means of reaching out and crying ; but, the cake once safe in his hands, he was prepared to carry out the clapping-movement.

It is clear that in both of these cases there is a distinction between an act which the child has learnt to perform in a given situation and the use of this act in an *instrumental* fashion in this situation. The child's adoption of conventional words (or other symbolical acts) is very far from being the mere reproduction of movements which he can perform, whenever he comes across a situation in which he has learnt to perform them. The new movement must, in fact, be made a more efficient tool for the child than his own accustomed act, before he will replace the latter. Once, however, this superior efficiency of the conventional word is borne in upon the child, the way is open to its adoption as an instrument in place of his own.

These factors of initial resistance to change and subsequent rapid acceptance of it are of the greatest importance in the child's development, both at the present stage of his first adoption of conventional words, and also at the later stage of further conventionalisation of their use (see Chapter XII, p. 215).

(*e*) *What is referred to at this Stage ?*—Finally, we have to notice that when the child first uses and responds to adult words referentially, he is referring not so much to an object— a thing within the situation—as to the situation as a whole. At this stage words are far from being simply names, means of the static representation of objects. A word that the child speaks is to be regarded rather as one means by which he responds to a situation, as an essential part of his total reaction to it. If he says **mama** on seeing his mother, or **tiktik** on seeing the clock, or **goga** on seeing the chocolate, he is not simply labelling a thing seen. He is expressing his affective and conational state as well as making sounds that are linked up with the particular situation : and when he speaks these sounds it is his way of dealing with the situation.

This is true even in the special case where we train the child to give " names " to things or persons, to say *Mama* for instance in answer to such a question as *Who am I ?* Casual observation of this would suggest that the child is using the word very much as an adult would use it, as a name for a particular person, but closer enquiry shows that this is very far from the truth. Stern, for instance, found (KSp 19) that when his daughter Hilde at 1;1 first learned to say *Mama* in reply to *Wer bin ich ?* her answer was the same whoever asked the question—her mother, her father or the nursemaid. Six weeks later, when the child had learnt the word *papa*, she used it indiscriminately on seeing either of her parents, and on being asked *Wer bin ich ?* by her father, she replied on one occasion *pa-ma*. In the same way, Lindner's daughter, having learnt at 0;10 to say *mama* and *papa* " correctly ", still throughout the following month often said *mama* on seeing either of her parents (B 335). A striking instance is that of Nice's daughter, a child slow in learning to speak ; having begun to say *mamma* for her mother at 1;7, she soon after-wards extended it to include her father and then used it in this undiscriminating way until she was as old as 2;6 (CT 107). In all these cases the child's spoken word is hardly at all a label for the person before him ; it is the performance of an act by which he is dealing with the situation, and it will also express his affective and conational state aroused by the situation. Only to a slight extent will it be linked with the sight of the person, and only as time goes on does this last factor become dominant, so that ultimately the word is used as a means of referring to this person.

An exactly similar state of affairs is to be observed when a child responds to a word. Here again the word, for instance *mama*, is far from being simply a name for the person by whom or in the presence of whom it is spoken. The fact is rather that the word arouses a specific activity from the child, and that at the outset this activity is hardly at all directed towards a particular person. This is illustrated by K's confusion at 1;1,6, Appendix IV (5), pp. 308-9. Having learnt at 1;0,6 to respond appropriately to *Give mama crustie*, a month later he gives the crust to his *mother* on hearing *Give daddy crustie* and immediately afterwards to his *father* on hearing *Give mummy crustie*. A corresponding observation is reported by Guillaume of his son at 1;0 (DP 6). When he is told *Donne à papa* he gives what is in his hand to his father, but does this also when he is told *Donne à maman*; a moment later being again told *Donne à papa* he puts the object into his own mouth. Clearly in these cases the heard phrase is a stimulus to the performance of an act, and only to a very slight extent does the occurrence of a particular word within the phrase result in the direction of this act towards a particular person or object. The development of this objective direction is a slow process.

Further, we can in general say this, that even when a word has become a means of directing the child's activity more definitely towards a particular object, the word has not simply the function of a name for this object. Take, for instance, K's inhibition in the use of the word *mummy* at 1;5,8 and at 1;6,13, Appendix IV (5), page 311. At this time he was obviously speaking the word and responding to it with some directed reference to his mother. Yet we see that he was prevented from speaking the word or responding to it merely as a label representative of her. It seems reasonable to say that the fact that this word had for him so full an affective and conational background prevented the restriction of its use in a simple objective way. For a long time past when he had heard *mama*, his reaction must have been widespread and deep; so too when he had said the word, this must have been only one factor in a full and stirring activity. The restriction of the use of such a word until it becomes the name of a person is a slow process. Early signs of this narrowing of reference are the child's use of a particular word when he sees a picture of the corresponding object—for instance, K's use of **mama** at 1;6,15 or of **tita** at 1;6,11 (p. 312) ; or the use of a word in the absence of the object, for instance, K's **ha** for honey at breakfast time when he was 1;4,17 (p. 303) ; or the response to a word in the absence of the object, for instance, K's action on hearing *Where's ballie?* at 1;1,5 (p. 304). This process of narrowing of reference we take up in the following section.

Here we have found, in our study of the growth of meaning, that we have not to show how it is that a word, spoken or heard, becomes immediately attached as a label to a thing, but rather how it is that the experience of speaking or hearing language comes to have objective reference to a thing, and so ultimately to name it.

Summary of the Process.—The instances we have given from K's behaviour certainly justify us in accepting Meumann's general formulation, subject to the modifications suggested by Stern, Delacroix and Lorimer. The child's experience, both in uttering specific words and in responding to them, has at the outset an affective-conational basis, as well as some direction of his attention towards objective elements of the situation. This objective direction gradually becomes more prominent.

We have found that there is no simple and clear division between what is contributed to this development by the child on the one hand and by the adult on the other. It might be supposed from Meumann's original statement that when a child first utters his own words, his behaviour is purely affective and conational, and that only when an adult brings a word before him does his response become objectively directed. If this were true, a child's first cry of **mama** would be nothing but an expression of his affective state and accompanying striving; and on the other hand, his response to such a word as *ballie!* or *tick-tick!* nothing but direction of his attention to a specific object.

The observations we have considered lead us to the conclusion that while there is some truth in this account, it is too simple to embrace all the facts.

On the one hand, it appears that the utterance of a given sound-group, from a very early stage, and before adults have intervened, already may be accompanied by the rudiments of objective reference. In the words of Stern (KSp 182), the child's early utterance is not merely " a gleeful shout or a cry of distress; it is a striving towards something, an avoidance of something, a delight in something ". The truth of this is illustrated in our series of observations of K's word **mama.**

On the other hand, we have been able to show that the child's immediate response to a heard word is not simply objective reference. In the first place, a word such as *ballie!* or *tick-tick!* includes within it those intonational features to which the child has long responded in an affective and conational manner. Further, the situation to which the child's attention is drawn, itself evokes affective and conational responses from him, and these must rapidly come to be evoked by the accompanying word. Finally, the objective reference which the heard word does bring about through training, is certainly not narrowly directed to one specific portion of the situation : as we have seen, the child's response consists rather in the initiation of an act which certainly may involve a particular object but which only in the course of time becomes definitely directed towards that object.

The child's utterance of conventional words and his response to them, proceeding as they do side by side, combine to bring about a further increase of reference. When the child utters a word he not only uses it instrumentally, bringing about some reference by others, but he also tends to respond to it himself as he has previously done when it was spoken by another— that is, by reference to some portion of the situation. The part, in fact, played by a word in the child's behaviour is throughout determined by his affective and conational responses characteristic of the situation as well as by its physical features. Thus the reference that he makes will not at first correspond to that made by others in using the same words. This correspondence—which is essential if the child's language is to acquire a fully symbolical function—is the result of a further process which, beginning even before the child first uses and responds to adult words, extends throughout the period of his education. In the section which follows we shall study the earlier stages of this process.

SECTION IV

THE APPROACH TO THE CONCEPTUAL USE OF SPEECH

CHAPTER X

THE MASTERY OF CONVENTIONAL FORMS

WE have now to consider the further conventionalisation of the child's speech ; his adoption of the forms of adult language and his use of them with their current functions. In the present chapter we shall study the conventionalisation of form, in the following chapters that of function.

The strange transformations which adult words undergo when spoken by the child have often been described, and are well summarised by Stern (KSp, Chapter XVIII). But since, for the most part, they have been treated very much in the way of philological curiosities—interesting perhaps as showing occasional similarities with the changes that have occurred in the history of language—it is not very surprising that, as Stern points out, the study of them has borne very little fruit.

Yet it is evident that the forms of the child's language may be considered from quite another point of view. The child is engaged in mastering a complicated form of skill, and the patterns of sound that he utters in the effort to use the words that he hears around him should throw light upon the development of this mastery. We are indeed confronted with a highly interesting problem of the psychology of education ; the manner in which the child proceeds to the control of the forms of language : a process in which he learns to submit to the rigours of a social institution, and at the same time masters an instrument of the first importance to himself.

Further, it is not as though the development of form were to go on independently of the development of function. Throughout our study of the growth of language we have seen that the forms that the child uses are intimately related to their functions in his behaviour. It is to be expected that a study of each of the two processes will throw light upon the nature of the other.

We have found that the uses to which the child puts his early words are to be explained by recognising that he begins with a repertory of sounds which soon become a means of social behaviour, and endeavours to adapt this behaviour to his growing needs, under the influence of the language used by the society around him. The development of form is surely a parallel process. For the acquisition of adult words is not simply an accumulation of vocabulary by a speechless child. A new word is not just dropped into his repertory, like a ticket into a box, to be reproduced when needed. The child begins with a repertory of his own noises, and as time goes on these approximate more and more to the noises that he hears. The manner in which the child speaks his early conventional words is due to a convergence between his own primitive utterance and the conventions of the mother tongue. Looked at from this point of view, baby-talk ceases to be a queer collection of imperfectly-articulated words, and is seen to bear the clear marks of the child's progress towards the ultimate mastery of conventional language.

The Data.—Many of the generalisations which have been attempted concerning the form of children's language have been drawn from the statistical study of vocabularies. Tracy (LC), for instance, gathered together those of 21 children of ages ranging from 9 to 30 months ; while Stern's remarks (KSp, Chapter XVIII) were based in a similar fashion upon the records of at least 26 children. Where the forms have been noted with due attention to their phonetic characteristics, some results of importance may emerge from this method : for instance, we are enabled—as we saw in Chapter VIII, page 125, to make a general statement of the form of the first few words normally spoken.

But this method is certainly inadequate when we come to deal with the problem now before us : the relation of the forms of children's language to the process of their mastery of the conventional mother tongue. For this, once more, we need studies of individual children, recording their pre-conventional sounds, their attempts at conventional words, and the corresponding adult forms used within their hearing. Accounts of this kind, it need hardly be said, are almost entirely lacking. A very good one is that of Deville, to which we have already referred ; all his records being given in an accepted phonetic script—that of Littré. Stern's account of his daughter Hilde is the fullest I know of a German-speaking child ; but since Stern—as he himself tells us—is not a phonetician, it is not always easy to be certain which sounds he means to indicate ; further, he does not always give the corresponding adult word. To these two records I add here my own account of K ; we thus have before us surveys of a French, a German and an English child.

Characteristics of the Child's Language when Conventional Words are acquired.—Conventional words, at the moment when the child first utters them, are already invested with a form due to the primary characteristics of his speech ; they are almost entirely front-consonantal and they are to a large

TABLE V

INITIAL CONSONANTS OF WORDS ACQUIRED AT SUCCESSIVE PERIODS, COMPARED
WITH ADULT SPEECH

Subject.	Age.	No. of words beginning with consonants.	Percentage of consonants.				
			Front.		Middle.		Back.
			I p, b, m, f, v.	II t, d, n.	III l, r.	IV j, s, z, ʃ, ʒ.	V k, g, h.
Hilde Stern . .	0;10–1;6	53	49	19	4	9	19
	1;9–1;11	117	32	20	10	15	23
Adult German .			37	16	10	16	21
Deville's daughter	0;11–1;6	141	50	37	2	8	3
	1;11	101	47	21	4	22	6
Adult French . .			37	17	12	16	18
K	0;9–1;9	69	51	25	0	7	17
	1;10–2;0	102	42	20	4	10	24
Adult English. .			35	20	11	12	22

For the classification of consonants, see p. 259.

extent reduplicated. As we have already seen in Chapter VIII (p. 125), of the earliest half-dozen words of 27 children, 75 per cent. contain only front-consonants and 46 per cent. are reduplicated.

In the cases of the three children we are here specially studying, a fuller analysis is possible : we are able to trace the further conventionalisation of form from this first stage.

Table V gives my analysis of the initial sounds of words beginning with consonants in the records of the three children. In each case I have taken the first batch of words as recorded :

141 from Deville—his first complete list ; the 53 words spoken by Hilde by the time she reached the same age, 1;6 ; and the first 69 words spoken by K (he had spoken only 25 words by 1;6, being thus somewhat retarded compared with the two girls). Then in each case I have taken the last hundred or so words recorded in the child's second year ; and finally I have made an estimate of the proportions of initial consonants in English, French and German, the first from Jones's *Pronouncing Dictionary*, the second from *Le Petit Larousse*, the third from Cassell's *German-English Dictionary*. The consonants are arranged in percentage groups according to the point of phonetic origin—a note on the classification is given in Appendix III, page 259.

TABLE VI

PROPORTION OF REDUPLICATED WORDS AT SUCCESSIVE PERIODS

Subject.	Age.	No. of reduplicated words.	Total vocabulary.	Percentage of reduplicated words.
Hilde Stern	0;10–1;6	22	64	34
	1;9–1;11	12	119	10
Deville's daughter . .	0;11–1;6	46	174	27
	1;11	18	113	16
K	0;9–1;6	9	30	30
	1;10–2;0	7	105	6

It will be seen that in each case the front-consonants of the earliest words are considerably in excess of the corresponding proportion in adult speech, the deficiency in the case of the English and the German child being mainly in the middle-consonants, and in the case of the French child in the back-consonants as well. By the end of the second year the proportions are much nearer those of the adult language, although still the French child has rather further to go than the others.

Turning now to the question of reduplication, I have calculated from the records of these three children the proportion of reduplicated words, first in the vocabulary acquired by 1;6 and then again in the last hundred or so acquired in the second year. The figures are given in Table VI ; and from these it is clear that by the end of the second year in each case the high proportion of reduplicated words has greatly diminished. I have not attempted to calculate the proportion of reduplicated words in the three adult languages : obviously here, as in the initial consonants, an approximation to the conditions of conventional speech will have taken place.

Relation between the Child's Speech and the Adult Language. —The child, we see, comes to the acquisition of adult words with a system of speech which has marked characteristics of its own, both in phonetic constitution and in intonational form. Phonetically, it consists of a limited group of sounds, mainly front-consonants ; intonationally it tends to consist of single or reduplicated syllables. In what way does the child make use of this speech in his advance upon adult language ?

To deal first with his acquisition of the consonants and consonant-compounds of conventional speech, we may say that there are three moments of importance in the history of every acquisition : the time when the sound or combination appears in the child's speech, the time when he first attempts to imitate it as it occurs in an adult word, and the time when he succeeds in this imitation. If we can observe these events in the life of individual children, it will give us some indication of the relation between the child's own repertory and the language that he is attempting to master.

In Table VII, I show the results of my analysis of the records of the three children here studied, the full details being given in Appendix III, pp. 260–9. I have also plotted the results in Fig. I, from which the general course of development emerges in a very interesting way. In all three cases the child begins with a few sounds (mainly, as we have seen, front-consonants) and for some months confines himself to the imitation of the corresponding forms of the adult language, imitating these successfully, and ignoring the rest. There comes a time (1;6 in the case of Hilde Stern and K, three months earlier in that of Deville's daughter) when the child begins to be more ambitious, using his slowly-increasing repertory of sounds for a wider and wider range of those of the adult language, and failing naturally to imitate all of these accurately. Finally, as the number of sounds which he can attempt reaches its maximum and his own repertory continues to grow, he becomes more equal to the task before him. The beginning of this final stage is just

172   CONCEPTUAL USE OF SPEECH

indicated in the case of Deville's daughter, and clearly shown
in the case of K.

In a word, the child begins by ignoring the sounds that he

TABLE VII

CONSONANTS AND CONSONANT COMPOUNDS

Relation between Child's Repertory and Adult Speech

Age.	Hilde Stern.			Deville's daughter.			K.		
	Sounds attempted.	Sounds in use.	Sounds successfully imitated.	Sounds attempted.	Sounds in use.	Sounds successfully imitated.	Sounds attempted.	Sounds in use.	Sounds successfully imitated.
0;9				2	2	2	2	2	2
0;10	2	2	0	2	2	2	4	4	4
0;11	7	6	5	7	7	7	4	4	4
1;0	10	9	8	8	8	8	7	7	7
1;1	10	9	8	9	9	9	9	9	9
1;2	13	12	11	13	12	10	9	9	9
1;3	18	17	13	22	18	16	9	9	9
1;4	28	29	21	41	28	24	13	13	13
1;5	34	32	26	44	30	26	17	17	16
1;6	49	44	39	59	33	29	22	20	18
1;7	66	55	51	69	35	30	25	22	20
1;8	71	59	56	81	40	34	32	27	25
1;9	83	62	58	89	43	37	40	31	26
1;10	89	65	60	95	50	41	51	37	34
1;11				100	59	53	61	45	39
2;0							74	54	49
2;1							80	60	54
2;2							87	66	60
2;3							93	73	65
2;4							98	78	71
2;5							98	79	71
2;6							98	79	71
2;7							99	81	73
2;8							99	85	77
2;9							100	90	82
2;10							100	90	82
2;11							100	90	82
3;0							100	92	84

cannot make, then for a long period he attempts them, but
unsuccessfully ; finally he reaches the stage of mastering them.

It is evident that the most interesting period for us is the
middle stage : it is here that the great crop of baby-talk
appears. For in the first stage the range of the child's forms
tends to be limited and the forms themselves closely imitative

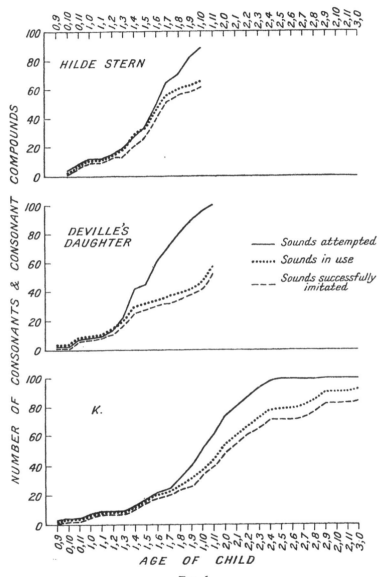

FIG. 1.

of what is heard—a process aided by the adult practice of bringing more frequently before the child only those words which the latter is capable of saying. But in the second stage the child, beginning to feel his feet, makes wild dashes at tasks that are still really beyond his powers. He now uses a limited repertory of his own sounds in the attempt to cope with the manifold variety of the adult language. Finally, as he does become capable of what he attempts, his efforts become less interesting, perhaps, to the psychologist, but less trying for his mother.

Characteristics of the Middle Period.—The middle period, then, is marked by the following features. The child continues to elide some sounds ; for others he substitutes his own. And this substitution may be of two kinds : either total replacement of the heard sound, or its assimilation to a neighbouring sound. Thus we arrive at the three most characteristic features of baby-talk : elision, substitution and assimilation.

(i) *Elision.*—From the very outset of his acquisition of adult words the child, as we have said, merely omits consonants— usually initial or final ones ; he says, for instance, **titta** instead of *tick-tack*. Gradually another—and perhaps more interesting—form of elision begins to appear : when the child, attempting the consonant-compounds of the adult language, omits one of the consonants. By consonant-compounds I mean such groups of consonants as appear regularly in conventional language—for instance, **pr, kl, kw,** groups that frequently are " felt " by adult speakers to be single sounds rather than compounds. The effect of elision on these is to produce such forms as *feisch* for *fleisch* (Hilde Stern), *tou* for *trou* (Deville's daughter) or **ki:m** for *cream* (K).

Stern (KSp 335) gives what is obviously the correct explanation of the first kind of elision, the omission of initial or final consonants : the accented portion of the heard word stands out for the child and it is this which he reproduces before he has acquired the skill to manipulate a succession of vowels and consonants. As for the second kind of elision—where one element of a consonant-compound is omitted—Stern will attempt no generalisation, for, as he says, there seems to be no regularity as to which of the two consonants will be omitted : for *fleisch* some children say *leisch*, others *feisch*.

But this elision in consonant-compounds is undoubtedly worthy of our close study, for as we shall show, it throws considerable light upon the child's mastery of conventional forms.

The first thing that we have to notice about these consonant-compounds is that the whole problem is misconceived if we ask which of the two elements is elided, the first or the second. For this is to regard the compound as a static model which the child perceives before him, whereas the fact of the matter is rather this : here is a pattern of vocal behaviour which the child undertakes, and the elements of which he may be capable of producing separately, but which he finds it difficult to produce in combination. Thus, if we analyse our three records we find that of a total of 266 compounds undergoing elision, 237 (or 89 per cent.) occur after the child has shown himself capable of making both consonants separately. (I analyse the full records in Appendix III, pp. 270–4, the 29 exceptional cases being marked with an asterisk.)

Further, when we examine the compounds with an eye to their phonetic form—that is to say, noticing which vocal movements are required to perform them—we find this : that they may be classified into two main groups. The first group are those which consist of a front and middle or back and middle consonant, for instance

**pl, sp, bl, br, fl, tr, dr, sn,
kl, sk, kj, gl, gr.**

The second group are those which consist of a consonant (front, middle or back) and the consonant **w, v,** or **ɥ, for** instance,

pw, bw, sw, lw, kw, gw, ʃv, pɥ.

These two groups together constitute the great majority of those undergoing elision ; thus of the 266 compounds before us no fewer than 245 (or 92%) belong to either of these two classes (see Table VIII).

If now we ask which of the two consonants in the compound is elided, a simple generalisation may be made for each of the two groups. Where we have a front or back consonant together with a middle consonant, it is the middle consonant which is elided. Where we have a consonant together with **w, v** or **ɥ**, the child produces a front consonant : this may be called " fronting ".

No fewer than 218 cases out of the 245 conform to these

generalisations, i.e. 89 per cent. (see Table VIII). The details are given in Appendix III, pages 275–7.

How are we to explain these facts ? The general principle is this : that in attempting to produce the subtle differences of the adult consonants the child tends to replace them by cruder and more familiar vocal movements. He is indeed very much in the position of a child learning to dance, who is able to produce many of the steps one by one, but who makes clumsy " sketchy " movements when called upon to combine these steps.

Take first the compounds consisting of a front or back consonant together with a middle consonant. Here the child

TABLE VIII

ELISION IN CONSONANT COMPOUNDS

Name of child.	Total no. of cases of Elision.	Kinds of compounds in which Elision occurs.			Nature of Elision.				Totals.	
		A Back or front and middle.	B w (v, ɰ) com- pounds.	C Others.	A Back or front and middle.	Elision of middle.	B w (v, ɰ) com- pounds.	Front- ing.	No. of A and B cases.	No. of Elision of A middle and front- ing.
Hilde Stern	45	33	4	8	33	23	4	2	37	25
Deville's daughter	140	91	39	10	91	86	39	36	130	122
K . . .	81	77	1	3	77	70	1	1	78	71
Total . .	266	201	44	21	201	179	44	39	245	218

has to pass rapidly from contact at the back or front of the mouth to contact in the middle, or from middle to back or front, and then in each case pass to the next consonantal position through the vowel position. For instance, in saying **kri:m** the child has first to make back contact for **k,** then middle contact for **r,** then pass through the vowel-position for **i:** in order to make lip contact for **m.** What happens is that the child makes a broad sketchy movement, omitting the more subtle features of the pattern : he makes the two out-standing contacts clearly, back and front, and slurs over the middle consonant. We hear the result as **ki:m.**

Exactly the same principle, that of the substitution of broad movements for more subtle ones, holds good in the case of the compounds with **w, v** or **ɥ**. But here the persistence of well-established acts shows itself in another form : **w** or **v** or **ɥ** is a front consonant, and when the child attempts to utter it in conjunction with another consonant, a species of assimilation takes place : the whole compound is reduced to a single front consonant. Thus the child will say *fatz* for *Schwanz* (Stern), or *mano* for *moineau* (Deville), or **fi:t** for *sweet* (K), presenting in each case a front consonant for the **w** or **v** compound.

We shall see these general tendencies again exemplified as we pass to the other characteristics of the child's speech.

(ii) *Substitution.*—Perhaps no feature of baby-talk has received more attention than the child's substitutions of consonants for those that occur in the adult language. We have already noticed such cases as Hilde Stern's *didda* for *tik-tak* and *dedda* for *Berta* ; other instances are *badon* for *ballon* (Deville's daughter) and **da** for *again* (K).

Stern (KSp 335) in dealing with this problem points out that although many generalisations—" laws of sound-change "—have been attempted, none has been successful in the sense that it enables us to predict which sounds children in general will substitute for those that they hear. There appear to be, in fact, wide individual differences. This cannot be gainsaid, but in looking for " laws of sound-change " we may be putting the wrong problem.

Why should we expect to find that a given consonant of the adult language is replaced in all children alike by another specific consonant ? It is true that such regular substitutions characterise the history of language, but these, it must be remembered, are the cumulative effect of changes in the speech of innumerable individuals, an " average " embodied in the written word. In the case of children, it must satisfy us for the present if we can find some uniformity in the *process* of development, underlying all the differences of detail. With this aim before us, we can certainly make a generalisation which is true, at least, for the three children here studied, and one which might reasonably be true of all children : that a child's substitutions of consonants depend upon the order in which these have appeared in his development.

The records of our three children are full enough to enable us to trace the order in which sounds appeared, once the child began to attempt conventional words.

This is shown in Table IX, where the date is given of the

TABLE IX

Order of Appearance of Consonants in Conventional Words

Age	Hilde Stern					Deville's daughter					K.				
	Front		Middle		Back	Front		Middle		Back	Front		Middle		Back
	I	II	III	IV	V	I	II	III	IV	V	I	II	III	IV	V
0;9	p[2] b[3]	d[1]				w[1]					m[1] p[2]				
0;10															
0;11	m[5]				h[3]	p[2] m[2]	n[4] t[5]				b[3]	n[3] d[5]			
1;0															
1;1	v[6]					b[6]									k[6] h[7]
1;2				s[7]					ʃ[7] s[8]		f[8]	t[9]			
1;3		ts[9]	l[9]	f[8]			d[9]		j[10]						g[10] ŋ[12]
1;4		t[11] n[13]	r[13]	j[13]	k[11] g[13]	f[13]		l[15] r[12]	z[16]	g[11] h[14]			l[14]	j[11] ʃ[13] s[15]	
1;5	f[17]			z[18]	x[20]	v[17]			ʒ[18]		v[16]		r[17] ʒ[19] z[20]		
1;6				c[19]	ŋ[21]						w[18]				
1;7							n[19]			k[20]					
1;8															
1;9												θ[21]			
1;10															
1;11															
2;0															
2;1												ð[22]			
2;2															
2;3															
2;4															

The Index figures indicate the order in which the consonants appear; the numbers I, II, III, IV, V refer to the classes of consonants, as given on page 259.

first appearance of each consonant, whether initially, medially or finally, from the time when the child first begins to use conventional words.

The first point to emerge from this is that substitution is not usually a matter of replacing a consonant that the child cannot make by one that he can. On the contrary, in the great majority of cases the three children were already able to produce the consonant now attempted. This is shown in Table X, where I give my analysis of all the cases of substitution recorded by Stern and Deville and of those in my own

.TABLE X

SUBSTITUTION OF CONSONANTS

Name of child.	Total Number of cases.	Where replaced consonant is		(a) Where replaced consonant is in child's repertory.				(b) Where replaced consonant is not in child's repertory.		
		(a) in child's repertory.	(b) not in child's repertory.	No. of cases.	Substitution			No. of cases.	Substitution	
					by earlier cons.	by later cons.	doubtful.		by existing cons.	by new cons.
Hilde Stern	35	30	5	30	23	6	1	5	4	1
Deville's daughter	210	164	46	164	116	41	7	46	44	2
K . . .	110	94	16	94	85	9	0	16	15	1
Total . .	355	288	67	288	224	56	8	67	63	4
Percentage	100	81	19	100	77	20	3	100	94	6

record of K up to the age of 2;3, the full details being given in Appendix III, pp. 278–93. Here, out of a total of 355 cases, no fewer than 81 per cent. consist of attempts upon consonants already in the child's repertory.

Taking now these cases where the child attempts a consonant already present in his repertory, we find that of 286 substitutions, 77 per cent. consisted in replacing the attempted consonant by one which had appeared *chronologically earlier* in the child's history, while in only 20 per cent. of the cases did he substitute a sound chronologically later. (The remaining 3 per cent. are doubtful, because the records do not enable us to say which of two consonants occurred the earlier.)

In the second group, where the child attempts a sound not already present in his repertory, we find that of 67 cases no fewer than 94 per cent. consist of substitutions by some sound that he has already produced, while only in the remaining 6 per cent. does he utter a consonant which he has never before produced.

In brief, the rule is this : substitution occurs when the child *replaces a heard consonant by one relatively more familiar,* one which has been longer established in his repertory. The child, when confronted with the necessity of carrying out a new, or relatively new, pattern of action, often produces one which has become more habitual to him.

Now this generalisation certainly does not enable us to predict which substitutions will occur among children in general. There are, however, two points that seem hopeful. In the first place, the children we have here studied belong to different linguistic communities, and it is not improbable that their individual differences are in some measure due to this. It is not unlikely that children of parents speaking the same language produce their consonants in a particular order, and thus their substitutions would tend to be uniform.

Further, even in the cases of the three children before us, it is evident that the range of substitutions is by no means unlimited. Certain consonants appear to interchange more frequently than others. Thus, in the records of these three children, we find that we can group the great majority of substitutions into three classes : the substitution of front for front consonants or middle for middle : the interchange of **t** or **d** with **k** or **g** ; and that of the dentals (**t, d, ts, ð** or **θ**) with the sibilants (**s, z, ʃ,** or **ʒ**). These groups comprise no fewer than 89 per cent. of all the cases, as Table XI shows. The full details are given in Appendix III, p. 294. And although these groups may seem rather broad, it must be remembered that the speech-sounds of children are far less precise than those of adults, and that one might quite reasonably speak of a consonant of the **t**-type or of the **k**-type.

It is noteworthy that, apart from the special cases of the second and third groups just mentioned, the interchange of consonants from widely separated points of articulation hardly occurs at all. To a very large extent the child when he replaces a consonant does so by uttering a sound at the same point of articulation or one very near it. And it is also interesting to notice that while the *direction* of substitution is not always the same in different children, it is frequently the same consonants that are involved ; thus while Deville's daughter usually substituted **s** for **ʃ**, in the case of K only the reverse substitution occurred ; similarly **t** for **k** occurred in the former child, the reverse in the latter.

The fact that we can limit the range of substitutions in the manner shown in Table XI rather suggests that with more data at our disposal it might begin to be possible to make clear generalisations as to their occurrence in detail.   At present we have to content ourselves with recognising that the chief factor is the replacement of a comparatively unfamiliar consonant by one more securely established in the child's repertory.   And even this generalisation is more illuminating than

TABLE XI

KINDS OF SUBSTITUTION OF CONSONANTS

Name of child.	Front for Front and Middle for Middle.	t or d with k or g.	t, d, ts, ð, or θ with s, z, ʃ or ʒ.	Others.	Total no. of cases.
Hilde Stern . . .	21	0	1	13	35
Deville's daughter .	88	61	47	14	210
K	92	5	2	11	110
Total	201	66	50	38	355
Percentages . . .	57	18	14	11	100

any law of "sound-change", for it points out the psychological similarity between the acquisition of the forms of conventional language and the development of skilled behaviour in general through imitation of the acts of others.

(iii) *Assimilation.*—The child's assimilations of adult words fall into two groups named by Stern "general" and "special". In general assimilation, words which are very diverse in the adult language are adapted by the child so as to conform to a single general pattern.   In special assimilation a particular sound is changed by the influence of a neighbouring sound in the same word.

(a) *General Assimilation.*—We have already come across one form of general assimilation in reduplication ; for a large proportion of the child's reduplications are not imitated from similar adult words, but imposed by the child himself.   Thus, of the 32 cases of reduplication which I recorded of K up to the age of 2;3, 15 had no corresponding reduplication in the adult word : while of the 88 cases recorded by Deville 55 (62 per cent.) also belong to this category.[1] The full lists are given in Appendix III, pages 295–6. It is evident that the child tends to assimilate adult words to a general pattern of reduplication.

The cases of general assimilation mentioned by Stern (KSp 339) are those in which the child assimilates diverse words either by beginning or ending them all in the same way. Thus his son Günther tended to begin different words with either *h* or *ch* (phonetically **x**) ; for instance *hāta* for *Vater*, *hēdel* for *Mädel*, *chotto* for *Lotto*, *chasser* for *Wasser*. In other cases mentioned by Stern the child ended diverse words with the same syllable, for instance, *aich* or *ere* ; saying *onkaich* for *Onkel*, *verschiedere* for *verschieden*. A well-known instance of this not mentioned by Stern is the tendency in some children to end words with **i**, as in *doggie*. This was very marked in the case of K, occurring in 72 words up to the age of 2;3 (15 per cent. of his total vocabulary). And in 30 of these 72 words (42 per cent.) there was no **i**-ending in the corresponding adult word : the child, for instance, said **gʌgi** for *another* and **ʃʌti** for *supper*.

In all these cases, just as in reduplication, the child reduces diverse words to the same pattern. This pattern may be due to some idiosyncrasy of the child himself (as perhaps in the case of Günther Stern's *h* and *ch*) or it may first have arisen in imitation of adults (as perhaps in the case of K's **i**-endings). Whichever be its source, the particular pattern of action, once established, tends to dominate subsequent acts, with the result that the child's speech at this stage tends to be more uniform than the adult language upon which it is based.

General assimilation, then, like substitution, shows the dominance of earlier-established habits over the later acquirement of new forms of vocal skill.

(*b*) *Special Assimilation.*—The process by which one consonant may be affected by another neighbouring one has often been commented upon, particularly since it occurs in the history of language as well as in the development of children.

---

[1] I cannot give the proportion in Hilde Stern's case, as Stern does not always mention the adult word.

Here again discussion has mainly centred upon the relative positions of the two consonants in the adult word : two classes of assimilation have been distinguished which Stern (KSp 340) names " proleptic " and " metaleptic ". In prolepsis a consonant is affected by one that succeeds it, for instance *Zucker* becomes *kucker*; in metalepsis a consonant is affected by one that precedes it, for instance *peitsche* becomes *peipe*. For each of these cases, Stern adds, there is a psychological basis : in prolepsis there is a species of anticipation—the coming consonant affects the one now being uttered. In metalepsis we have something in the nature of perseveration : the consonant just uttered affects the one now in process of utterance.

All this cannot be doubted. But an additional question arises. What is the relation between the sound which exists in the adult word and that to which the child assimilates it : between **g** and **d**, for instance, when he says *dade* for *regarder* ? Meumann, to whom we owe so many fruitful ideas suggested, Stern tells us, that in prolepsis at any rate, back consonants tend to be replaced by front ones ; as Stern adds, this generalisation is inadequate to cover all the cases. But Meumann's clue is still worth following up ; and when we examine the records of " special " assimilation we find, here as before, that in the great majority of cases the substitution is determined by the chronological relation which exists between the two consonants in the history of the child's development. In general, we can say this : of the two sounds in the adult word, *the one which comes later in the child's history is assimilated to the one that comes earlier*, even if he can pronounce both (see Table XII, and for details, Appendix III, pp. 297–9). This generalisation holds in 77 per cent. of the cases recorded of our three children. Once more we find the dominance of earlier-established vocal habits over those that occur later in the child's linguistic history. " Special " assimilation may indeed be regarded as a form of substitution ; where the child, attempting to utter two consonants of an adult word, doubles the dominant one. To this extent we see also the effect of the child's general tendency to reduplicate.

Uniformity of Children's Language.—It is clear that as a result of the characteristics we have described, a child's language will both tend towards uniformity within itself and also in relation to that of other children. Thus initial and final consonants will be elided, consonant-compounds will be rendered by single consonants, the diverse consonants of a word will be assimilated, and the whole word frequently take on a reduplicated form. These tendencies, coupled with that dominance of the front-consonants which we have already noticed (see p. 170), lead to a remarkable uniformity of speech

TABLE XII

ASSIMILATION

Name of child.	Total no. of cases.	Later sound assimilated to earlier.	Earlier sound assimilated to later.	Doubtful.	No. of cases where *both* sounds are already in use.
Hilde Stern . . .	11	8	3	0	11
Deville's daughter. .	82	65	16	1	71
K	29	21	8	0	26
Total	122	94	27	1	108
Percentage	100	77	22	1	88

among children brought up in communities speaking different languages. Nothing, for instance, could be more striking than to find such a word as **didda** (and its variants) recurring in the language of these three children, and with such an enormous range of meaning. (See Table on opposite page.)

The Parallel with Verbal Aphasia.—Our discussion of elision, substitution and assimilation has shown this : that these processes exemplify, in different ways, the same process—the persistence of earlier modes of functioning when the child finds himself under the need of using unfamiliar words in an instrumental way. In elision, when dealing with consonant compounds, he tends to make cruder vocal movements instead of the more complicated ones that the compounds demand—these cruder movements being of the kind to which he is accustomed in his own primitive speech. Thus he produces a broad alternation of front and back contacts to the exclusion or slurring of middle consonants. In substitution, again, he replaces an unfamiliar consonant by one more familiar, even though he may have shown himself already capable of uttering both. In general assimilation we find the dominance of a general pattern already well established, in special assimilation the dominance of particular consonants already well established. In brief, we see throughout the persistence of earlier established

Hilde Stern.		Deville's daughter.		K.	
Child's Form.*	Adult Form.	Child's Form.*	Adult Form.	Child's Form.	Adult Form.
didda	tik tak	dade	regarder	**dada**	dada
dedda	Berta	dadi	radis	**dədə**	Dempy
didelideli	(bell)	dada	(horse)	**din-din**	dinner
dada	(pointing)	dodo	(sleeping)		
du-du	scolding	dedon	édredon		
nä nä	nahen	nana	canard	**nana**	Nana
		nienie	papier	**nini**	Winnie
		nonon	ognon	**neini**	navel
		na	journal	**nu:ni**	balloon
papa	papa	papa	papa	**papa**	papa
puppe	puppe	papo	chapeau	**pʌpʌ**	{ powder-puff / puff-puff
pip pip	(bird)	papo	crapaud	**papa**	grandpa
put-put	(fowls)	popo	compôte		
		papié	papier	**pæpe**	paper
		pipi	pipi		
		poupé	poupée		
baba	(disgust)	baba	ball	**bæba**	baby
bā bā	(going out)	bubu	omnibus	**bibi**	bib
		babo	bravo	**biba**	creampot
tatei	(going to bed)	tata	{ café / tasse / canne	**tæta**	(going out)
				tæti	potato
				tætoun	telephone
				ti:tot	(nursery rhyme)
		tété	{ laitier / chef / thé / cotelette / secher		
		toté	{ ôter / cotelette		
		toto	{ couteau / œuf		
		taté	{ caché / saleté / corset		
		toton	{ saucisson / chausson / torchon		
		toti	coquille		
		titi	qui qui		
		toutou	coucou		

* As given by the observer.

modes of functioning in the effort to produce new acts. The child, spurred on to produce a series of sounds by a powerful incentive—the need to use them instrumentally—tends to make use of well-established familiar acts that have served his instrumental needs in the past.

Now it is of very great interest to notice that the defects which children's speech shows at this stage are very similar to those which occur in the speech of aphasics—the cases, for instance, described so strikingly by Head. He himself has drawn attention to this similarity : the speech of aphasics, he tells us (A 231) " sometimes closely resembles baby language ". The parallel was, in fact, first emphasised as long ago as 1882, by Preyer (MC 34), although its full significance has only recently become apparent as a result of Head's epoch-making work. But although such writers as Lorimer (GR 57) have recognised the similarity in a general way, no attempt has I think hitherto been made to show its bearing upon the specific forms of children's speech.

One caution is certainly necessary, as Head warns us (A 510) : we must be careful not to identify the main species of aphasia with definite stages of development in children. The point is rather this : we find in children's speech defects similar to those encountered in aphasia, and as we are dealing in both cases with language it is reasonable to ask whether similar effects may not be due to similar causes.

The exact parallel with the defective speech described in the present chapter is to be found in the form of aphasia named by Head, Verbal Aphasia, which he describes as a defect in the structure of words (A 229). In these cases the patient is usually well able to comprehend the words that he hears or sees, but when he comes to utter them he does so in a defective fashion, retaining the general pattern of the conventional word, but altering the actual sounds.

These three features also characterise the stage of language that we have considered in the present chapter : the child certainly " understands " the words that he utters, and the general intonational patterns of his words correspond in some measure to those of conventional words (subject to the persistence of reduplication), but he fails when he attempts to make the particular sounds.

The parallel holds even in detail ; in Head's cases we actually find clear instances of elision, of substitution and of assimilation. Thus his patient number 4 (A 221) elided initial consonants, saying *claration* for *declaration*; final consonants, saying *confine* for *confined*; and uttered a single consonant for a compound: *tenical* for *technical*. Another patient, number 17 (A 225) substituted **b** for **v,** saying *oboid* for *ovoid*; while in yet another case we find assimilation: *nines* for *lines* (number 13, A 231). Two examples of this last patient's speech are indeed, as Head says, closely similar to baby language [1]: *Tiff-rent from uffer 'um . . . kā tell oo, know zis 'un seems strong.* (Different from other one . . . can't tell you, know this one seems strong), and " *Here's lay, here handle, the man condukr, on the nines, shot seats on it. Zee passengers, two man, lady.*" (Here's lady, here handle, the man conductor, on the lines, it's got seats on it, three passengers, two men, lady.)

How does Head explain defects of this kind? He regards all aphasia as a disturbance of the functioning of the highly-complicated act of language; the effect of a lesion of the brain is that " more recent aptitudes suffer in excess of those acquired earlier in ontological history " (A 476). In a word, the aphasic, confronted with the difficult task of expressing himself through language, reverts to earlier-established modes of vocal behaviour.

Thus not only outwardly, but fundamentally also, baby-language and Verbal Aphasia are seen to be alike. The child as a result of his inexperience, and the aphasic as a result of his physical defect, tend to produce familiar, simpler, modes of vocal activity in their effort to make instrumental use of the complicated forms of human language.

In both cases the present act is subordinated to the pattern of established behaviour—the existing " schema ", as Head calls it (A 488). And since we have regarded the child's attempt at conventional forms as a problem of the acquisition of skill, it is interesting to observe that Bartlett accepts this notion of a " schema " as providing the most illuminating explanation of our behaviour in learning a game of skill—tennis or cricket, for instance. " Determination by schemata ", he says, " is the most fundamental of all the ways in which we can be influenced by reactions and experiences which occurred some time in the past " (R 201).

---

[1] This patient's main defect was Syntactical Aphasia, but he also suffered from marked Verbal Aphasia.

Thus the work of Head has helped us to corroborate what we have found to be the guiding principle throughout the present chapter. In acquiring the forms of adult words, the child's ability lags behind his attempts. He tries to use a wider range of sounds and their combinations than his repertory will permit, and this repertory influences his attempts. The result is baby-language.

So much is true of the forms of speech. We have now to see that a similar principle holds good of much of his further progress in acquiring its functions.

Chapter XI

THE EXPANSION OF MEANING

In the course of the last section we have come upon a marked characteristic of children's early use of words ; that both in response and in utterance they will apply a word to a wide range of situations extending far beyond those in which it was first acquired. K, for instance, came to respond to *Where's ballie ?* (0;10,27) by holding up a large coloured ball in place of the original small one ; and—in the development of an uttered word—he grew to say **tittit** (1;8,28) on seeing the church clock, having previously used this word for his father's watch.

Such extensions are so striking and obviously so important that they have never failed to obtain a good deal of attention. Perhaps the best known case is that reported by Romanes of a child in his first year who having learnt the word *quack* for a duck, applied it to the figure of an eagle seen on a coin, and then to coins in general. The Chamberlains tell us of their daughter (SC 265) that having at 1;7 learnt the word *mooi* with reference to the moon, she proceeded to apply it to cakes, round marks on the window, writing on the window, writing on paper, " round things in books ", tooling on books, faces, postmarks, and the letter O. Lindner (B 340–2) records that his wife had made a sledge (*schlitten*) out of a postcard for their daughter at 2;0. A month later, when the toy had long been destroyed, the child said *mama litten* on seeing a postcard delivered at the house, and some months after this again *litten* on seeing a letter. Numerous other instances of this kind of extension occur in the records of a host of observers : Sigismund (KW 111), Darwin (BI 293), Taine (AL 253), Jespersen (ND 116), Guillaume (DP 8, 18), Kenyeres (PM 194), Major (FS 316), Nice (CT 112), Pelsma (CV 354), Preyer (MC 117, 140), Sully (SC 163, OP 382), and Stern (KSp 189).

The records of most of these observers consist of a list of the various meanings which have been given by a child to one and the same word. Observations of this kind, valuable as

189

they may be as illustrations, do not throw much light on the actual process of extension. For this we need a fuller statement ; we need to know in some detail how the child behaved in using or responding to the word on successive occasions. Records of this kind are rarer ; the only ones in fact at all full enough for this purpose are those published by Ament in 1899 and Idelberger in 1903. To these I venture to add some of my own observations of K (Appendix V).

Extension as the Growth of Generalisation.—How are we to explain this wide use of words ? The most obvious view is that the child has begun abstraction and generalisation ; abstracting from diverse situations some features which they have in common, and thus grouping all these situations into the same class. Most of the things, for instance, named *mooi* by the Chamberlains' little daughter were circular in shape. The child extends the use of the word from the situation in which it was first acquired—seeing the moon—to other situations more or less like it.

There is obviously some truth in the view that here we have a clear step in the development of conceptual thinking— and this is a point which has been fully recognised, from the time of the early observers—Sigismund, Taine, Darwin and Romanes—right up to our own day. But no one to-day would, I think, be satisfied with this as a full explanation. At least three other factors must be taken into consideration. First we must recognise that this broad use of words does not begin at the moment when the child acquires conventional speech : it is a gradual development of his earlier linguistic activity. Secondly, it is not enough to speak of the objective similarity of situations for the child, neglecting the affective responses they arouse in him and their functions in his behaviour. Thirdly, we must not forget that the word itself is an instrument for the child, a tool, and that this certainly determines the manner in which it is used.

In these three ways we have to supplement the account given even by Stern (KSp 189). For although he refers to other factors, on the whole he confines himself to a summary of those kinds of *objective* similarity in diverse situations which will cause a child to extend a word from one to the rest.

I

The Early Wide Use of Sounds.—To take full account of the process it will not do to begin at the point where the child first acquires conventional words from the adult language. We must go further back into his linguistic history.   If, for instance, we find Stern's daughter Hilde in her twelfth month applying *puppe*—used first for her doll—to any one of a large number of her toys, we have to consider the possible connection between this behaviour and the sounds which she made while playing with these toys before she learned their conventional names.   For our study of children's language leads us to assert that its development is continuous, not—as some writers such as Bühler have maintained—a series of sudden steps.   The history even of the child's first conventional words does not begin at the moment when he acquires them ; they have their root in his earlier use of sounds.   In a real sense we can say that no word used by the child can be totally new to him ; every word has affinities with his earlier linguistic experience.

With a record of observations such as those of K, it is not difficult to trace the changes in the child's use of sounds, preceding his adoption of conventional words.   We find that even at the outset the child's sounds are used in a wide rather than in a limited way.   This is true both of his utterance of language and of his response to it.   As for his response to language, we found in Chapters IV and VII that when he hears a particular pattern of intonation and sound he will respond at first not always with the same movement but with any of a number of movements—all expressive of the same affective state.   And in the development of his utterance, we find in Chapter IX, page 151, that a particular sound such as **a** is called forth at first not by a particular situation, but by any one of a number—again alike in this, that they arouse the same affective state.

In tracing the development of such a sound we were able to observe these stages : first its use with varied intonations to express different affective states : secondly the increase of reference to a situation in the use of the same sound ; thirdly the adoption of a conventional substitute for the sound, such as **fa** (flower), or **pei** (aeroplane), this bringing with it a further increase of objective reference.

The next stage of development is that which particularly interests us here : the child extends the use of the conventional word to situations other than those in which it has been acquired. Thus K, having at 1:6,14 begun to use the word **fa** on seeing some hyacinths, used the same word on the following day for tulips, six days after this for irises, and again six days later (1;6,27) on being wheeled beneath a flowering cherry. Four months later, at 1;10,26, he said the same word on seeing a biscuit decorated with a flower in sugar, and again on seeing embroidered flowers on a pair of slippers (Appendix V, pp. 317–18).

A similar development took place in the case of the word **pei,** which the child used for the first time at 1;9,27 on seeing an aeroplane, in place of his customary ɛ ɛ (Appendix IV, p. 307). Next day he repeated the word on seeing not an aeroplane, but a child's kite.

Now the important point that emerges from these series of records is that it clearly is not possible to draw a hard-and-fast line at any particular moment in the child's development and say : Here the extended use of sounds begins. For while the child is still in the stage of uttering his own primitive sounds he already uses them in an extended fashion. K, for instance, used **a a** at 1;4,8 on smelling a handkerchief and again at 1;4,12 on smelling jonquils (Appendix IV, p. 306). Similarly, he used ɛ ɛ at 1;1,26 while reaching out for milk, at 1;4,1 for cake, and up to 1;8,16 for butter ; again he used the same sound at 1;8,10 for shoe, and at 1;9,15 for aeroplane (Appendix IV, pp. 305–7). About all these cases we could say, if we wished, that the child was extending his use of a sound in an extraordinary and striking manner : to mean two different pleasant smells, or to mean milk, cake and butter, or to mean aeroplane and shoe ; and this in fact is what such an observer as Idelberger says of his son's varied uses of the sound *a* (Appendix V, p. 315), a list which is cited by Lorimer (GR 59) as an instance of the unstable character of early " nominal relationships ".

But if we trace the child's development as I have done here it is clear that a sound such as **a** or ɛ is not a name for any one object, subsequently extended to another. It is simply a differentiation of the child's earlier use of a sound to express an affective state, a use which gradually becomes more definitely directed to the situation with which he is dealing, without however being attached to any one particular situation. And if we accept this, then it also becomes clear that when the child begins to use a conventional word such as **fa** for flower instead of his own primitive sounds, he is at first likely to use it just in the same extended manner as he has been using his own sounds. This point needs to be stressed, because when we find a child using adult words it is only too natural for us to imagine that he is using them as names for particular objects; but more careful observation makes it clear that he is using them not very differently from the way in which he was using his own primitive sounds not long since.

For instance, if we heard a child who has been accustomed to say **a** on seeing flowers, say this the first time he sees a branch of flowering cherry, we should probably regard this simply as an expression of the child's delight at seeing the beautiful thing, and of his desire to touch and smell it. It would hardly occur to us to say that the child has made a generalisation, extending the name **a** from its use for tulips and applying it now to cherry-blossom. But let us suppose that this happens at a time when—as in the case of K—he was already using the word **fa**; at once we feel that the child has shown himself capable of generalisation, that he has realised the similarity between the tulips and the cherry-blossom, and therefore uses the same name for them both.

Clearly we can easily overestimate the difference between these two stages—before and after the child adopts the conventional word. It is true that there has been some development of the kind we have discussed in Chapter IX : the word **fa,** because it has been adopted from the adult name for the flower, is rather more closely attached to that object than the child's own sound **a** had been. But even so, the use of a word, first for tulips and then for cherry-blossom, cannot be accepted purely as a case of objective reference to one thing, followed by extension of the name to another thing on a basis of objective similarity. For in neither case is the child using the word simply as a means of naming a thing, as a label to be attached to an object. Just as when the child said **a a** he was at the same moment drawing attention to the flower, expressing his delight at seeing it and possibly his wish to smell it, so now when he uses the learnt word **fa** this new utterance must retain something of the new functions of the earlier sound which it replaces.

Further, it is also brought home to us that this extension of the use of a word to apply to a new situation is something more than the evocation of a sound from a passive child. It is the child's own activity which brings about the extension. The flower which he sees is something to be grasped and smelt. And the word he utters is a means by which the attention of others may be drawn to this desirable thing (the declarative use), or their help secured in obtaining it (the manipulative use). Of course, it need hardly be said that I am not suggesting that the child will be aware of these functions ; only that they are likely to be present in a more or less rudimentary form. What I *am* suggesting is that because the word and the new situation each plays a part in the child's behaviour he will broaden his use of the word to apply to the situation.

Thus in tracing the course of the child's development preceding his adoption of conventional words, we see that objective extension is not to be regarded as beginning with this adoption, but that it is based upon the early use of a sound to express an affective state, first in a wide range of situations, and then with an increase of objective reference to these situations. This use develops under the stress of the child's need to bring other human beings into the situation, to obtain their help, or at least their company. Then, by the intervention of these other human beings, the original widely-functioning sound-group is replaced, in one situation after another, by a specific conventional sound-group. We next have to consider which features of these situations are likely to give rise to wide applications of words.

II

The Kinds of Similarity among Situations : Objective Similarity.—Stern (KSp 186–9) gives a comprehensive summary of the objective conditions under which the application of a word will be extended. He classifies the conditions of similarity between situations into three groups. First, the situations may be similar as a whole : secondly, there may be similarity of particular features : thirdly, the child's attention may shift from feature to feature, so that a word is applied to a new situation which has no resemblance at all to the original situation, but has some point of likeness to an intermediate situation.

(i) *Similarity of the Situation as a Whole.*—In Stern's first group of cases a word is applied from a customary situation to another one which as a whole objectively resembles it ; for instance, **pei** for an aeroplane and then for a kite, *mooi* for the moon and then for any round object. Many other instances could easily be given.

(ii) *Similarity of Particular Features.*—Stern's second group of cases are those in which the likeness is said to exist only in particular features of the situations. This may be illustrated by two cases from my own observations. The first is K's use of the word **kotibaiz.**

At 2;2,14 he was given a large toy abacus ; immediately on seeing it he said **kotibaiz.** It was impossible to tell whether the use of this word was due to a memory of a cot in which he had last slept more than a year since, and which had one or two rows of beads, or whether he was referring to the parallel wires of the abacus which resembled the parallel bars of his own cot. Two months later, at 2;4,12, he used the same word **kotibaiz** for two other objects : on first seeing a toast-rack (with parallel bars), and again for a picture of a building with fluted columns.

In the second case, having learnt to say ʃiː (sea) for the seashore, K subsequently said it on seeing a railway-track ; there was certainly a resemblance between the slope of the grassy sand-banks by the sea and the slope of the railway embankment (Appendix V, p. 319).

(iii) *Shifting from Feature to Feature.*—Stern's third group of cases are those in which the extended application of a word is due to particular features similar to those present in an earlier situation. Here Stern cites the instance from Romanes which we have already mentioned, where the word *quack* first used for a duck, ultimately came to be used for a coin. Similar cases are recorded by Idelberger (Appendix V, p. 315) ; the child, having used *wauwau* on seeing a dog or hearing the animal bark, later said it at the sight of a fur collar with a dog's head, then for a fur collar without a head, finally for buttons ; presumably he had seen buttons on the fur collars. It was the same child who used the word *baba* both for his father and for the sound of a bell ; the route this time being from his father to his father's trousers hanging on a hook, then for his father's portrait, then for an electric bell which his father had repaired, finally for the sound of any bell.

This threefold classification of Stern's certainly helps us to understand what we may call the objective side of the process—the various kinds of objective similarity among situations which may help to bring about the application of a word from one to another. But when we come to examine both Stern's own cases and others more closely, we find that this analysis is inadequate.

The Affective Aspect of Extension.—In the first place, Stern hardly lays sufficient emphasis upon the part played by the child's affective responses. It is true that he mentions affect (KSp 183, 195) as a factor which is likely to permeate all the varied applications of a word, but he makes no further reference to it in his detailed analysis. This neglect seems strange in the light of the importance that has been given to affect as one of the chief factors in determining the influence of past upon present experience, not only by the psychoanalysts but by English writers such as Ward, Stout and Bartlett : and all the more strange since Meumann—to whom Stern constantly refers—paid special attention to this point in his account of children's wide applications of words.

Meumann's view is this (EK 186) : that in cases where situations are only very slightly similar objectively, extension of a word may take place because the situations arouse in the child similar feelings and similar strivings. To apply this, for instance, to a case given by Stern ; his daughter Hilde at 0;11 extended the word *puppe* from her doll, to a toy rabbit and other playthings. Stern suggests from this that a general similarity of the most superficial kind may be enough to bring about extension ; but if we follow Meumann here we should say that the sight of a toy rabbit aroused the same feeling of delight and desire to play as the original doll had aroused ; and it was this affective-conational similarity which was powerful in bringing about the extension.

The truth is perhaps that Stern, making a somewhat conservative summary, is still mainly concerned with the cognitive factors in the process of extension, and sees this process mainly as a step in the development of abstract thinking ; but there is no doubt that Meumann was right : the more we pay attention to the conditions in which the wide applications of words take place, the more certain does the place of affect become. It plays an important part, as we have seen, while the child is still using his own primitive sounds, and it retains this function when he comes to replace them by conventional words. When, for instance, K said ʃiː for the first time (Appendix V, p. 319, entry 1;9,28) it was not a mere indication of the sea or sandhills; the child had been awakened by the thunderstorm and called out the newly-learnt word to express his terror at what he thought was the roaring of the sea. In the same way when he said **pei**, first for an aeroplane and then for a kite, it was surely partly because he felt the same delight (or perhaps fear or wonder) at them both. A few weeks earlier he would have said ɛ ɛ on seeing the new thing; now he uses the learnt word **pei** which, whatever else it may do, expresses his affective reaction just as his earlier sounds had done. Again, when he said **fa** on seeing the cherry-blossom, this must have expressed the peculiar pleasure aroused in him by the sight of a flower. Observations of this kind make it certain that affective similarity may be a very powerful factor in determining the wide use of words.

Functional Similarity.—If affective similarity has been neglected, this is even truer of functional similarity. Yet it is more than forty years ago that Dewey first drew attention to its importance, in his usual vigorous fashion (PI 65):

> The tendency to apply the same term to a large number of objects (" ball " to ball, orange, moon, lamp-globe, etc.) can be understood, I think, only if we keep in mind the extent to which the formal noun " ball " has really an active sense. " Ball " is " to throw " just as much as it is the round thing. I do not believe that the child either confuses the moon with his ball, or abstracts the roundness of it; the roundness suggests to him something which he has thrown, so that the moon is something to throw—if he could only get hold of it.

In a word, Dewey insists upon the importance of functional similarity in the situations for the child, that they do not merely exist statically for him, but are bound up with his activity. To this we shall have to add that they are also frequently bound up with the activity of those around him. Functional similarity of either kind may determine the wide use of words.

(i) *The Function of the Situation in the Child's Own Activity.* —This point is not absolutely neglected by Stern; he does note in passing what he calls an exceptional instance where the function of the situation becomes a factor in bringing about the wider use of a word. Hilde, he tells us (KSp 188), used *Nase* at 1;7 for the toe of a shoe, because she found she could pull this in the same way as she would playfully pull someone's nose. But we have to go further than Stern and point out that this is by no means an exceptional instance; functional similarity is as constant a factor as objective or affective similarity.

Take, for instance, Hilde's use of *puppe* for a wide range of playthings, including a doll, a toy rabbit and a toy cat; Stern recognises that these things are objectively unlike each other, and urges therefore that extension will occur when only a very superficial resemblance is present. But the fact is that a stuffed cat is really very unlike a doll, unless we remember that a child *plays* with both of them. Again, to go back to K's use of **fa** for tulips as well as cherry-blossom; the resemblance is certainly very superficial unless we remember that when he saw a flower he was usually invited to *smell* it.

It is equally necessary to emphasise this functional factor in these cases where the likeness is said to lie not in the situations as wholes, but in particular features of them. When K used ʃiː for the railway-track after having used it for the seashore, there can be no doubt that the word was evoked not only by the resemblance between the two slopes, but also by the fact that the child had enjoyed climbing the sandbank and that here was something else to climb. That this view is justified is shown by an observation of mine in this connection; a few days after the episode of the railway track the child was taken near a grassy bank; this time he said ʌpi ʃiː, using again the word ʌpi that he had constantly used when he wished to be taken over the sandbanks by the sea (Appendix V, p. 319).

It is interesting to notice that in some cases, the wide application of a word seems to rest almost entirely upon the existence of this functional similarity. Take, for instance, K's use of the word **da** (from the word *down*; Appendix V, p. 316). At 1;6,8 he said the word before climbing *down* from his mother's knee; a few days later he began to use the word frequently to indicate that he wished to go *up* stairs (1;6, 16–26). Here the circumstances show that the point of similarity was not a matter of direction, up or down, but that there was climbing to be done in both cases.

(ii) *The Function of the Situation in the Activity of Others.*—

In a further group of instances we have to take a broader view of this notion of functional similarity ; where the situations have a similar function, not in the child's own activity, but in the activity of some other person. For instance, among the extraordinary uses made by Idelberger's son of the word *wauwau* (Appendix V, p. 315) were those which included, first, a sewing-table and secondly a bath-room thermometer. Now the only possible point of resemblance between these two objects is this, that they are instruments used by someone. Again, Guillaume tells us (DP 18) that at 1;2 his son learnt the word *ato* (*marteau*) for hammer, and in a short time was applying it to a large variety of objects : button-hook, hand-mirror, comb, handbag, saucepan, hairpin, wooden spade, key, gun, box, belt, purse, ruler, puttees, basin, safety-pin, candlestick, coffee-mill, plate, spoon. Guillaume adds that it was never used for people, animals or food, but seemed to be equivalent to *machin* or *chose*, that is to say, an instrument used by some person.

No interpretation which relies upon the evocation of a word by the similarity of objective features can cover a case of this kind. We are bound to say that the word is the child's way of dealing with a complex situation, the similarity of which with another situation is now mainly this, that in each case some-one is using something, a person manipulating an instrument.

It is clear that to Stern's emphasis upon objective simi-larity we have to add the two other features emphasised by Meumann and by Dewey—affective and functional similarity. Together these three views give us a comprehensive view of the similarities of the *situations* among which a child may extend the use of a word. Now if we look at this summary two very interesting points stand out. The first is that while the traditional account emphasised by Stern gives a picture of a somewhat passive child from whom a word is wrung on successive occasions by similar situations, both Meumann and Dewey emphasise the place ,of the situation in the child's activity. And secondly, that all these three views alike deal only with one side of the process—the nature of the situations —and neglect the other side—the nature of the instrument which is applied to those situations, that is to say, the func-tion of the word used.

III

The Place of the Word in the Child's Behaviour.—Turning then to the instrumental aspect of words, we have to remind ourselves that throughout the child's development language is closely related to his activity : the heard word rouses him to activity, his spoken word is a means of supplementing his activity. And in both respects the child's first conventional words have a wider application than they have among adults.

Wide Range of Responses to Conventional Words.—The wide range of the child's responses to words has on the whole been neglected, although it undoubtedly plays an important part in his linguistic growth. An illustration occurs in my record of K's successive responses to the phrase *Where's ballie ?* (Appendix IV, p. 304). By 0;9,14 the child had learnt to turn towards and seize a small white ball on hearing this phrase. Repeated tests in the course of the next five weeks showed that this response was well established, but that it was also definitely limited to the one particular ball, for when at 0;10,21 a large coloured ball was in front of the child as well as his original small white one, it was always the latter he seized, never the former. Six days later, however (at 0;10,27), he took the next step ; on hearing the phrase, sometimes he seized the large ball, sometimes the original small one. The significance of the phrase had become extended for the child beyond the situation in which it was first learnt.

How are we to understand this step ? We must first recall that the child's initial response to the phrase *Where's ballie ?* was not simply an awareness of the ball, or even merely the turning of his attention to it. His response consisted rather of a series of movements involving the ball—turning towards it, seizing it and presenting it to the speaker, receiving in return a smile and a word of approbation. The phrase in fact had acquired the function of initiating a certain activity centring about the ball.

Now we say that the meaning of the phrase *Where's ballie ?* has become extended for the child when, in response to it he deals with another ball in the same way as with the original one. This happens, no doubt, because the two balls are similar " things " for the child—he recognises objective similarity between them. But we must also point out—taking our cue from Dewey—that the balls also become more similar as things because the child finds that he can use them in the same way. In a word, objective similarity and functional similarity foster each other.

This of course will happen quite independently of language. K, for instance, at 1;2,19 picked up a clothes-brush and began to brush his hair with it. There was undoubtedly some resemblance between the brush and the child's own hair-brush —both were long and slender, with handles, and brown in colour ; but the clothes-brush was twice the size of the hair-brush, and had black bristles instead of white. It is certainly reasonable to say that the child used the clothes-brush as he had used the hair-brush because they were rather alike in appearance, but we must also add that they became still more alike for him when he found he could use them in the same way.

What part then is played by language in this process ? A phrase such as *Where's ballie ?* does this : it incites the child to seek similarity between the new situation and earlier ones. On hearing the phrase, the child is put into a condition of readiness to perform the specific movements, and looks round for the appropriate object with which to perform them. The large coloured ball, because it is objectively similar to the small white one, prompts the child to make the same use of it ; thus the adult's word helps to increase the objective and functional similarities of the two situations for the child.

At the same time it increases their affective similarity. The phrase is spoken in a familiar voice. It has regularly been the prelude to the smile and the word of approbation which has followed the right response. These qualities of the heard phrase are carried over into the new situation, giving it an affective similarity with those in which it has customarily been heard. When in the past someone has said *Where's ballie ?* in an interrogative manner, the experience has been satisfactorily completed for the child by his doing something with a ball ; now when he hears this phrase with its characteristic intonation in a new situation, affective similarity will incite him to complete the experience in the same way, and he will be the readier to see the new ball as a fit object to take the place of the original one.

In brief, the heard phrase serves this purpose ; it helps to rouse the child to the objective, affective and functional similarities of successive situations. No doubt the situations would have something of these similarities apart from the heard phrase, but the introduction of this has the function of directing the behaviour of the child to them. The heard phrase thus helps to stabilise similarity of behaviour towards successive situations.

The Wide Application of Spoken Words.—Turning now to the child's own speech, we find that its instrumental functions—the declarative and the manipulative—characteristic of his own primitive sounds persist and develop further when he takes over conventional speech. He uses the word as a tool, as a social instrument, a means of bringing others within his circle of activity. In the declarative use he attracts their attention to an object or situation, in the manipulative use he demands that they shall do something for him with it.

Now a conventional word is different from the child's own primitive sounds in these two ways : it is supplied by others, and it tends to be closely limited to the particular situation in which it first occurs. Both these characteristics would at first sight appear to be likely to work against the wider use of a word, different as this is from the child's own cry—a natural mode of activity, only very loosely linked to any particular situation.

Yet, as we know, the application of an acquired word may be as wide as that of the child's own sounds ; the acquisition of conventional words may actually foster rather than hinder the tendency towards extension. This is partly because the conventional word, supplied though it is by others, is yet not wholly conventional : it has some " natural " features ; and partly because its very linkage with a particular situation makes it so much more efficient a tool that it is readily adopted by the child as a substitute for his own pre-conventional cries.

(i) *The Natural Features of the Acquired Word.*—The child who uses a conventional word is very much in the position of Köhler's chimpanzees ; having learnt to use a stick to bring in a banana they soon began to use it for reaching other things. It would be unwise to push the analogy between language and this kind of tool too far ; but there is one point of comparison to which I think attention should be drawn for the light which it throws upon our problem here. Just as the stick which the chimpanzee seizes is in some respects natural to him and in some respects suggested by others, so too is the child's word both natural and conventional.   The chimpanzee's stick we may call natural to him in that it is a development of his reaching movements, a means by which he lengthens his arm ; and—in Köhler's experiments at any rate—it is in a sense conventional in that he is put in the way of using it by the human beings around him.

Similarly, the child's word is obviously conventional : it is supplied by his adult environment ; what is perhaps not so often realised is that it is also natural to him, in that it is a development of his own expressive cries.   This is true both of its form and its function.

As for the form of his earliest acquired words, it has been the theme of Chapters VIII and X to show how closely related these may be to his own sounds.   The child when he adopts adult words adapts them to his own forms of speech.   We see this both in their intonation and in their patterns of sounds. As for the intonation, the child uses the same tones in speaking his first conventional words as he has used in his own primitive speech ; and as for the patterns of sound, there is no doubt that if we examine children's earliest conventional words— such as **mama, papa, baba, dada, atta**—we find in them the clear marks of the child's own earlier expressive cries.

Much the same can be said of the *function* of these earliest words.   For some time before the child adopts adult words he has been using his own cries in declarative and manipu- lative ways and with some reference to the situations before him.   When he is presented with an adult word linked to a situation, he proceeds—if the situation is important to him— to use this word declaratively or manipulatively.   The child's use of an adult word will thus be partly conventional, sug- gested by those around him ; and partly natural, along the lines of his own linguistic habits.   As I have already put it, every new word that the child acquires has its roots in his linguistic past.

Now I think it is clear that in so far as these words are in some measure a development of the child's own cries they will retain within them that tendency to be extended to a variety of situations which we noticed as characteristic of the child's earliest, pre-conventional use of sounds.

(ii) *The Conventional Features of the Acquired Word.*—But on the other hand, it might be urged, the word is strongly conventional in form ; further, it is presented to the child in a conventional manner, that is, closely linked with a situation in a manner not natural to the child. An adult, for instance, says *dolly* on giving the child the doll. What effect will the conventional features—form and function—of such a word have upon the process of extension ?

A good deal of light is thrown upon this problem by a very interesting experiment carried out by Schäfer with quite another object in view (see Chapter VII, pp. 113–15), and the significance of which for our present topic has not, I think, been discussed before. In this experiment Schäfer happened to teach his son a purely conventional gesture—handclapping ; and linked it in a purely conventional manner with a particular situation—the presence of food. The child, who was of the age when the earliest conventional words are usually acquired (0;10), was trained first to make the movement, and then to make it in response to the phrase *Mache bitte bitte*. When this was well established, Schäfer proceeded to build up a connection between the movement and the presence of food. From the record of the experiment (see Appendix V, p. 322) it is clear that a particular act, however conventional, may, if brought into relation with a situation of importance to the child, become an instrument of dealing with this situation and then ultimately be applied to other situations.

At the outset, it was difficult to establish the connection between the movement and the particular situation—the presence of cake—but once this was accomplished the child began to make it when he wanted different varieties of cake, then when he wanted a letter, then for a box, a piece of string and a book. The conventional movement rapidly acquired a wide instrumental function for the child.

Comparison of this with a child's wide instrumental use of a word suggests that even if a word were wholly conventional, its connection with a situation being imposed on the child from without, it would not remain something which the situation wrings from the child ; it would become in the end a means by which he attempts to deal with a situation. But the words which the child acquires from the adult language are, as we have seen, natural as well as conventional for him ; thus the instrumental function given them by social training is fostered by their primitive instrumental character, in that they are a development of the child's own primary expressive sounds.

Thus, both independently of training by others and also as a result of it, the child will come to use a conventional word instrumentally in situations other than those in which it was first acquired.   This is seen in both instrumental functions of language—the declarative and the manipulative.

Declarative Extension.—To illustrate declarative extension we may again refer to one of Idelberger's records (Appendix V, p. 315) the child in his thirteenth month used *baba* on seeing his father and then applied it to a picture of men in a tailor's catalogue, and again to the sound of a carriage-bell heard in the street.   This last extension, Idelberger tells us, was due to the fact that the child's father had recently mended an electric bell.   Obviously the connecting link here is the child's father—this is the point of similarity among these diverse situations ; but are we to say that the child is merely abstracting this similarity and naming it ?   There is no doubt that we should have to follow Meumann and admit that something of the child's affective response to his father was also being expressed when he said *baba* on seeing the picture or hearing the bell.   And if we admit this we must go further and recognise that while the child was expressing his feelings, he was also at the same time drawing attention to the object which aroused them and communicating these feelings to others.   In place of an earlier expressive cry, he has come to use a conventional word in a fully declarative way.   And because the child can use this conventional word declaratively he will—for a time at any rate—tend to use it with a wide application.

For a conventional adult word is obviously a much better instrument of declaration than the child's own expressive cries. Compare what happens before and after he acquires one of these words.   In the pre-conventional stage, were he to see a new thing, the picture for instance, which arouses in him something of the same feeling as the sight of his father, at the most he could reach towards it and say ɛ ɛ.   But now he can say **baba** !   And because this word is much more closely linked with the original situation—his father—than ɛ ɛ could have been, the efficiency of the process of declaration is enormously increased.   For in adult life, a word normally refers to a situation ; thus when the child uses a conventional word, his hearers will be more likely to turn their attention to the situation than when he merely used an expressive sound.

And the more clearly their behaviour shows this to the child, the greater the incentive for him to extend the use of this instrument to further situations. In brief, as the efficiency of declaration increases, it brings with it a corresponding incentive to extension.

It is in this way that we are to understand many of those cases where a child applies a familiar word to a new situation, calling upon us not to deal with the situation, but to attend to it. In some of these instances, the place of affect may be considerable—as for example when K called out ʃiː on being awakened by the thunderstorm, or fa on seeing his flower-embroidered shoes (see pp. 197, 192). In other cases, affect may be less strong, as when K said **kotibaiz**—seeing in the abacus the bars of his own familiar cot (page 195) ; or Idel-berger's son *wauwau* for a dog, a fur, a coat, and for buttons, or again for a sewing-table and a thermometer (Appendix V, p. 315) ; or Guillaume's daughter *ato* for a hammer and for a saucepan (p.199). But in none of these cases is it adequate to say that the spoken word is merely a mark of recognition ; it is clear that the child is both expressing the feeling aroused in him by the situation, and drawing attention to it, with the result that the bystander is brought into his circle of activity.

Thus the child's earlier need to declare the presence of an object, and to express the feeling aroused in him by it, persists and becomes an important factor in bringing about the extension of words. As before, the child finds himself con-fronted with new situations which rouse him to speech : but now instead of using one of his own primitive cries he uses a tool which he has found effective in a similar situation. Urged then by this declarative impulse, he uses an acquired word, and in doing so extends its use. The need for declaration has helped to bring about extension.

Manipulative Extension.—Much the same may be said of those cases of extension in which the manipulative use of a word is the dominant factor. Now the child is not merely expressing the affective state aroused in him by an object, or drawing attention to it ; he is also signifying his need to obtain possession of some thing, or engage in some activity.

Before the child acquires conventional words, his own sounds, as we have seen, often have this double function ; they express his needs and also serve to secure satisfaction of them by enlisting the help of others. Now when he learns conventional words, both of these functions become more effective because the child is able to refer so much more adequately to the object of his concern.

This incentive of manipulation thus becomes a powerful factor in bringing about extension of learnt conventional words. Take for instance K's use of the word **goga,** his imitation of the word *chocolate* (Appendix IV, p. 313). Having learnt to say it at the sight of chocolate when he was 1;6,9, the child subsequently used it on a number of occasions both declaratively and manipulatively. For instance, he would reach up to a drawer where chocolate was often kept, rattle the handle and say repeatedly **goga, goga.** The most interesting case occurred about two months after the child had first learnt to say the word (1;8,18) ; finding his mother's hat box, he produced one of her hats from it, saying urgently **goga, goga.** I am a little afraid that some writers on children's language would have found this to be a strange case of similarity between chocolate and a hat. But the fact of the matter is, the child's mother had on a few occasions before this put on the hat before going out with him, saying sometimes : " Come on, I shall buy you some chocolate ! " One has to confess that K's behaviour was only too similar to that of the terrier who lays his master's cap at his feet as an indication that his evening run is now due, with the difference that by using the word **goga** K was able to make his intention enormously more definite.

Clearly in a case like this, it is the manipulative function of the word which more than any other factor helps to bring about its extension to a new situation. Much the same can be said of the case of *litten*, cited from Lindner at the beginning of this chapter. The child, it will be remembered, learnt at 2;0 to use the word in imitation of *schlitten* which her mother said on making a sledge for her out of a postcard. Some time later the child said *mama litten* on seeing a postcard brought to the house and again subsequently on seeing a letter. On these last two occasions the child can hardly be said to have been naming the card or the letter ; it was rather that she was reminded of the card out of which the sledge had been made, and was now demanding that the new card or letter should be treated in the same fashion. The same analysis might be made of many of the other examples given in Appendix V. K's use of **da,** for instance (Appendix V, p. 316, entry

1;6,16), on seeing the stairs was not simply a way of naming them, or even a way of showing that he realised they could be climbed ; it was rather a means by which he indicated that he wanted to be allowed to climb. Again, when he said ʃi: on seeing the embankment (p. 319, entry 1;9,29), this was his way of indicating that he wished to be taken over it, just as two days previously he had used ʌpi to express the same need. And to take one more case from my own observations, the child having repeatedly said æg on seeing an egg, one morning said it on seeing the breakfast table laid for the meal (p. 317, entry 1;7,29). This was clearly not a way of naming anything before him, but almost certainly his manner of indicating that he wanted an egg.

If an interpretation of this kind must be made when we have some knowledge of the circumstances in which the words were used, one is tempted to apply the same reasoning to cases where the circumstances have not been recorded, for instance, the extraordinary extensions which appear in the observations of Ament and Idelberger. In this way a case such as the use of *mimi* (*minni*) by the former's niece (Appendix V, p. 314) to indicate a cat, a rabbit, and a champagne-bottle becomes at once more intelligible. In the first place, it seems that Ament has confused two words which happened to have the same *form*—the child's use of *mimi* (or *minni*) for the cat from her 578th day and her use of *mimi* for milk from her 609th day. The former use became extended, probably in a declarative way, to include other animals, a rabbit as well as a cat. The latter use, imitated from the word *Milch*, and used as an expression of the desire to drink, was naturally evoked when the child saw a cup of chocolate or even a bottle of champagne.

Of course, it is evident that in some cases both the manipulative and the declarative functions of a word may determine its wider uses. A good example of this occurs in one of Guillaume's records (DP 8) : at 1;0 the child learned to say *blablab* for the act of vibrating his lips against his fingers ; the word was then used for " mouth, particularly that in a child's portrait, then for any portrait, any drawing, a picture postcard, a printed or written page, a newspaper, a book, the act of reading or the desire to read ". Here objective and probably affective similarity runs from situation to situation throughout the series ; in the later applications functional similarity also begins to play some part ; and while most of the extensions may have been impelled by the declarative need, in the last situation at any rate the manipulative need is also present.

I think that it is clear that the instrumental use of a word in the child's behaviour—its declarative or manipulative function—may be of the greatest importance in determining the wider applications of his words. We have to recognise that in the child's early use of conventional words objective reference is comparatively slight, and that even throughout the child's second year it is only one of several factors in his use of language. The notion that the child learns a conventional word as a " name " for an object or situation, subsequently extending it to other cases, is thus seen to be totally inadequate. The impulse to use words widely is already present before the child acquires conventional words, and is a factor which works in conjunction with the growth of objective reference.

It is indeed through insisting too strongly on the use of words as names, and failing to recognise their declarative and manipulative functions, that the child's wide uses of words have been made to appear so strange and haphazard. We adults constantly tend to lay stress upon the function of the word as a name, and when we find the child using one of these " names " in a wide range of situations, we are struck by his unconventional applications of it. But the assumption that the word has for the child the same function of naming that it has for us is quite unjustified by actual observation. Words come to play the part of names in the child's language only gradually, and during a long period, at the outset of which he is already making wide applications of their use. Instead, therefore, of saying that the name of an object becomes extended to refer to other objects, it is much truer to say that the wide application of a word leads to its becoming the name of one or a group of objects.

These wider uses we have found to be determined by factors which, already present at an early stage of the child's linguistic history, continue to manifest themselves strongly when he begins to use fragments of adult speech. They are first, his response to the objective, affective and functional similarities of diverse situations, and secondly the urge to use language as a declarative or manipulative social instrument.

CHAPTER XII

FURTHER PROGRESS IN CONVENTIONAL USE

WE now have to study the process by which the child, from
using acquired words in this wide fashion, comes to use them
more nearly in the conventional manner current in the community about him. In the present chapter we shall outline
the actual process as it is observed in children, and then
consider this in the light of modern accounts of the growth of
conceptual thinking.

It is clear that the process of conventionalisation does not
consist simply in imposing a vocabulary upon a passive child.
He has at first a repertory of his own, which owes as much—
both in form and in function—to his primitive modes of
expression as it does to the influence of the community around
him. Under the stress of the forces which we have described
in the preceding chapter, he extends and limits the applications of his words in ways at first different from those current
in this community. In time he learns to conform to their
usages ; to extend the use of a word only where they extend
it and to limit its use where they limit it. Our use of speech
reflects the lines of cleavage that we make in the world about
us : one word we apply to a particular " thing ", enabling us
to preserve its identity ; other words we use to group things
together, to distinguish characteristics which they have in
common or relationships we find between them. Education
largely consists in familiarising a child with these lines of cleavage
and with the uses of language which preserve them for us.

The Child's own Discrimination.—In a similar fashion the
child's use of words reflects the lines of cleavage that he makes
in his own little world. Some words he uses more widely than
we do, others more narrowly. And these two processes, we
find, are due to the same factors—those which we have distinguished in the preceding chapter : the need to use language
in an instrumental way, declaratively or manipulatively, and
the presence of objective, affective and functional similarities
in diverse situations.

Take, for instance, a case that we have already discussed : Hilde Stern's use of the word *puppe* at 0;11 (KSp 19). This covered a very wide range of her playthings, but was never extended to one of the most favoured of these, a little bell, which remained without a conventional name until at 1;6 it was christened *didelideli*. The child was using the word *puppe* more widely than the adult equivalent " doll " and yet less widely than the adult equivalent " toy ". It is evident that her refusal to extend the use of the word to include the bell was due to the presence of objective, affective and functional differences.

The first of these is recognised by Stern when he says that the bell had a different appearance (*Format*) from that of the child's other toys. But there can be no doubt that this explanation, taken by itself, is inadequate. Just as we cannot fully understand extension without taking into account other factors besides objective similarity, so too we have to look beyond mere objective dissimilarity if we are to understand the child's limitation of the use of a word. Clearly the objective appearance of a plaything is by no means the most important aspect of it for a child : it also arouses an affective response in him—he loves it—and has a definite function for him—he plays with it. Because Hilde could caress and play with her toy rabbit and toy kitten as with her doll she extended the same word *puppe* to include them all ; but from this very same cause she did not extend it to include the bell, a plaything which must have aroused quite a different affective response in her, its functions for her being so different. The same factors that caused her to extend the use of the word to many other playthings besides her doll also caused her to stop short at the little bell.

Something of this indeed seems to be in the mind of Stern himself when he later mentions in passing (KSp 195) that a child will limit the name *puppe* to a particular object, because he stands in a special relationship to it—he keeps the name for that one and only doll which is his most beloved plaything. Further on Stern adds that in the same way the child will keep the word *mama* for that one person who specially satisfies his desires. There can be no doubt that these affective and functional characteristics are at least as important as objective features in bringing about both widening and narrowing in a child's use of words.

Personal and Social Factors.—It is the current usage of
society which determines whether a word is being used by a
child too widely or too narrowly. The word *puppe*, for
instance, was used too widely by Hilde ; but if under similar
circumstances an English child had learnt the word *toy* for her
doll and then refused to extend its use to include a bell, another
plaything, it would have been too narrow a use. This point
is illustrated very clearly in K's response to the word *mummy*—
a case exactly parallel to the typical instance of *mama* mentioned by Stern. As we saw in Chapter IX (pp. 155 and 161),
the child would not respond to the word *mummy* when it was
used merely to denote the objective appearance of his mother,
her reflection, for instance, in a mirror (Appendix IV (5), p. 311,
entries 1;5,8 and 1;6,13). Here, since the word had become
linked up for the child with situations vitally important for
him and capable of arousing strongly affective and conational
responses, it was difficult for him to accept the word in mere
play, and extend its application because of a merely objective
likeness.

In cases such as this, the child's linguistic development is
the story of the subordination of affective and conational
factors to the objective standards imposed upon him by his
adult environment. The barrier which his private attitudes
erect around a word and its linked situations are broken down
by social pressure. He learns to use the word *mummy* more
widely, to apply it to his mother whatever the circumstances,
and then to limit it again to denote the special relationship
which exists between him and her. So the process of limitation and extension goes on until at last there comes the day
when he even uses the word *Mother* to denote an abstract
relationship in which he himself may play no personal part.

The same ultimate goal of conformity is reached—perhaps
by a slightly different route—where the child's early uses of a
word are too wide instead of too narrow. To take another
typical case from Stern (KSp 195), Hilde at first used the word
papa with reference to all men alike ; it was only at 1;7 that
she began to confine its use to her father, using *onke* (*Onkel*)
for other men. Here the effect of social pressure was to limit
the use of the word, as the first stage in the process which
ultimately led to conformity with current usage.

In both these cases—whether the child's initial uses be too
wide or too narrow—the main factors in the process of con-

ventionalisation are the same. First there are the objective, affective and functional characters of the various situations confronting the child, secondly the child's instrumental needs in using his words, and thirdly the constant effect of social pressure, supplying new words and approving or disapproving of the child's use of them. We have now to see how these factors work together in the actual process of conventionalisation.

The Process as Observed.—Once more we need a continued record of a child's uses of language, together with some account of the circumstances in each case. Perhaps the nearest approach to this is to be found in the work of Ament (SD), where the successive " meanings " of a large number of the child's words are given, with dates ; and although unfortunately there is little detail of the circumstances, we can see the main line of change. By bringing together his records of various words,[1] I have been able to make out the diagram in Fig. 2, which gives an interesting picture of the uses of the word *mammamm* and its substitutes. I shall use this first to study the process as a whole, and then for points of detail refer to my own observations of K.

At the beginning of this period, on the child's 354th day, she has the one word *mammamm* which she uses alike for solid food and for her sister who feeds her. On the 513th day the use of the word is extended to include liquid food (which presumably up to this time has been referred to only by primitive cries or by gestures). On the 571st day the child's sister receives a new designation *desi*, while the original word *mammamm* is now (in the form *momi*) extended to include her mother. On the 597th day, the new word *brodi* enters, with reference to bread, *mammamm* remaining with reference to other solid food. On the same day the child begins to call her mother *mama*. There is no need to continue the story further ; new words enter, some to be limited, others to be extended, until at last the child has seven words—all used in a comparatively conventional way—instead of the original one word with its unconventionally wide usage.

It is quite clear that this process is never a matter of merely adding new words to the child's own slender repertory. The process is, rather, parallel to the child's adoption of his first conventional words, with this difference : that while at the

[1] See Appendix V, p. 314.

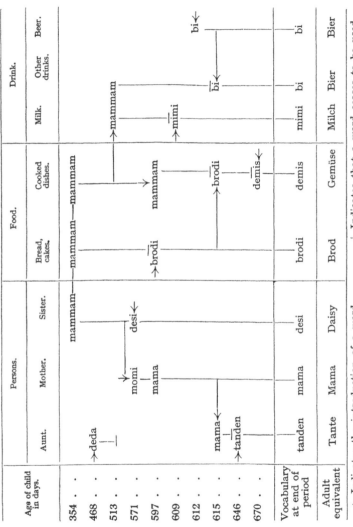

Fig. 2.—Development of Meaning of *mammam* and its substitutes (Ament's Niece).

→ Indicates the introduction of a word.

⊥ Indicates that a word ceases to be used.

earlier stage (as we saw on p. 153), the conventional words are superimposed only upon the child's own primitive cries, at the stage we are now considering a new word is often imposed upon and substituted for some of the applications of a conventional word already in use. And—in the same way as at the earlier stage—adult usage meets with some resistance and also receives some reinforcement from the child's own linguistic habits.

The pressure of this resistance at the earlier stage—when a conventional word is superimposed upon a child's own cries— is shown in the little experiment with K described on p. 158. There we saw that when the child was able and willing to repeat the word *Cakie* merely in imitation he would not use this word when he desired cake, but reverted instead to his own primitive sounds ɛ ɛ. Something of the same resistance is encountered at the later stage, when the adult endeavours to introduce a new word in place of the conventional one already known to the child. Even though the child may imitate the adult word when encouraged to do so, he will not necessarily use the word spontaneously when again faced with the new situation ; he will often revert to a more familiar word. Take, for instance, this example from the series of observations of K given in Appendix V, page 320, and shown as a diagram in Fig. 3. The child had for some time past been accustomed to say **tiː** on seeing animals of various kinds. At 1;11,24, seeing a horse in the street, he said **tiː** ; his father immediately added *horse*. Next day, while he was out walking with his mother, who had heard of this incident, they came upon a child riding ; she said : " *There's a little girl riding on a . . .,*" and K responded quite correctly **hɔʃ**. When she repeated her remark he replied in the same way—the new word seemed well established. Yet the following day, when he was again out with his mother and saw a horse, he reverted to the older word **tiː** (1;11,26). His mother again repeated the word *horse*, which he imitated, and this—in the form of **hɔʃ**—now became well established, as may be seen by the child's application of it to a large dog at 2;0,10.

What incentives are there for the child to overcome his tendency to make use of a familiar act and adopt a new one in its stead ? There must, it is clear, be a concurrence of influences both from within himself and from the adults about him. His discrimination of objective, affective and functional

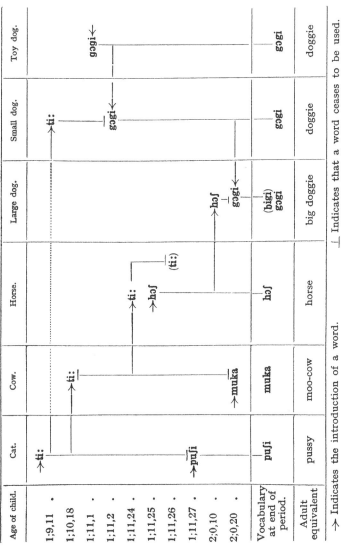

FIG. 3.—Words used to refer to animals (K).

→ Indicates the introduction of a word.   ⊥ Indicates that a word ceases to be used.

characters will develop partly as a result of his own growth and partly under social pressure.

Objective Discrimination.—This is the factor which has been the most emphasised in the past : as the child becomes more aware of objective likenesses and differences in the things around him he extends the uses of his words in some directions and limits them in others.

The child learns, in fact, to differentiate between some situations and to group others together. This discrimination, the foundation of further progress in the conventional use of words, itself arises out of the child's earlier progress in objective reference. As long as a child uses words as a means of expressing his affective-conational responses to situations as wholes, these words will inevitably be applied more widely and more narrowly than in adult usage. For the affective-conational likenesses and differences will rarely correspond exactly to objective ones. But when the child begins to use a word to apply to a specific portion of a situation, then the way is open to his acceptance of the objective distinctions current among adults. In the case of Ament's niece, for instance, as long as *mammamm* expressed the child's desire to obtain drink, and therefore referred to the whole act of drinking, it could be applied alike to all drinks ; but the new word *mimi* (acquired on the 609th day in imitation of *milch*) being closely linked—from the moment of its adoption—with a particular liquid, would not quite so easily be applied to other situations merely because they involved the act of drinking.

The process must, however, frequently meet with resistance from the child—unwitting, no doubt. His tendency to deal with a situation as a whole rather than with a mere object within it often remains strong. This is illustrated by Miss Sullivan's account of Helen Keller at the time immediately preceding the famous *water* episode, and which indeed seems to have been generally neglected in the over-emphasis which has been given to that event. On March 20th, 1887, Miss Sullivan writes :

> Helen has learned several nouns this week. " M-u-g " and " m-i-l-k " have given her more trouble than other words. When she spells " milk " she points to the mug, and when she spells " mug ", she makes the sign for pouring or drinking, which shows that she has confused the words. She has no idea yet that everything has a name (Keller SL 312).

Miss Sullivan says that the child confused the words and had no idea that everything has a name, but the truth seems to be rather that the child was using the two words for the same whole situation, not yet linking each of them with some objective feature of it. " Mug " and " milk " alike meant the whole act of drinking.

A fortnight later (April 5th) the difficulty still persisted, and then, records Miss Sullivan, the child indicated that she wanted to know the name for water. Having spelt out this word for her, it occurred to Miss Sullivan that the new knowledge might be used for " straightening out the mug-milk difficulty ". She took the child out into the garden to the pump, and it was then that the famous episode occurred : the child was suddenly helped to realise that the various " words " she had been taught, referred to *objects* within situations and not widely to situations taken as wholes.

In this case there seem to have been three stages : first, a growing discrimination between the object and the situation in which it occurred (for she " asked for " the name of water) : secondly, the adoption of a word, *water*, to apply narrowly to the object rather than widely to the situation ; and thirdly, the realisation that words may have this narrower function. Without stressing the parallel too strongly, one may reasonably suppose that these processes also go on in the life of a normal child. Just as Helen Keller had begun to direct her attention upon the object " water " within the total experience of drinking, before she had a name for this object, it seems reasonable to suppose that the normal child will also begin to discriminate between different drinks and the total situation in which each is embedded. And just as Helen Keller was helped in this discrimination by being given the word *water*, so Ament's niece would be helped to a further discrimination between milk and other drinks by being given the word *mimi* for the former and *bi* for the latter.

So much then seems to be clear, that the child's growing discrimination between objects and their situations renders him ripe to use words of objective reference when they come ; and the use of these words fosters in turn the use of them in conformity with adult standards. The process is clearly one in which there is interaction between the development which takes place within the child himself and the effects of adult intervention.

An illustration of this may be found in the final entries of the records of K summarised in Fig. 3 from Appendix V, page 320. The child, having learnt by 1;11,26 to say **hɔʃ** on seeing a horse, extended the word a fortnight later (2;0,10) to apply to a St. Bernard dog : a large dog was a **hɔʃ**. It is safe to say that this usage received no social sanction. But when ten days later, seeing the St. Bernard again, he said **bigi gɔgi,** this was certainly approved. It is clear that the conformity to adult usage arose partly from the child's own growing discrimination and partly as a result of adult intervention. To call a St. Bernard a **hɔʃ** is not allowed, but it may be called a **gɔgi.**

The Affective Aspect.—The growth of affective discrimination in the child's use of words shows the working of similar factors : some resistance by the child and some welcome to adult intervention.

With regard to affective resistance to adult usage, it is only rarely that we have a clear example that reveals it—one, for instance, like that in which K refused to allow the extension of the word *mummy* to include his mother's reflection in a mirror. But one may suspect its presence in many other cases. Thus, in the series from Ament given in Figure II, we find that the use of the word *mama* was extended by the child to include her aunt on her 615th day ; an extension, one would say, due at least as much to affective similarity between the two persons as to any objective or functional likeness. Now—even in the absence of any record of Ament's—we can be pretty sure that this extension can have received little or no adult sanction ; we do in fact know that the child had frequently heard the word *tante* long before this, for as early as her 468th day she had adopted it in the form *deda*, a word which became obsolete after her 513th day. Yet she preferred her own extension of *mama* for a whole month, only adopting the word *tante* in the form of *tanden* on her 646th day.

On the other hand, it is equally clear that the discrimination ultimately suggested by adults between the mother and the aunt must have been reinforced by a growing affective discrimination in the child herself. No child well on in her second year, as this child was, can fail to experience different emotions towards her mother and an aunt.

We may surely regard this as typical of many cases : since the affective discriminations made by adults are not merely arbitrary, but correspond to those likely to be made by a child living under the same conditions, so adult intervention will often meet with welcome from the child's own growing discriminations.

The Functional Aspect.—More than any other factor, it is the functional differences between things which determine the discriminative use of words by adults. In the main we group things for practical rather than for æsthetic or scientific purposes. When we name a sphere a *ball* we are distinguishing it from spheres in general by its function for us, and we go on in the same way to distinguish a football from a tennis ball.

The same tendency, we have seen in the preceding chapter, is very marked in the case of children, leading them to extend and limit the application of their words, according to the function of the situation dealt with. Thus again we have some resistance to adult usage, as well as conformity with it.

Take again the series we have cited from Ament, page 214. By the 513th day, *mammamm* stands for everything that may be consumed, food and drink alike, whatever their detailed objective and functional differences. Then the word *brodi* enters for bread and cakes (597th day), and for a while this group is distinguished from all other food, solid or liquid. But now the child achieves by herself a much more important distinction : she discriminates between the acts of eating and drinking when on her 615th day she extends the word *brodi* to cover all solid food. This is done in the face of adult usage, for (although we have no record of Ament's on the point) it is reasonable to assume that the word *Brod* (from which she derived *brodi*) was certainly not the current word for cooked dishes. Finally—with adult aid this time—she makes a further distinction, retaining *brodi* for bread and the like, and adopting *demis* (from *Gemüse*) for cooked dishes (670th day) ; an important difference between these being the manner in which they are eaten.

Thus once more we see the child approaching conformity to adult conventions by a process of extensions and limitations in which his growing discrimination is fostered by his acquirement of words, and these in turn foster further discrimination. Things become alike or different for him as he handles them or as they enter into his activities, and the use of words helps to stabilise these likenesses or differences. The child, for instance, begins to distinguish between bread which is taken up in the hand, and cooked dishes which are eaten with a spoon ; then enters the adult word *demis* and helps to fix this distinction. Which of the two factors is the more dominant —the child's own growing discrimination or adult intervention—cannot be estimated.

Although on the whole the growth of functional discrimination runs parallel with that of objective or affective discrimination, it would appear to differ from these in offering slighter resistance to adult intervention : the child's own functional discrimination runs to meet adult usage. For the child lives in a world of things made by adults to be handled in certain ways, and which are named accordingly, and as the child learns to handle these things he inevitably paves the way for the functional distinctions and groupings which the adult language embodies. One might well say that it is not so much what the child perceives or what he feels that determines the growth of the conceptual use of language, but what he does.

The Instrumental Aspect.—The child's need to use language declaratively and manipulatively, which plays so important a part in determining his initial wide uses of words, remains an equally important factor in the further process of conventionalisation.

It is clear that once a word has been given a wider use because of an instrumental need, this extension will tend to resist further change, and thus hinder the adoption of a new word. It is only under a certain amount of pressure that a child will take over a new word to do the work which a familiar one is already doing.

For an example of this in the declarative use of language, we may refer once more to our example from K (Fig. 3).

The child, already in possession of **ti:** for dog, cat and cow, is confronted (at 1;11,24) with a horse. The need to declare himself, to draw attention to this striking thing, is strong : at once he produces the familiar instrument, saying **ti:**. Now enters the interfering adult and remarks : *horse*, which the child duly imitates next day as **hoʃ**. Yet on the third day, when he sees a horse once more, it is the older word, not the new one, which is produced ; the child again says **ti:**. But the adult is persistent ; once more he says *horse*. This time he is only too successful, for when a fortnight later the child sees a large St. Bernard he says **hoʃ,** showing that not only has he adopted the word but is using it declaratively beyond its original application (see Appendix V, p. 320).

A parallel example in the manipulative use of a word may also be taken from observations of K (Appendix V, pp. 320–1). By 1;7,8 the child was using the word **bɔ** (box) either for boxes in general or for his toy bricks which were usually kept in a box.   In the course of the next week (by 1;7,15) he showed clearly that he could respond correctly to both the adult words *box* and *bricks*.   Yet for the next three months he himself continued to use the word **bɔ** for both box and bricks : and it was only at 1;10,4 when he was moved by the urgent desire to possess some bricks that he first used the adult word.   He was away from home and had not seen his own bricks for a fortnight.   His mother said to him : " *Baby, come and buy some bricks* " ; immediately he repeated **biki biki** eagerly.   Eighteen days later we find him using the word spontaneously in a manipulative way.

Thus the child's instrumental use of a word may lag far behind his comprehension of it.   Although he constantly hears and understands the word *bricks*, he will go on using **bɔ** when he wants his bricks, because this is the instrument which has become effective for him.   Why then, we may ask, should he ever change to a new tool, **biki** ?   The answer seems to be that usually it is just at the moment when the child has an urgent declarative or manipulative need that the adult comes in with a new word and so impresses it upon the child (as in the cases of **hɔʃ** and **biki**) ; sooner or later the child comes to realise that the conventional tool is more efficient than his own non-conventional one—in other words, the social instrument is more efficient than his private and personal one.   It is more efficient in this sense, that it does its work of *communication* more efficiently : the conventional word is immediately accepted by the listener, as his response shows ; whereas the child's own personal usages—arising out of his personal attitudes to situations—are received much more slowly, usually either with amusement or disapproval, often with bewilderment and sometimes without any response at all.

In brief, we may sum up as follows the effect of the child's instrumental needs upon his use of conventional words in a conventional way.   The need to deal declaratively or manipulatively with a new situation impels the child to say a word ; he extends the use of a familiar one to meet this situation.

The adult frequently intervenes, supplying a new word, and —if the child adopts it—making it by his responses a more efficient tool than the child's own familiar word. As the process recurs the child comes to realise that the conventional use of words is more efficient than his unconventional use of them.

The whole process is, of course, also influenced by other factors : by the child's growing discrimination—objective, affective and functional : by the strength and constancy of adult intervention, and even by the degree to which an individual child naturally tends to conform to those about him.

We have thus reached the point at which the child begins to enter into the conventional use of the mother tongue ; it is left to us to consider briefly the theoretical implications of this step.

The Conventional Nature of Conceptual Thinking.—We have suggested that the forms of conceptual thought into which the child ultimately grows are not only determined by the " nature of things " in themselves, but also by the usages of the society around him. In fact, it would seem that the child achieves his conceptual grasp of the nature of things largely through conformity with these conventional usages.

Does this mean that our conceptual grasp of things—the lines of cleavage with which we divide up the universe— depends upon the society in which we live ? There can be no doubt that this idea has recently been gaining ground. The point has been very well brought out by Hocart (PL) in discussing the conceptual differences which are found to characterise different communities. The existence of these differences might be taken to mean that the " savage " is not capable of the higher forms of generalisation habitual to a cultivated European ; in the words of Stout, to whom Hocart refers, " the savage mind . . . has not pushed its analysis far enough to be able to reconstruct certain complex concepts out of simpler " (AP ii, 231). Hocart agrees that, as Stout says, among the Fijians there are two words *tooe* and *taoe* both represented in English by the word *your*—which seems to show that they are not so capable of generalisation as we are. He points out, however, that in the same language the two English words *in* and *on* are both represented by the one word *e*. In brief, it is not that the Fijians are less capable of generalisation than we are, but that their generalisation is differently directed.

The truth, says Hocart, is that the distinctions made by any community depend upon the manner in which its members need to deal with the situations before them—the practical significance of these situations for them. Our words reflect the functions of the things with which we deal. Among the Solomon Islanders, for instance—a community studied by Hocart—there are nine distinct names for the coconut, signifying different stages in its growth, but no word corresponding to our general term " coconut ". On the other hand, they have only one word which covers all four meals of the day— breakfast, dinner, tea, supper—but no special name for each of these. It is of practical importance to them to distinguish the nine stages of the coconut but not to discriminate between " dinner " and " tea ".

A particularly striking instance is the distinction made by the Islanders between the *vino* and the *ngari*, which to Europeans seem merely to be smaller and larger specimens of the same nut.

> We found that from trifling differences sprang a host of momentous ones—technical, commercial and religious ; the seasons of the two species do not coincide ; they are gathered differently, because the branches of the *vino* will bear a man, and the *ngari* will not ; they are cracked differently because the *ngari* is larger, and in one island this was the object of a taboo ; they are preserved differently ; the *vino* is pounded and made into a package, then smoked, the *ngari* is smoked in the shell ; the *vino* coming early supplies the offerings of the first fruits, while the *ngari* being abundant, is used for the later smoked-nuts festival ; in certain diseases the one is tabooed as food and the other not ; the two, in fact, are only identical in the kitchen, and therefore they have but one word for the roasted kernels or puddings of either.

Distinctions of this kind, which grow out of the practical necessities of a community, remain the fundamental conceptual distinctions of that community. We may say, in fact, that a concept is a means of preserving distinctions which are of practical importance in the life of a community ; and that a conceptual term in language is an instrument for dealing with one's environment in accordance with these distinctions.

This view of the nature of a concept and of a conceptual term is reflected in the work of such recent writers on language as Malinowski and de Laguna, in Head's work on aphasia and in

Spearman's work on the growth of cognition. Head's study of aphasia leads him to insist that "a name is a descriptive label employed to designate some aspect of an event, selected for special attention with a view to subsequent behaviour" (A 526). And Spearman concludes that it is more in keeping with the facts of the growth of cognition to take the view, not that a concept is an "essential character" of things, but that it is "any apprehended character which has somehow become stably fixed in the usage of a person or a society" (NI 263).

It is clear then that the view which we have found to be most consistent with observations of children—that concepts are determined by social behaviour—also emerges from a study of primitive communities, of the pathology of language and of the growth of cognition in general.

Genesis of Conceptual Thinking.—We have also found it necessary to describe the process as something more than the growth of cognitive discrimination : the whole development is complicated by other factors. And once again we are able to find corroboration in the work of Spearman, whose account of the growth of cognition is generally held to be the most penetrating in recent psychology.

Stern's Account.—Let us compare what he says with the view recognised by Stern (KSp 189, 195). This writer distinguishes two main lines of development : the first leading to a concept of an individual thing (*Individualbegriff*), the second to a concept of a class of things (*Gattungsbegriff*).

In the first case, the child is led to his concept of an individual thing or person by noticing that certain items—which together make up the "thing"—stand out together again and again from many varied situations. For instance, although the child's mother appears to him in many different circumstances, doing different things and dressed differently, she remains throughout them all the same person for him, and thus at last the concept of his mother as an individual person arises for him and becomes established throughout all the different events in which she may appear.

In the second process the child is led to his concept of a class by noticing that the features of a situation as a whole reappear in other situations ; when, for instance, a child uses the word *papa* for all men, there may be considerable differences among them, but he attends only to the general likeness. At first, says Stern, this is no more than a mere grouping of things or situations side by side (*Pluralbegriff*)—there is as yet no notion of a class ; gradually by a continued process of discussion with those about him, the child acquires an abstract general notion corresponding to such a word as *father*, that this embraces a certain class of persons standing in a definite relation to others. This final stage rarely begins before the child's fourth year.

Now although this account accurately describes some of the main features of the child's development, it does not quite cover the actual facts which may be observed in children and which we have summarised in the preceding chapter. Several points merely implied by Stern need to be more fully stressed. First, it is not made clear why sometimes a small group of items claim the child's attention, leading to an " individual " concept, while at other times he is concerned with the broad features of a situation, leading to a " class " concept. Secondly, although the two processes described by Stern undoubtedly occur, in actual fact they do not run side by side but alternate in the development of a single concept. Stern himself points out that his daughter Hilde first used the word *papa* in a wide way for all men (as a *Pluralbegriff*), and then limited it to her father (an *Individualbegriff*). But there may be more alternation than this : thus Idelberger's son first used *baba* for his father alone ; then more widely for objects closely connected with his father, and at the same time for all men ; then ultimately, no doubt, he came to use either this or a substitute narrowly again for his father (Appendix V, p. 315). Here we have in succession, first a concentration of the child's attention upon his father, as standing out from the whole situation, then a broadening of his attention to embrace the main general features of the situation, so that *baba* is used for any man as well as this particular man ; and again a concentration of attention upon the particular features which distinguish his father, so that *baba* (or a substitute) is finally used for this person and for no others.

Spearman's Account.—As far as I know, only Spearman— of all writers upon the growth of cognition—has taken into consideration this fact of the child's alternation between concentration and broadening of attention, and attempted to discuss its cause. Following up his definition of a concept, which we have already cited, he bases his account of the development of conceptual thinking both upon the introspections of adults in the course of experimental work and also in some measure upon personal observations of children. He names three processes (NI 266), which turn out to be roughly parallel with Stern's three main lines of development (leading to an *Individualbegriff*, a *Pluralbegriff*, or a *Gattungsbegriff*) but are described as intermingling in much more subtle a manner. First, we have the process of attending to a limited group of items—this Spearman calls Disintegration : secondly, that of attending to the broadly similar characters of situations as wholes—this he calls Confusion : thirdly the final process of abstraction—this he calls the Eduction of Relations and Correlates under the influence of social training.

Something of this kind might be regarded as implied by Stern. Where Spearman goes beyond the latter is in insisting upon these two points : first, that the whole course of development is determined by the lines of the child's " constant biological needs " ; secondly, that in the development of a particular concept, two of the fundamental processes or even all three may enter at different times. And in both of these respects he is more closely in accord than Stern with the results of observation of children.

The former point—that concepts grow up along the lines of the child's biological needs—we have so constantly stressed that little more need be said here. Stern certainly hints at it when he says that it is the child's *affective* attitude which causes the particular group of items constituting his " mother " or his " doll " to emerge clearly from the whole situation of which it forms a part. But Spearman is ready to go much further than this ; he points out that biological factors are at work throughout : in Disintegration they determine that a particular character shall emerge ; in Confusion it is biological necessity which causes the child to deal in the same way with diverse situations only broadly alike ; and finally, biological needs will determine eduction of relations and of correlates, both at the more primitive levels when concepts are beginning to develop, and also later when, faced with unfamiliar situations, the child has consciously to seek concepts with which to deal with them.

There can be no doubt that if we take such cases as the *mammamm* series of Ament's niece, or K's use of **ti:**, Spearman's account is amply corroborated ; particularly when we point out that the function of language is to subserve bio-

logical needs, and that these may be of two kinds : manipulative—the need to master a situation practically ; and
declarative—the need to master it by affective communion
with others. Thus in the process of Disintegration, once the
child has begun however dimly to be aware that some food
is solid and some liquid, the manipulative need to obtain one
or the other more readily will spur him on to adopt a distinctive term such as *brodi* for one of them. Again, in the
process of Confusion, if the child expands the use of a word
such as *mammamm* to include his aunt as well as his mother,
it is in the effort to secure a satisfaction, declarative or manipulative, which both can equally well supply. And it is clear
also that in the development of more abstract concepts, through
the processes of Eduction of relations and of correlates, the
same two incentives will be at work, leading the child to more
and more subtle distinctions and groupings.

To come now to Spearman's second point, that all three
processes—Disintegration, Confusion and Eduction—may enter
into the development of a single concept. First of all, he
suggests, there must be Disintegration ; on this Confusion
may supervene, to be followed possibly by a further period of
Disintegration, and this in turn by a period of training in which
Eduction plays the chief part. The truth of this analysis is
well illustrated by the development of a child's use of the
word **mama** corresponding to the growth of his concept of
mother—as seen, for instance, in our observations of K or in
Ament's of his niece. At first (Appendix IV, pp. 308–11) K uses
the cry **mama** when in a state of mild discomfort : already
there would seem to be a slight Disintegration of this state of
discomfort from the rest of the situation. Soon, by the
process of training that we have described in Chapters VIII
and IX, the attention of the child begins to be directed towards
his mother while he is uttering the cry—a further development
of Disintegration. Upon this there supervenes a period of
Confusion, during which the word **mama** may be applied
to a wide range of situations into which the child's mother
enters—or other persons objectively, affectively or functionally
resembling her. The ease with which this process takes
place appears to depend on the strength of the previous process of Disintegration. In the case of Ament's niece, for
instance, the word **mama** seems to have been extended without
difficulty to include the child's aunt as well as her mother (see

p. 314), but in the case of K, on the other hand, the Disintegration ("along the lines of the child's biological needs") had been so strong, that the word became strictly limited to certain situations in which his mother appeared and was not extended to others, for instance, the sight of her in a mirror. But even in this case, the process of Confusion at last occurred : the word was applied to include the portrait of another woman.

Arising out of this process of Confusion, there would normally follow a further period of Disintegration of the special characteristics which distinguish the child's mother, both from other people, and from all the varied situations in which she appears. This is the point at which most children will have arrived during their second year ; the word is now said to be used as a name for the child's mother.

There follows upon this a further period of training, under social influence, during which the processes are certainly largely the eduction of relations and correlates. It is now that the concept of "mother" (and the application of the corresponding word) becomes both extended in some directions and limited in others until at last it squares with the socially accepted concept. On the one hand, its scope is limited in that it no longer includes every woman, or indeed every woman that satisfies the child's needs, but is applied now only to a certain person who stands in a special relation to him ; on the other hand it is extended to include the whole class of such persons, those who bear this particular relationship to others. Then it is extended further still, to include any living creature which stands in this particular relationship to another, until ultimately there develops the bare abstract concept of motherhood, as we find it in the notions of Motherland or Mother Nature.

It is important to notice that in the course of such a development, the processes of Disintegration and Confusion do not correspond in any simple fashion with the contractions and expansions of the use of a word. Thus a process of Confusion may give rise to a word's contracted use : for instance, a child's experience of all the various situations in which his mother appears may help to limit the use of the word **mama** to her. On the other hand, a process of Disintegration may give rise to a word's expanded use ; for instance, the example given by Spearman of the child of two who having learnt the word *ho* (hot) when touching a can of hot water, used it later when pointing to a steaming pie (NI 267).

It is clear that Spearman's account, as a whole, applies with the greatest exactness to the development of concepts and of the use of conceptual terms in children. The processes of Disintegration, Confusion and Eduction which he describes show themselves in the contractions and expansions characteristic of the growth of language. If, in dealing with children here rather than with adults as he does, we must add anything to his account it is this : that in children the process of development is less dominantly cognitive in nature, other factors playing a larger part—the child's affective responses, his use of language as an instrument, and the presence around him of an adult community bent on training him. With these necessary additions to Spearman's analysis we are enabled to give an adequate account of the early stages of the development of concepts.

Having thus brought the child to the threshold of the conventional use of the mother tongue, we may here end our survey of his early linguistic development.

APPENDICES

THE SOUNDS UTTERED SPONTANEOUSLY BY CHILDREN IN THE COURSE OF THEIR FIRST YEAR

TABULATED FROM DATA IN PREYER (MC), STERN (KSp) AND HOYER (LK); TOGETHER WITH THE WRITER'S RECORD OF A BOY, K

PREYER'S SON

Age.	When in a state of discomfort.		When in a state of comfort.	
	Sounds.	When uttered.	Sounds.	When uttered.
0;1,0	uä	During crying.		
0;1,15			amma (among other sounds)	Child in a comfortable posture.
0;1,16			tahu ,, ,,	,,
0;1,18			gö, örö ,, ,,	,,
0;1,23			ara ,, ,,	,,
0;2,0			örö, ärä, very frequent	,,
0;2,8	ma, often repeated	During crying		,,
0;2,9	nei nei ,, ,,	,, ,,		,, ,,
0;2,10			la, grei, aho, ma, among other sounds	,, ,,
0;2,13	mömm, ngo, often repeated	Child was hungry	Of all those mentioned above, only örö was now frequent.	
0;2,14				
0;2,15			ra-a-ao	In comfort.
0;2,20	nä, näi-n	During general discomfort and hunger.		
0;2,22			habu	In contentment.
0;3,0			a-i, uåo, åoå, åaa, oåo	,,

233

PREYER'S SON (*continued*)

Age.	When in a state of discomfort.		When in a state of comfort.	
	Sounds.	When uttered.	Sounds.	When uttered.
0;3,14	lŏ na	During crying	ntŏ, ha	In comfort.
0;3,21	nannana, nă-nă, nanna	In refusal.		
0;4,0	uă, and variants; amme-a	During screaming.		
0;5,0			k, gŏ, kŏ	While child was yawning.
0;5,14			ŏgŏ, maŏe, ha, ā, o-ich, brrr-ha; also a peculiar labio-lingual sound between b and d	During "crowing," or while he was lying comfortably on his back.
0;6,0	mă, uă, lă	In crying	ŏrrŏ	In a state of comfort.
	p	Very rarely, in screaming	p	Very rarely, in a state of comfort.
0;7,0]			ŏrrŏ, nteo, mija; also the labio-lingual sound	In the course of "Lallen".
0;8,0			māmă, mă, ămmă	While listening to music.
			nana, ŏrrŏ, apa, ga-au-a, acha	In a state of comfort.
0;9,0			ndăe, băe-băe, ba-ell, arrŏ, ma, pappa, tatta, babba, tătä, pa, uvular r	All uttered when the child was comfortable.
0;10,0			dadada	When comfortable.
0;11,0	anananana, uttered with an expression of longing	When something was eagerly desired	atta, hŏdda, hatta, hatai	With the meaning that something had disappeared.
1;0	nana	Denoting that something was desired.		
	mama	Referred to mother, but uttered also without this reference	mama	Referred to mother, but uttered also without this reference.

HILDE STERN

Age.	When in a state of discomfort.		When in a state of comfort.	
	Sounds.	When uttered.	Sounds.	When uttered.
First few days	ähä	Chief sounds made in crying.		
0;1,14			krä krä	After feeding.
0;2,0			erre	In comfort.
0;2,14			ekche, ekche, together with sounds noted above. Beginning of repetitive chains	Most frequently after feeding.
0;7,14			rrrr (uvular)	Uttered with apparent pleasure.
0;8,0			p	(?) It is not clear whether this was uttered in comfort.
0;8,14			ä, a	In comfort.
0;9,0			da, pa, ja, neinei, ää	In the course of " Lallen ".
0;10,14			didda	The child had learnt to make this sound on seeing the clock.

GÜNTHER STERN

Age.	When in a state of discomfort.		When in a state of comfort.	
	Sounds.	When uttered.	Sounds.	When uttered.
First few days	ä, ähä	In crying.		
0;2			ähä, erre	After a feed; or when being played with.
0;3				Trains of "Lallen" began to appear.
0;5			a, dadada	In the course of "Lallen".
0;7	äbuä, uwä, papapa	In discomfort. The last-named group of sounds were rare	bababa, dadada, tä tä tä, äbuä, hä, pu, papapa	In the course of "Lallen".
			pupupu	In the course of play.
0;8	mamama, mememmem	These sounds appeared during illness, when the child was crying.		
0;9			da	Had learnt to use this in game of hiding his face.
0;11,14			papa	Seemed to utter this on seeing his father; Stern is doubtful.

HOYER'S SON

Age.	When in a state of discomfort.		When in a state of comfort.	
	Sounds.	When uttered.	Sounds.	When uttered.
Immediately after birth	â	While crying.		
0;0,11	uâ, uâ (u consonantal)	,, ,,		
0;0,21	â	In hunger.		
	uâ; also nasalised	In pain.		
	mãã, nasalised	In discomfort.		
0;1,20			Bilabial r, with organs relaxed	In a state of comfort.
			ğ	,, ,,
0;3,0	m	While crying	ağğ	,, ,,
			ma	In milder comfort.
0;4,28			ğ	With joyful expression on face, on seeing parent.
0;5,8			b, p, g, m; accompanied by vowels	In comfort.
0;6,3			a (long drawn out)	Expressive of pleasure.
			Beginning of repetitive chains	

HOYER'S SON (*continued*)

Age.	When in a state of discomfort.		When in a state of comfort.	
	Sounds.	When uttered.	Sounds.	When uttered.
0;7,22			am am am	On seeing that his rice was sprinkled with sugar.
0;7,24	awa awa	Usually followed by weeping.		
0;9,24	ááá, with distinctive intonation	When a person he needs is not forthcoming.		
0;10,13			daí (adult word *daj* means "give")	Expressive of mild desire for an object.
0;10,20			kxxx	Expressive of wonder at something novel.
0;10,31			tata or t'ai	When tearing something, with pleasure.
			kxxx	When he sees the floor being swept.
0;11,20			prrr (bilabial)	When pulling at a string.
0;11,27			tam (adult word *tam* means "there")	When asked where an object is; points.

THE BOY, K

Age.	When in a state of discomfort.		When in a state of comfort.	
	Sounds.	When uttered.	Sounds.	When uttered.
0;0,14	ŭɛ ŭɛ, ɛ, a, ŭa, lɛ	All heard in course of crying.		
0;1,10			ga (once only, doubtful)	After a feed.
0;1,11–13	le, lɛ, la, ne, nɛ, na, ŋe, ŋɛ, ŋa	In the course of crying; or while he was being washed.		
0;1,14			g (occasionally)	Lying on his mother's lap, quite comfortable after a feed.
0;1,20			g (repeated about 12 times, at intervals of about 2 secs.)	On his mother's lap after a feed.
0;1,27			g (preceded or followed by a vowel)	After a feed. Makes many other grunting sounds.
0;2,2	ɛ, ŭɛ, ŋɛ, lɛ, jɛ, jɛ, ŭa, ŋɛ, ja, la	In various states of discomfort	g rather more palatal, almost j / r palatal	After a feed; other grunting sounds.
0;2,3			As above, continuous for about 20 mins.	After a feed, lying in his cot.
0;2,6			ələ, ŭɛ, ɛə, xɛ	After a feed. Also a number of silent lip-movements.

THE BOY, K (continued)

Age.	When in a state of discomfort.		When in a state of comfort.	
	Sounds.	When uttered.	Sounds.	When uttered.
0;2,10			ŋgɑi, ai, ga, ɛɛ, ɡɛɡɛ, ge, gi, gɛi	After a feed; [also lip-movements.
0;2,12	ŋgɛ̃, nɛ̃	While crying at night.		
0;2,20			ɛɛɛ, ɡɛɡɛ	After a feed.
0;3,21		No new sounds observed during this month	Chains of "babbling", often with variety of intonation, giving a tune *	After a feed.
0;4,0		No new sounds observed during this month	Chains of babbling, as above	After a feed.
0;4,2			ɛɛɛ, staccato cries, with "happy" intonation	When his mother approaches him.
0;5,1			bub bub, repeated about 12 times	After a feed.
0;5,2			ppp, as a "burred" lip-sound, repeated several times	After a feed.
0;5,4			bub, bub ; p p	After a feed.
0;5,6	bub	In course of crying, while being washed.		
0;5,7			ha (twice) very guttural	After a feed.

* This was the first occurrence of repetitive chains of babbling: I had made a special note of their absence at 0;1,27, at 0;2,20, at 0;2,24 and at 0;3,12.

THE BOY, K (*continued*)

Age.	When in a state of discomfort.		When in a state of comfort.	
	Sounds.	When uttered.	Sounds.	When uttered.
0:5,13			m m m, during a chain of babbling	After a feed.
Seventh month and eighth month	No observations at all were made during these two months.			
0:8,20	mammam, m m m	When he *mildly* lacks something (in a tone of mild distress)	mammam, in the course of babbling	When quite comfortable.
0:8,26	axa, æ æ, æxæ, mæm mæm, mʌm	Crying, when in a state of discomfort.		
0:8,28			axa, axa, mæm mæm, mʌmi. In course of babbling	After a feed.
0:8,29			dada, merely articulated, but in a whisper	Seizing his father's finger.
0:9,3			mʌm mʌm, bæ bæ, also burring lip-sounds	When comfortable. When playing.
0:9,6			mʌmmam, in a very contented tone	Lying in his mother's arms, looking up at her.
0:9,7			mama, ə ə ə, gəgə	Comfortable, after a feed.
0:9,8			papa,† mama merely articulated, not uttered aloud	When sitting alone, quite comfortable ; playing.

† *Note on* papa. It is tolerably certain that this word was never heard by the child before he began to use it himself, and quite certain that nobody about him used it as a name for his father. As soon as he had uttered it, his parents decided to continue not to say it ; nevertheless he uttered it several times subsequently, once or twice with apparent reference to his father. The word had disappeared from the child's speech by the end of his first year.

I.S.

R

THE BOY, K (*continued*)

Age.	When in a state of discomfort.		When in a state of comfort.	
	Sounds.	When uttered.	Sounds.	When uttered.
0;9,9	məmə, alternating with brief cries of a a a	When evidently very uncomfortable	mama, mɛmɛ, in course of babbling. papa, in a whisper. pr, br, bɛ, jə, ŋə, in course of babbling	Quite contented. Reaching out towards his father. Before falling asleep, threshing about in his cot.
0;9,16	mʌm mʌm	Several times, in tone of discomfort, followed by weeping	baba, papa, aaa, with characteristic "crowing" intonation	When quite comfortable. When pleased.
0;9,29			mamama	In play, while reaching for his ball.
0;10,4			aaa, in tone of delight	When seeing someone of whom he is fond.
0;10,5			papa, whispered	On being taken up by his father.
0;10,18			dada, repeated several times	When lying comfortably in his cot.
0;10,28-29	aaa, in a tone of slight distress a, loudly, in a tone of rage	When trying to get at his toy dog, which was beyond his reach. When reprimanded.		
0;11,0	No new sounds recorded		No new sounds recorded.	

SOUNDS UTTERED IN IMMEDIATE IMITATION BY CHILDREN DURING THE FIRST YEAR

TABULATED FROM DATA IN STERN (KSp), HOYER (LK), GUILLAUME (IE),
VALENTINE (PI) ; TOGETHER WITH THE WRITER'S OWN RECORD OF K

(C = Child ; M = Mother ; F = Father ; A = Adult)

HILDE STERN

Age.	General Progress.	Imitation, or similar behaviour.		
		Circumstances.	Adult.	Child.
1¼ mths.	Said *krä krä* in state of comfort.			
2 ,,	Said *erre erre* in state of comfort.			
2½ ,,		C silent in contented mood	erre erre	erre erre.
2¾ ,,		As above	krä krä	krä krä.
		(Stern says that, in general, imitation lapses after these early responses ; KSp 162.)		
7½ ,,		Similarly for longer strings of these sounds	hä hähä	hä. hähä.
8 ,,		C lying contentedly in cradle	papa	p . . . p . .
		On one occasion, above episode was followed by *Lallen*, in which C said *papapa*. When A again spoke to C, correct imitation occurred :	papa	papa.
8¼ ,,		This kind of conversation (*Unterhaltung*) could be carried on for several minutes.	a or ä	Similar sound.
9 ,,			High-pitched whistle	High-pitched shriek.

HOYER'S SON

Age.	General progress.	Imitation, or similar behaviour.		
		Circumstances.	Adult.	Child.
1st wk.	C smiled when contented.			
3rd ,,	C crying : A spoke to him, and he ceased crying.			
0;1,23			Smiled	Smiled.
0;1,24		Hoyer refers to this as *Nachahmung*	Smiled and spoke	Smiled and spoke.
0;2,0		Sounds chosen from C's repertory. This kind of imitation persisted for about a month, then lapsed	au, g, ă	Somewhat similar sounds.
0;8,10		C did this frequently and gleefully	â â â	Similar sounds.
		For several weeks after this, when sounds were made to C, he watched mouth of A, but remained silent as a rule. When he did reply, his sounds were unlike those of A. If the sounds were drawn from his own repertory, often responded with similar ones.		
0;9,26		Imitation of this kind ; not very frequent	mama papa	papa. t'at'a.
0;10		Imitation still not frequent or accurate.		
0;11		Imitation increasingly frequent and accurate		

GUILLAUME'S SON

Age.	General progress.	Imitation, or similar behaviour.		
		Circumstances.	Adult.	Child.
0;0,4	General movements in response to sounds.			
0;0,5	Turning of head in response to sounds.			
0;2,0			Spoke	Spoke.
0;2,11–19		Sounds from C's own repertory	ghe, pou, re When A repeated sounds, C responded similarly.	Fixed his eyes on A; smiled.
0;2,20		Conditions as in last entry : but on one occasion C replied as follows :	pou	re.
0;2,23		Conditions as in last two entries, but very difficult to obtain vocal response from C. This difficulty persisted for about six weeks.		
0;3,2	C showed some recognition of a familiar voice.			
0;3,15	C turned to F on hearing *papa*.			
0;3,21	C responded by laughter to conversation of A.s.			
0;3,22		M spoke to C	papapa	Looked at speaker; made silent lip movements.

GUILLAUME'S SON (*continued*)

Age.	General progress.	Imitation, or similar behaviour.		
		Circumstances.	Adult.	Child.
0;3,24		C's intonation re-sembles A's	papa	a.
0;3,30			A singing	Responded with varied noises.
0;4,0		Sounds from C's reper-tory. C also imi-tated sound of a kiss	ata, atita	Similar sounds.
			Piano played	Made noises.
0;4,10		Response to A sing-ing, as 0;3,30.		
0;4,17			Spoke	Silent lip-move-ments.
0;4,22		As in last entry.		
0;5,0			bô	Similar sound.
0;5,2	Spontaneously said *atita*, *titit*, with some effort.			
0;5,6		These were sounds adopted by A from C's repertory.	ata, ta, atita	Similar sounds.
		Sound not yet in C's repertory	pa	Silent lip-move-ments.

No further systematic observations are given, but Guillaume makes the generalisation (IE 36) that vocal imitation does not clearly appear until the end of the first year.

VALENTINE'S SON, B

Age.	General progress.	Imitation, or similar behaviour.		
		Circumstances.	Adult.	Child.
0;0,15	" Suggestion of mouth opening in response to mine," but this may have been a coincidence.			
0;1,2 (32nd day)		Results of test : number of " croons " spoken by C per minute, with and without stimulus of croon by M :		

Results of test : number of " croons " spoken by C per minute, with and without stimulus of croon by M :

Minutes.	Without stimulus.	With stimulus.
1st . .	8	—
2nd . .	5	—
3rd . .	—	12
4th . .	—	9
5th . .	2	—
6th . .	0	—

Here B began to cry for food.

Age.	General progress.	Circumstances.	Adult.	Child.
0;1,4 (34th day)		Above experiment repeated : 1st ½ minute (without stimulus)—no response. 2nd ½ minute (with stimulus)—5 croons. Here the test was interrupted.		
0;1,8 (38th day)		This occurred about 20 times ; A's coo set C cooing repeatedly.	ar-roo	Similar sound.
0;1,9 (39th day)		C lying silent. A's coo sets C cooing rapidly for 2 or 3 minutes, smiling occasionally	ar-roo	Similar sound.
0;3,10 (100th day)		" During last week or two, if not much earlier, I believe smiles have led to smiles."		

VALENTINE'S SON, B *(continued)*

Age.	General progress.	Imitation, or similar behaviour.		
		Circumstances.	Adult.	Child.
0;3,25 (115th day)		C laughed in response to laugh of M or F.		
0;6,0		Valentine says that, in general, we obtain about this time " the attempt to imitate a particular sound or word, and not the mere making of any sound in response to sound ".		
0;7,3 (213th day)	C had said *da-da* distinctly during two previous days	On three occasions within an hour	da-da	da-da in a faint whisper.
0;7,7 (217th day)		C looked at A with great interest : imitation occurred after interval of 5 or 6 secs. Four times in all, at intervals of 5 to 7 secs. " This speaking seems quite different from his babbling, it is so deliberate, so suggestive of effort."	da-da ba-ba	da-da. da-da.
0;7,20 (230th day)		Test described in last entry failed.		
0;11,24 (354th day)		If A utters this at short intervals (2 or 3 secs.) C does not imitate. 5 or more secs. must be left for imitation to occur.	bow-wow	bow-wow.

Note.—Valentine gives the child's age in days ; for comparison with other records I have counted 30 days to a month.

OBSERVATIONS OF THE BOY, K

Age.	General progress.	Imitation, or similar behaviour.		
		Circumstances.	Adult.	Child.
0;1,10	By this time was smiling at A.s familiar to him.			
0;1,14	Says **g** in state of comfort.			
0;2,16	Smiles in response to A's smile.	F smiled and said : *Note.*—No response at all to word without smile, or unless C's eye is caught.	hullo	**lɔu** (not very certain).
0;2,19		C lying comfortable after feed, smiling. Results of experiment. Number of sounds made by him spontaneously and in response to F's word *hullo*, said at intervals of 10 counted.		
		Without stimulus of *hullo*. With stimulus.		
		1st min. . 2 sounds 2nd min. . 6 sounds 3rd ,, . 0 ,, 4th ,, . 5 ,, 5th ,, . 2 ,, 6th ,, . 7 ,, At end of 6th min. C seemed tired, cried a little. *Note.*—(i) *Hullo* was said with smile in each case. (ii) C's eye had to be caught. (iii) C's own sounds were nothing like *hullo*. (iv) Ten minutes later, F said *hullo* to C several times ; no response.		
0;2,20		F smiles, and says :	hullo, or one of C's own sounds	Sometimes responds with sound of his own.
		Note.—(i) C *never* responds to word unaccompanied by smile. (ii) *Never* unless his eye is caught.		
0;2,24		F smiles, and says :	hullo	Responds with own sound, sometimes repeatedly.

OBSERVATIONS OF THE BOY, K (*continued*)

Age.	General progress.	Imitation or similar behaviour.		
		Circumstances.	Adult.	Child.
0;3,12		C lying comfortable on F's knee after a feed	(i) Smiles (ii) Smiles and says **gu** (iii) **gu** without smile (iv) Smiles, lips in position for **gu**, no voice	(i) Smiles. (ii) Says **ŭɛ.** (iii) No response. (iv) Says **ŭɛ.**
0;3,22	Although previously tested many times, this is the first occasion when C responds to F's voice when he is out of sight, by ceasing to cry.			
0;4,2	Marked increase of response to presence of M; especially at feed-times. C stretches out arms and says ɛ ɛ ɛ	F does not smile, but says:	F smiles hullo	Smiles. No response.
0;4,4	C ceases to cry, on hearing voice of F; as in 0;3,22.			
0;4,18		F makes these sounds, from C's own repertory, with or without smile, after C's feeding-time. When any response occurs it does not resemble F's sound	ɛ, ŋɛ, ɛgɛ	Usually no response.
0;4,26		Observations as in last entry.		
0;5,1	C says **bub-bub** in babbling	When C is babbling, F says: This is repeated with other sounds from C's repertory; no response	**bub-bub**	No response.

OBSERVATIONS OF THE BOY, K (*continued*)

Age.	General progress.	Imitation or similar behaviour.		
		Circumstances.	Adult.	Child.
0;5,4	C says **p,p** in babbling	M smiles and says : C merely looks back at her	**m-m-m ;** **bub-bub ;** **p,p**	No response. ,, ,,
0;5,6		C lying comfortable. F says : M says :	**bub ; ε ;** **gε ; ŋε.** **bub,** 30 times	No response. One response.
0;5,14 to 0;8,20		No definite observations during this period. On latter date, M smiles and says :	cuckoo	Smiles only.
0;8,28	C says **dada** when comfortable	F later says : C merely looks back intently	**dada**	No response.
0;9,5	C's definite response to *No !*			
0;9,6	Waves hand in response to *Say Goodbye !*			
0;9,6 to 0;10,23	Responds suitably to : *ballie, daddy, nannan,* etc.			
0;10,23	Brushes his hair with a hair-brush.			
0;10,29	Responds appropriately to *doggie*			
1;0,0		M says : This happened five out of six times.	**bø**	**bø.**
1;0,1		M says :	**bø** **gø**	**bø.** **mø.**
1;0,5		M says :	**bø, ba**	Similar sounds.
1;0,6		M says : In both cases, test repeated six times	**ba** **bu-bu-bu**	**ma.** **bø-bø.**

OBSERVATIONS OF THE BOY, K (*continued*)

Age.	General progress.	Imitation or similar behaviour.		
		Circumstances.	Adult.	Child.
1;0,15		M speaking to C	bø gø gø dø	bø bø gø (3 times). dø (8 times).
1;1,8		M says : C accompanies his response with usual hiding movement	Peep-bo	ɛbo.
1;1,11		C was being undressed. He said : Whereupon A said : But further attempts by A brought no response	 Peeky-bo.	ɛbɔ. iːkibɔ.
1;1,15		M said : C turned in direction of F while saying this	Where's Daddy ?	dada, dada.
1;1,20	F put cloth over C's head, who pulled it off, saying iːpba.			

APPENDIX III

THE DEVELOPMENT OF FORM

1. CHILDREN'S EARLIEST WORDS:

the first (up to six) given in each case by Stern (KSp 172), together with those of Hilde and Günther Stern (KSp 18,85), and those of K

Observer.	Child's form.	Adult form or meaning.
Stern (Hilde) . . .	papa	Papa.
	mama	Mama.
	didda	tik-tak.
	dedda	Berta.
	hilde	Hilde.
	puppe	Puppe.
Stern (Günther) . .	mama	Mama.
	papa	Papa.
	da	da.
	ta ta	ta ta.
	puppe	Puppe.
	das	das.
Stern (Eva) . . .	āta	Vater.
	papa	Puppe.
	hap	hap.
	wauwau	wauwau.
Preyer	hatta	hatta.
	da	da.
	papa	Papa.
	bät	bitte.
	dakkn	danke.
Ament	mammamm	Mama.
	deda	Tante.
	li	Willi.
	mra	Irma.
Lindner . . . . (daughter)	papa	Papa.
	mama	Mama.
	auf	auf.
Lindner . . . . (son)	mm	(noise of cart).
	da	da.
	bap	(for various food).
	gack	Gasse.

253

1. CHILDREN'S EARLIEST WORDS (*continued*)

Observer.	Child's form.	Adult form or meaning.
Idelberger	dada baba ada obba wauwau	(cry of pleasure). Vater. (going out). hoch*gehoben*. wauwau.
Tögel	de baba babap wauwau obala	da. Vater. (food). wauwau. (when lifted).
Stumpf	papn-mapn kn ⎫ gagn ⎭ ha tn	(food). (signs of satisfaction). (addressing a bird). (" out ! ").
Schneider . . . . (daughter S)	da mē mē	(pointing). mehr ! mehr !
Schneider . . . . (daughter F)	da take take ida bitte	danke ! (dancing). Ida. bitte.
Strümpell	adē ssi-ssi	adieu ! (tea-urn).
Sander	dida wauwau	tik-tak. wauwau.
Meringer . . . . (daughter G)	baun	bauen.
Meringer . . . . (son J)	ba bu huhu	Ball. Blumen. Hund.
Meringer . . . . (daughter M)	ama dada awa wawa äbl	Mama. da. Wasser. weh. Säbel.
Oltuscewski . . .	papa njanja daj pa ta nie	(eating). (nursemaid). daj (give). (good-bye). (yes). (no).

1. CHILDREN'S EARLIEST WORDS (*continued*)

Observer.	Child's form.	Adult form or meaning.
Gheorgov . . . . (son 1)	dza	daj (give).
	fa	pfui.
	lea	chleb (bread).
	ča	čaj (tea).
Gheorgov . . . . (son 2)	de	(in play).
	ade	adieu !
	di	(addressing a horse).
	zj zj	(It is hot !).
	boc	(to poke).
Shinn	da	there !
	nanana	(cry of protest).
	mamama	(mother).
	mgm	(all gone !).
	kha	(cry of disgust).
Major	hi	(expression of longing).
	babee	(child himself).
	titit	(hearing the clock).
	baw	ball.
	ack	hat.
Deville	papa	papa.
	mama	mama.
	non non	non.
	oua oua	oua oua.
Rasmussen . . .	mama	mad (food).
	ar	far (father).
	buar	mor (mother).
	wauwau	wauwau.
Pavlovitch	mama	mama.
	tata	(father).
	bébé	(reflection in a mirror).
	baba	(grandmother).
	ett	Rosette (dog).
K.	**mammamm**	(When mildly lacking something ; later for mother.)
	nænæ	(looking at maid).
	dada	dada (father).
	ɛbɔ	Peep-bo !
	kæke	cakie.

2. ANALYSIS OF CHILDREN'S EARLIEST WORDS

Observer.	Total number.	Containing		Others.	Polysyllabic words.		Mono-syllabic words.
		only front cons.	one front cons.		Redupli-cated.	Non-redupli-cated.	
Stern 1 . . .	6	5	1	0	5	1	0
,, 2 . . .	6	5	1	0	4	0	2
,, 3 . . .	4	3	1	0	2	0	2
Preyer . . .	5	3	2	0	1	2	2
Ament . . .	4	2	1	1	2	1	1
Lindner 1 . .	3	3	0	0	2	0	1
,, 2 . .	4	3	0	1	0	0	4
Idelberger . .	5	5	0	0	3	2	0
Tögel . . .	5	4	1	0	3	1	1
Stumpf . . .	5	2	0	3	1	1	3
Schneider 1 . .	2	2	0	0	1	0	1
,, 2 . .	4	3	1	0	1	2	1
Strümpell . .	2	1	0	1	1	1	0
Sander . . .	2	2	0	0	2	0	0
Meringer 1 . .	1	1	0	0	0	0	1
,, 2 . .	3	2	0	1	1	0	2
,, 3 . .	5	4	1	0	2	3	0
Oltuscewski . .	6	5	1	0	2	0	4
Gheorgov 1 . `.	4	3	0	1	0	0	4
,, 2 . .	5	3	1	1	1	0	4
Shinn . . .	5	3	1	1	2	1	2
Major . . .	5	3	0	2	2	0	3
Deville . . .	4	4	0	0	4	0	0
Rasmussen . .	4	2	1	1	2	1	1
Pavlovitch . .	5	5	0	0	4	0	1
K	6	5	0	1	4	0	2
Total	110	83	13	14	52	16	42
Percentage . .	100	75	12	13	46	15	39

3. EXAMPLES OF EARLY FRONT-CONSONANT FORMS

Meaning.	Form.	Adult language.	Reference.
Mother	mama	English French German, etc.	
	babab	German	Ament SD 78.
Nurse	amme	German	
	nana	English	
	njanja	Slavonic	Oltuscewski GE 21.
	bäbe	German	Ament SD 79.
	tété	French	Taine AL 254.
	dedda	German	Stern KSp 19.
Aunt	muhme	German	
	deda	German	Ament SD 79.
Grandmother. . . .	amma	Scandinavian	Jespersen ND 155.
	baba	Slavonic	Oltuscewski GE 21.
Food	mum	English	Darwin BI 293.
	mem	German	Stern KSp 356.
	mama	German	Preyer SK 307.
	am	French	Taine AL 257.
	nana	French	Stern KSp 357.
	pap	English	
	papa	Slavonic	Oltuscewski GE 21.
		German	Stumpf EE 7.
	wawa	English	Keller SL 7.
Bed, sleep	nana	Spanish	Jespersen ND 159.
	nanna	Italian	Jespersen ND 159.
	bye-bye	English	
	baba	German	Stern KSp 373.
	teitei	German	Stern KSp 373.
	dodo	French	Deville ND.
Father	papa	English French German, etc.	
	baba	German	Idelberger KS.
	tata	Slavonic	Hoyer LK.
	dada	English, etc.	
Ball	ba, baw	English German	Major FS 319. Meringer LS 212.
Clock	titta		K.
	didda	German	Stern KSp 18.

3. EXAMPLES OF EARLY FRONT-CONSONANT FORMS (*continued*)

Meaning.	Form.	Adult language.	Reference.
Dog	wauwau oua-oua bow-wow	German French English	Deville ND 340.
Pointing	tatta da tem	German English German French	Stern KSp 366. Shinn BB 225. Stern KSp 174. Taine AL 254.
Giving	da dsa daj	English Slavonic Slavonic	 Gheorgov AA 335. Gheorgov AA 336.
Thanking	nana ta da	English English English German	Tracy LC 120. Stern KSp 174.
Going out	pa tata haita ade dada	French German Slavonic English German, etc. Slavonic Slavonic German German	Deville ND. Preyer SK 363. Oltuscewski GE 21. Preyer SK 308. Kenyeres PM 194. Oltuscewski GE 20. Ament SD 85. Stern KSp 369.

4. NOTE ON THE CLASSIFICATION OF CONSONANTS

The consonants of English, French and German do not fall into clearly-defined groups—apart from the obvious class of labials and labio-dentals. The classification of the rest must depend partly upon the portion of the tongue used, partly upon the portion of the roof of the mouth touched or approached by it : the quality of the sound articulated is influenced by both of these factors.

In the following classification I have arranged into five main groups the many smaller classes recognised by phoneticians, e.g. Pillsbury and Meader : *The Psychology of Language* (1928) ; and G. N. Armfield : *General Phonetics* (1931).

Group.	Sounds.	How formed.
I. Labials and Labio-dentals	p, b, m, w, ɥ (French), f, v	Lip against lip, and teeth against lip.
II. Tip-dental . . .	t, d, n, ɲ, θ, ð, ts, tʃ, dʒ	Tip of tongue against teeth (or gum-ridge).
III. Tip-alveolar (rolled and lateral)	l; r (English)	Tip of tongue against gum-ridge (with modification for rolled or lateral formation).
IV. (a) Blade-alveolar palatal (sibilants)	s, ʃ, z, ʒ	Blade of tongue against gum-ridge, front of tongue raised towards palate.
(b) Blade-palatal .	j; c (German)	Blade of tongue against hard palate.
V. Back-palatal (and uvular and glottal)	k, g, x, ŋ ; R (uvular, French and German); h	Back of tongue against soft palate or uvula ; also h made in glottis.

These again may be classified into three broader groups :

Front (groups, I, II) : Lip, lip-teeth, and tip of tongue against teeth.

Middle (groups III, IV) : Tip or blade of tongue against gum-ridge or hard palate.

Back (group V) : Back of tongue against soft palate ; also uvular and glottal.

5. RELATION BETWEEN CHILD'S AND CONVENTIONAL CONSONANTS

Note.—The sounds (in the second column) are given in phonetic symbols : the words as recorded by the observer. Figures after sounds : 1 = initial, 2 = medial, 3 = final.

HILDE STERN

Age.	Sound.	I. Attempted adult form (child's form in brackets).	II. In use.	III. Successfully imitated.	Total No. I.	II.	III.
0;10	t 1	tiktak (didda)					
	t 2	tiktak (didda)					
	d 1		didda				
	d 2		didda		2	2	0
0;11	p 1	puppe	puppe	puppe			
	p 2	puppe	puppe	puppe			
	b 1	Berta (dedda)	bu	bu			
	d 2	Hilde		Hilde			
	h 1	Hilde	Hilde	Hilde	7	6	5
1;0	b 2	baba	baba	baba			
	m 1	mama	mama	mama			
	m 2	mama	mama	mama	10	9	8
1;1					10	9	8
1;2	v 1	wauwau	wauwau	wauwau			
	v 2	wauwau	wauwau	wauwau			
	s 1	ss-ss	ss-ss	ss-ss	13	12	11
1;3	ps 3	knaps (atzatz)					
	ts 2		atzatz				
	ts 3		atzatz				
	tsv 2	eins-zwei (eischei)					
	l 2	Paula (ala)	ala	ala			
	s 2	assa	assa	assa			
	ʃ 2		eischei				
	k 1	kuh (muh)			18	17	13
1;4	p 3	pip pip	pip pip	pip pip			
	n 3	morgen (mon)	mon	mon			
	t 2	bitte	bitte	bitte			
	tʃ 1		tschetsche				
	tʃ 2	etsch etsch (tschetsche)	tschetsche	tschetsche			
	tʃ 3	etsch etsch (tschetsche)					
	r 3	hier	hier	hier			
	j 2		kille				
	k 1		kikiki	kikiki			
	k 2	kikiki	kikiki	kikiki			
	k 3	quack-quack (gagack)	gagack	gagack			

5. RELATION BETWEEN CHILD'S AND CONVENTIONAL CONSONANTS (*continued*)

Age.	Sound.	I. Attempted adult form (child's form in brackets).	II. In Use.	III. Successfully imitated.	Total No. I.	II.	III.
1;4 (*con.*)	g 1		gagack				
	g 2		gagack				
	kw 1	quack-quack (gagack)					
	kw 2	quack-quack (gagack)			28	29	21
1;5	f 1	Fuss (fu)	fu	fu			
	ps 2	hepsi (ssi)					
	t 3	putput	putput	putput			
	ts 2	Katze (mitze)		mitze			
	z 1	so	so	so			
	g 2	Auge		auge	34	32	26
1;6	pf 2	Apfel (apfe)	apfe	apfe			
	fl 1	Flasche (fasche)					
	c 2	pichel	pichel	pichel			
	c 3	Milch (milss)					
	t 1		talj	tir			
	d 1	didelideli		didelideli			
	n 1	nasse	nasse	nasse			
	l 1	Lampe	lampe	lampe			
	l 3		nickel				
	j 1	ja	ja	ja			
	s 3	das	das	das			
	ʃ 2	Flasche (fasche)		fasche			
	ʃ 3	Fleisch (feisch)	feisch	feisch			
	ʃl 1	Schlüssel (schlüchel)	schlüchel	schlüchel			
	ʃt 1	Stuhl (stulj)	stulj	stulj			
	ʃt 2	Bürste (bösche)					
	g 3	Tag	tag	tag	49	44	39
1;7	m 3	Arm (ahm)	ahm	ahm			
	f 2	offen (offe)	offe	offe			
	pf 1	pfui (feu)					
	ps 1		psi				
	ps 3		ziepzieps	ziepzieps			
	bl 1	Blume (psi)					
	d 3	Kind	kind	kind			
	n 2	Kind	kind	kind			
	ts 1	ziepzieps	ziepzieps	ziepzieps			
	ts 3	butz		butz			
	l 3	Ball	ball	ball			
	r 1	rrrr	rrrr	rrrr			
	r 2	Garnrolle (kulle)					
	z 2	Gemüse (miesse)					
	ʃ 1	Schuhe (schuä)	schuä	schuä			
	x 2	Kuchen (kuchel)	kuchel	kuchel			
	x 3	Buch	buch	buch			
	kn 1	Knopf (nat)					
	kr 1	Kragen (kaje)			66	55	51

5. RELATION BETWEEN CHILD'S AND CONVENTIONAL
CONSONANTS (*continued*)

Age.	Sound.	I. Attempted adult form (child's form in brackets).	II. In Use.	III. Successfully imitated.	Total No. I.	II.	III.
1;8	ps 2		papsel	papsel			
	tr 1	trinken (tinke)					
	r 2		ferdele	ferdele			
	g 1	gute		gute			
	ŋ 2	Klingling (gingging)	gingging	gingging			
	ŋ 3	Klingling (gingging)	gingging	gingging			
	kl 1	Klingling (gingging)			71	59	56
1;9	f 3	Muff	muff	muff			
	pf 3	Kopf (kupp)					
	br 1	Brust (busst)					
	tsv 1	zwei (ssei)					
	dr 1	drei (dei)					
	nts 3	Schwanz (fatz)					
	sl 1		slafe				
	st 2	Fenster (finzer)					
	st 3	Brust (busst)	busst	busst			
	ʃp 1	Spiegel (pickel)					
	ʃv 1	Schwanz (fatz)					
	ʃr 1	Schreibe (scheischeibe)					
	gr 1	Gretchen (gĕtzen)			83	62	58
1;10	tj 2		atje				
	dj 2	adieu (atje)					
	z 2		läsen	läsen			
	ʃm 1	Schmutz (mutz)					
	ʃn 1	Schnee (nee)					
	ʃr 2	ein Schreck (n'scheck)					
	ks 3	knix (nix)	nix	nix			
	gl 1	Glocken (luck'n)			89	65	60

DEVILLE'S DAUGHTER [1]

Age.	Sound.	I. Attempted adult form (child's form in brackets).	II. In use.	III. Successfully imitated.	Total No. I.	II.	III.
0;9	w 1	oua-oua	oua-oua	oua-oua			
	w 2	oua-oua	oua-oua	oua-oua	2	2	2
0;10					2	2	2

[1] The child's forms are in Littre's system of notation, as given by Deville.

5. RELATION BETWEEN CHILD'S AND CONVENTIONAL CONSONANTS (*continued*)

Age.	Sound.	I. Attempted adult form (child's form in brackets).	II. In use.	III. Successfully imitated.	Total No. I.	II.	III.
0;11	p 1	papa	papa	papa			
	p 2	papa	papa	papa			
	m 1	mama	mama	mama			
	m 2	mama	mama	mama			
	n 1	non	non	non	7	7	7
1;0	t 2	atata	atata	atata	8	8	8
1;1	b 1	bam	bam	bam	9	9	9
1;2	t 1		ta				
	s 2	merci (si)	si	si			
	ʃ 1	Charles (ta)					
	ʃ 2		chi (merci)				
	k 1	coucou (toutou)					
	k 2	coucou (toutou)			13	12	10
1;3	b 2	bébé	bébé	bébé			
	m 3	pomme (pom)	pom	pom			
	f 2	café (tata)					
	d 1	dodo	dodo	dodo			
	d 2	dodo	dodo	dodo			
	n 2	domino	domino	domino			
	ɲ 2	oignon (nomon)					
	l 1	la (na)					
	j 2	crayon (o-i-o)	o-i-o	o-i-o	22	18	16
1;4	p 3	hop	hop	hop			
	f 1	fichu (pipu)					
	f 3	ouf	ouf	ouf			
	pj 1	pied (pé)					
	pl 2	parapluie (pi)					
	br 1	brosse (bo)					
	bw 1	boire (ba)					
	t 1	torchon (toton)		toton			
	t 3	porte (popo)					
	n 3	chausson (toton)	toton	toton			
	tr 1	trou (tou)					
	nj 1		niénié				
	nj 2	panier (niénié)	niénié	niénié			
	l 1		l'eau	l'eau			
	r 1		r				
	s 1	sécher (tété)					
	s 3	tasse (tata)					
	z 1		zou (jouer)				
	z 2	musique (moni)					
	ʃ 2	sécher (tété)					
	g 1	Guesde (ghé)	ghé	ghé			
	h 1	hop	hop	hop			
	kl 1	clef (tété)					
	kr 1	crochet (kr)	kr	kr	41	28	24

5. RELATION BETWEEN CHILD'S AND CONVENTIONAL CONSONANTS (*continued*)

Age.	Sound.	I. Attempted adult form (child's form in brackets).	II. In use.	III. Successfully imitated.	Total No.		
					I.	II.	III.
1;5	l 2	lolo	lolo	lolo			
	r 2	Marie (ma-i)					
	g 2	Gugusse (gugu)	gugu	gugu	44	30	26
1;6	v 1	verre (ve)	vize	ve			
	pj 2	papier (papé)					
	pl 1	pleut (peu)					
	pw 1	poisson (paton)					
	fl 1	fleur (peu)					
	fr 1	fraise (te)					
	vr 1	vrai (ve)					
	dj 1	Dieu (deu)					
	r 1	radis (dadis)					
	z 3	Louise (vize)	vize	vize			
	ʒ 1	Jules	Jules	Jules			
	ʒ 2	bougie (bodzi)					
	sj 2	assiette (tate)					
	sp 2	asperge (apè)					
	kɥ 1	cuillère (boié)			59	33	29
1;7	pr 1	prêter (pe)					
	bw 1		boiia				
	bl 1	blanc (ba)					
	mw 2	tramway (mame)					
	vj 2	serviette (baje)					
	vw 1	voilà (boiia)					
	vw 2	revoir (ava)					
	tr 2	entrer (ate)					
	ʒ 2		abajou	abajou			
	sk 2	biscuit (beti)					
	ʃw 2	mouchoir (pata)					
	kl 2	éclair (te)			69	35	30
1;8	f 1		fin	fin			
	f 2		afin	afin			
	br 2	embrasser (apaté)					
	mj 2	lumière (mè)					
	vj 1	viande (van)					
	tj 1	tien (tian)	tian	tian			
	tw 1	toi (ta)					
	dr 1	drapeau (papô)					
	nw 1	noir (na)					
	nw 2	entonnoir (ana)					
	ɲ 1		gnognon				
	ɲ 2	oignon (gnognon)	gnognon	gnognon			
	sɥ 2	essuyer (afi)					
	gr 1	grand (da)					
	gɥ 2	aiguille (vi)			81	40	34

5. RELATION BETWEEN CHILD'S AND CONVENTIONAL
CONSONANTS (*continued*)

Age.	Sound.	I. Attempted adult form (child's form in brackets).	II. In use.	III. Successfully imitated	Total No. I.	II.	III.
1;9	pr 2						
	mj 2	après (apè)	mié	mié			
	mw 1	moineau (mano)					
	fw 1	fois (fa)					
	vr 2	ouvrir (avi)					
	dj 1		Dieu	Dieu			
	dj 2	adieu	adieu	adieu			
	rj 1	rien (ie)					
	sw 1	soif (fa)					
	ʃj 1	chien (tie)			89	43	37
1;10	pj 2		papie	papie			
	pw 1		poi	poi			
	vw 1		voi				
	d 3	amande (amam)					
	dr 2	André (ade)					
	ɲ 3	cygne (sim)					
	rw 2	tiroir (voi)					
	s 1		sose				
	ʃ 1		chaché				
	ʃ 2			chaché			
	ʃ 3	manche (mam)					
	sj 2		matasion	matasion			
	k 1		ki (crier)				
	kr 2	écrire (ti)			95	50	41
1;11	b 3		diab				
	bj 1	bien	bien	bien			
	bl 1		bleu	bleu			
	bl 2	table (tab)					
	bw 1			boi			
	mw 2		amoi	amoi			
	vj 1		vieux	vieux			
	vw 1			voilà			
	vw 2		avoi	avoi			
	dw 1	doit (doi)	doi	doi			
	tr 3	quatre (tat)					
	z 2		beze	beze			
	ʃ 1			chao			
	zw 2	besoin (bezan)					
	k 1			kaka			
	k 2		kaka	kaka	100	59	53

5. RELATION BETWEEN CHILD'S AND CONVENTIONAL CONSONANTS (*continued*)

K

Age.	Sound.	I. Attempted adult form (child's form in brackets).	II. In use.	III. Successfully imitated.	Total No. I.	II.	III.
0;9	m 1	mama	**mama**	**mama**			
	m 2	mama	**mama**	**mama**	2	2	2
0;10	p 1	papa	**papa**	**papa**			
	p 2	papa	**papa**	**papa**	4	4	4
0;11					4	4	4
1;0	b 2	peep-bo (ɛbɔ)	ɛbɔ	ɛbɔ			
	n 1	nana	nana	nana			
	n 2	nana	nana	nana	7	7	7
1;1	d 1	dada	dada	dada			
	d 2	dada	dada	dada	9	9	9
1;2					9	9	9
1;3					9	9	9
1;4	b 1	bath (bɑ)	bɑ	bɑ			
	k 1	cakie (**kæke**)	kæke	kæke			
	k 2	cakie (**kæke**)	kæke	kæke			
	h 1	honey (**hɑ**)	hɑ	hɑ	13	13	13
1;5	f 1	fire (**fff**)	fff	fff			
	t 1	tick-tick (**titta**)	titta	titta			
	t 2	tick-tick (**titta**)	titta	titta			
	sk 2	biscuit (**bik**)					
	k 3		bik		17	17	16
1;6	fl 1	flower (**fɑ**)					
	dʒ 1	jar (**dʒɑ**)	dʒɑ	dʒɑ			
	tʃ 1	chocolate (**gɔga**)					
	g 1	garden (**ga**)	ga	ga			
	g 2		gɔga				
	kr 1	creampot (**biba**)			22	20	18
1;7	j 2	Here-you-are (**i:juɑ**)	i:juɑ	i:juɑ			
	gr 1	Grannie (**gɑ**)					
	ŋ 2	uncle (**ʌŋkə**)	ʌŋkə	ʌŋkə	25	22	20
1;8	n 3	din-din	din-din	din-din			
	l 2	Eileen (**aigu**)					
	l 3	school (**ku:l**)	ku:l	ku:l			
	j 1	yes (**jeʃi**)	jeʃi	jeʃi			
	ʃ 1	shoe-shoe (**ʃʃ**)	ʃʃ	ʃʃ			
	ʃ 2	shoe-shoe (**ʃʃ**)	ʃʃ	ʃʃ			
	sk 1	school (**ku:l**)			32	27	25

5. RELATION BETWEEN CHILD'S AND CONVENTIONAL CONSONANTS (continued)

Age.	Sound.	I. Attempted adult form (child's form in brackets).	II. In use.	III. Successfully imitated.	Total No. I.	II.	III.
1;9	v 1		vɔki				
	w 1	walk (vɔki)					
	pl 1	plane (pei)					
	pr 1	pretty (piti)					
	fr 1	frock (vrɔki)					
	vr 1		vrɔki				
	θ 2	bathie (bɑ:ti)					
	tʃ 2		(water) fɔtʃi				
	s 1	six (si)	si	si			
	sl 1	sleep (si:)					
	kl 1	clean (ki:)			40	31	26
1;10	m 3	home (hɔum)	(hɔum)	hɔum			
	f 2	telephone (tætoun)	(Humphrey) hʌfl	hʌfl			
	v 2	lavatory (lædəti)					
	br 1	brickie (biki)					
	fr 2	Humphrey (hʌfl)					
	d 3	cold (koud)	koud	koud			
	ð 2	another (gʌgi)					
	tʃ 1		(chip) tʃiti	tʃiti			
	tʃ 2	picture (pitʃi)		pitʃi			
	l 1	lavatory (lædəti)	lædəti	lædəti			
	r 1	rain (rei)	rei	rei			
	g 2	doggie (gɔgi)		gɔgi	51	37	34
1;11	w 1		wi:wi:	wi:wi:			
	w 2	wee-wee (wi:wi:)	wi:wi:	wi:wi:			
	mj 1	music (muɲi)					
	t 3	mend-it (meɲit)	meɲit	meɲit			
	dj 1		djiɲki				
	dr 1	drinkie (djiɲki)					
	dʒ 3	porridge (pɔidʒ)	pɔidʒ	pɔidʒ			
	s 2	pussy (puʃi)					
	s 3	lettuce (jetis)	jetis	jetis			
	z 2	music (muɲi)					
	z 3	nose (nouʒ)					
	ʃ 3		(nice) naiʃ				
	ʒ 3		(nose) nouʒ				
	st 3	toast (tou)	ǀ		61	45	39
2;0	p 3	soap (ʃoup)	ʃoup	ʃoup			
	f 3	off (ɔf)	ɔf	ɔf			
	fr 1		(three) fri:				
	v 3	stove (touv)	touv	touv			
	bl 1	blankets (bæŋkets)					
	fl 1		(flannel) flænti	flænti			
	θ 1	thank-you (fæŋku)					

5. RELATION BETWEEN CHILD'S AND CONVENTIONAL CONSONANTS (*continued*)

Age.	Sound.	I. Attempted adult form (child's form in brackets).	II. In use.	III. Successfully imitated.	Total No. I.	II.	III.
2;0 (*con.*)	ө 3	teeth (**ti:ʃ**)					
	tʃ 3	reach (**ri:t**)					
	өr 1	three (**fri:**)	(throw) **өrou**	**өrou**			
	l 2		(hullo) **ʌlou**	**ʌlou**			
	z 3		(matches) **mætiz**	**mætiz**			
	ʃ 3	wash (**wɔʃ**)		**wɔʃ**			
	ʒ 2		(scissors) **ʃiʒiʒ**				
	ʒ 3	lounge (**lauʒ**)		**lauʒ**			
	k 3	hide-seek (**haiʃi:k**)		**haiʃi:k**			
	kj 2	thank-you (**fæŋku**)					
	gl 1	glass (**ga:ʃ**)			74	54	49
2;1	tl 2	mantlepiece (**mæŋkupi:ʃ**)					
	tʃ 3		(fetch) **fetʃ**	**fetʃ**			
	sk 3	ask (**a:sk**)	**a:sk**	**a:sk**			
	sp 1	speak (**pi:k**)					
	st 2	downstairs (**dautæө**)					
	st 3		(just) **dʌst**	**dʌst**			
	t 1		(stairs) **ʃtæөʒ**				
	g 3	fog (**fog**)	**fog**	**fog**			
	ŋ 3	getting (**getiŋ**)	**getiŋ**	**getiŋ**	80	60	54
2;2	v 1	very (**vedi**)		**vedi**			
	v 2		(over) **ouvə**	**ouvə**			
	ð 1	there (**jeiə**)					
	ð 3	with (**wiv**)					
	tr 1	trousers (**tauzəz**)					
	nj 1	new (**nu**)					
	r 2	Harold (**hærəld**)	(Harold) **hærəld**	**hærəld**			
	s 2		(dressing-gown) **desiŋgau**	**desiŋgau**			
	z 2		(trousers) **tauzəz**	**tauzəz**			
	kl 2	Buckley (**bʌkli**)	**bʌkli**	**bʌkli**			
	gj 1		(great) **gjeit**		87	66	60
2;3	b 3	Bob (**bʌb**)	**bʌb**	**bʌb**			
	pj 1	pianos (**panu:z**)					
	bj 1		(bless-you) **bjesju**				
	dr 1		(draw) **drɔ:**	**drɔ:**			
	dʒ 2	Roger (**wodʒə**)	**wodʒə**	**wodʒə**			
	nj 1		(new) **nju**	**nju**			
	sn 1	snow (**tou**)					

5. RELATION BETWEEN CHILD'S AND CONVENTIONAL CONSONANTS (*continued*)

Age.	Sound.	I. Attempted adult form (child's form in brackets).	II. In use.	III. Successfully imitated.	I.	II.	III.
2;3 (*con.*)	sw 1	sweet (fi:t)					
	ʃt 2		(yesterday) jæʃtədei				
	kr 1		(screw) kru:	kru:			
	gr 2	hungry (hʌngi)			93	73	65
2:4	ð 1		(there) ðær	ðær			
	ð 3		(with) við	við			
	r 3	there (ðær)	ðær	ðær			
	sl 2	asleep (əʃi:t)					
	sm 1	smoked (poukt)					
	st 2		(Mr.) mistə	mistə			
	3 2	treasure (tæʒəs)		tæʒəs			
	kr 2	unscrew (ʌŋkru:)	(unscrew) ʌŋkru:	ʌŋkru:	98	78	71
2;5	ʃt 3		(cost) kɔʃt		98	79	71
2;6					98	79	71
2;7	br 1		(bread) bred	bred			
	kl 1		(clothes) klouz	klouz			
	kw 1	queen (kri:n)			99	81	73
2;8	pr 1		(pram) præm	præm			
	bl 1		(blue) blu:	blu:			
	sk 1		(school) sku:l	sku:l			
	sp 1		(speaking) spi:kiŋ	spi:kiŋ	99	85	77
2;9	θ 2		(everything) evriθiŋ	evriθiŋ			
	sk 2		(biscuit) biskit	biskit			
	sl 1		(slipping) slipiŋ	slipiŋ			
	sl 2		(asleep) əsli:p	əsli:p			
	st 1	strawberry (stɔ:beri)	stɔ:beri	stɔ:beri	100	90	82
2;10					100	90	82
2;11					100	90	82
3;0	ð 2		(weather) weðə	weðə			
	gr 1		(green) gri:n	gri:n	100	92	84

6. ELISION : HILDE STERN

Age of Child.	Child's form.	Adult form.
1;7	**l** lalansch	**pl** plansch plansch.
1;9 1;9	**p** pickel pitze	**ʃp** Spiegel. Spitzenschleife.
1;5	**s** ssi-ssi	**ps** hepsi.
1;9 1;10	**b** busst bennt	**br** Brust. brennt.
1;10	**r(l)†** lief	**br** Brief.
1;9 1;10	**m** mutzen meckt's	**ʃm** schmutzig. schmeckts.
1;6 1;6	**f** fasche feisch	**fl** Flasche. Fleisch.
1;8	**t** tinke	**tr** trinken.
1;8 1;10	**t** fettig dott	**rt** fertig. dort.
1;11	**r(v)†** weppe	**tr** Treppe.
0;11	**d** dedda	**rt** Berta.*
1;10	**r(s)†** ssinken	**tr** trinken.
1;9	**t** siete	**st** siehst du.
1;9	**s** ssäne	**ts** Zähne.
1;9 1;10	**s** hüssn kassen	**st** husten. Kasten.
1;6	**ts** otze	**rts** Schürze.
1;7	**t** talj	**ʃt** Stall.

Age of Child.	Child's form.	Adult form.
1;6	**ʃ** bösche	**st** Bürste.
1;7 1;10	**d** dei dinne	**dr** drei. drinnen.
1;10	**n** nee	**ʃn** Schnee.
1;8	**k** kala	**kl** Clara.
1;8	**k(g)†** ging ging	**kl** klingeln.
1;7 1;8	**k** kaje katze	**kr** Kragen. kratzen.
1;10	**l** luck'n	**gl** Glocken.
1;9	**g** getzen	**gr** Gretchen.
1;9	**v(f)†** fatz	**ʃv** Schwanz.
1;9	**s** ssei	**tsv** zwei.
1;10	**v** wieback	**tsv** Zwieback.
1;3	**ʃ** ei-schei	**tsv** eins-zwei.*
1;9	**n(t)†** top	**kn** Knopf.
1;9 1;10	**n** neifen nix	**kn** kneifen. Knix.
1;0	**l** läft	**ʃl** schläft.*
1;9 1;10	**ʃ** scheischeibe n'scheck	**ʃr** Schreibe. Schreck.
1;9	**p** top	**pf** Knopf.
1;7	**f** feu	**pf** pfui.

* = Compound attempted before the child can produce both sounds separately.
† With substitution.

ELISION : DEVILLE'S DAUGHTER [1]

Age of child.	Child's form.	Adult form.	Age of child.	Child's form.	Adult form.
	p	**pl**		**k(p)†**	**kr**
1;4	api	parapluie.	1;8	papô	crapaud.*
1;6	peu	pleuvoir.			
1;6	pu	plus.		**p(b)†**	**pl**
1;8	peu	pleurer.	1;9	beian	pliant.
1;8	apan	rantanplan.	1;11	beié	plier.
1;9	pata	placard.			
1;10	épuché	éplucher.		**b**	**bl**
1;10	pa	place.	1;7	ban	blanc.
1;10	pum	plume.	1;10	beu	bleu.
1;11	patô	plateau.	1;11	tab	table.
1;11	pin	plein.			
	p	**pr**		**b**	**br**
1;7	pè	prêter.	1;4	bo	brosse.*
1;8	pan	prends.	1;6	babo	bravo.
1;9	apè	après.	1;7	baté	bracelet.
1;9	pum	prune.	1;7	ba	bras.
1;9	apeti	sapristi.	1;7	bo	broc.
1;10	pè	prêt.	1;8	bu	brûler.
1;11	aposé	approcher.	1;10	beio	Briolle.
1;11	puno	pruneau.	1;11	bozé	brosser.
			1;11	bou-ia	brouillard.
	p	**pj**		**f(b)†**	**fr**
1;4	pé	pied.	1;9	abodi	refroidir.
1;5	papè	papier.	1;11	bozé	frisé.
	f(p)†	**fl**		**k(b)†**	**kr**
1;6	peu	fleur.	1;9	beion	crayon.*
1;7	pé	sifflet.			
	f(p)†	**fr**		**m**	**mj**
1;7	pon	front.	1;8	mè	lumière.
1;8	pata	François.			
	b(p)†	**br**		**m**	**fl**
1;8	apaté	embrasser.	1;10	manè	flanelle.
	p	**sp**		**p(f)†**	**pl**
1;6	apè	asperge.	1;11	fa	place.
			1;11	fam	planche.

[1] See note, p. 262.

* = Compound attempted before the child can produce both sounds separately.

† With substitution.

ELISION: DEVILLE'S DAUGHTER (*continued*)

Age of child.	Child's form.	Adult form.	Age of child.	Child's form.	Adult form.
	f	**fl**		**s**	**sk**
1;8	feu	fleur.	1;6	s	biscuit.*
1;9	fé	souffler.			
				z†	**sk**
	f	**fr**	1;10	zaié	escalier.*
1;8	fa	froid.			
1;8	fon	front.		**t†**	**kr**
1;9	foté	frotter.	1;8	tin	crin.*
1;11	fosa	François.	1;10	totodi	crocodile.*
			1;10	ti	écrire.*
	v†	**pl**	1;11	tèm	crême.
1;11	veian	pliant.			
				d	**dj**
	v†	**bj**	1;6	deu	Dieu.
1;9	vè	bière.			
				d	**dr**
	v	**vr**	1;10	adé	André.
1;6	vè	vrai.	1;10	dedon	édredon.
1;9	avi	ouvrir.			
				d†	**gl**
	t†	**fr**	1;10	da	glâce.
1;6	tè	fraise.			
				d†	**gr**
	t	**tr**	1;8	da	grand.
1;4	tou	trou.*	1;9	do	gros.
1;7	até	entrer.	1;10	dôgnou	grenouille.
1;10	otu	Autruche.			
1;10	to	trop.		**k**	**kr**
1;11	taté	étrangler.	1;10	ki	crier.*
	s†	**tr**		**r**	**kr**
1;10	son	citron.	1;4	r	crochet.*
1;11	osu	Autruche.			
				p	**pw**
	t†	**kl**	1;6	paton	poisson.
1;4	tété	clef.*	1;9	pa	poids.
1;4	to	cloche.*	1;9	pa	poire.
1;7	tè	éclair.*	1;9	pao	poireau.
1;9	tou	clou.*	1;9	pa	pois.
1;9	toum	clown.*			
1;11	tè	clair.		**p**	**pɥ**
			1;10	pi	puis.
	t†	**sk**			
1;4	té	biscuit.*			
1;11	taié	escalier.*			

* = Compound attempted before the child can produce both sounds separately.

† With substitution.

ELISION : DEVILLE'S DAUGHTER (*continued*)

Age of child.	Child's form.	Adult form.	Age of child.	Child's form.	Adult form.
	b	**bw**		**t**	**tw**
1;4	ba	boire.	1;8	ta	toi.
1;6	ba	bois.	1;9	ta	étoile.
1;8	ba	bôite.			
				t	**trw**
	b†	**vw**	1;10	ta	trois.
1;7	ba-ié	voilette.			
1;7	boia	voilà.		**d**	**drw**
1;8	aba	revoir.	1;10	da	droit.
1;8	batu	voiture.			
				n	**nw**
	b†	**kɥ**	1;8	na	noir.
1;6	boié	cuillère.*	1;9	na	Chinois.
	m	**mw**		**t†**	**sw**
1;7	mamé	tramway.	1;8	pata	François.
1;9	manô	moineau.			
1;10	ma	moi.		**s**	**sw**
			1;10	pasa	François.
	m†	**pw**			
1;9	magné	poignée.		**t†**	**ʃw**
			1;7	pata	mouchoir.
	f	**fw**			
1;9	fa	fois.		**s**	**ʃw**
			1;10	fosa	mouchoir.
	f†	**sɥ**			
1;8	afi	essuyer.		**z**	**zw**
			1;11	bezan	besoin.
	f	**kɥ**			
1;10	fi	cuisse.		**m†**	**kɥ**
			1;11	meni	cuisine.
	v	**vw**			
1;7	ava	revoir.		**j**	**lj**
1;8	vala	voilà.	1;9	aié	collier.
1;8	va	voir.	1;10	zaié	escalier.
	t†	**vw**		**j**	**rj**
1;11	tolé	voilette.	1;7	éiè	derrière.
	v	**krw**		**s**	**sj**
1;11	vazé	croisée. †	1;10	meseu	monsieur.
			1;11	asè	assiette.
	v†	**gɥ**	1;11	sè	Lucienne.
1;8	vi	aiguille.	1;11	posé	poussière.
	t	**tj**		**t**	**sj**
1;4	tété	laitier.	1;7	tatè	assiette.
			1;7	peteu	monsieur.
			1;8	peté	poussière.

* = Compound attempted before the child can produce both sounds separately.
† With substitution.

ELISION : K

Left panel

Age of Child.	Child's form.	Adult form.
	p	**pl**
1;9	pei	aeroplane.
1;9	pʌ	plug.
2;0	pi:	please.
2;1	pei	play.
2;2	pæʃ	splash.
2;2	pi:zd	pleased.
	p	**pr**
1;9	piti	pretty.*
2;1	pæm	pram.
2;2	pezəntz	presents.
	p	**pj**
2;3	pa:nuz	pianos.
	p	**sp**
2;1	pi:k	speak.
2;2	pæŋk	spank.
2;2	potiz	spots.
	b	**bl**
2;0	bæŋkets	blankets.
2;2	bæk	black.
	b	**br**
1;10	biki	bricks.*
2;2	bekfəs	breakfast.
2;2	bɔ:t	brought.
2;3	bidʒ	bridge.
2;3	bʌʃ	brush.
	f	**fl**
1;6	fa	flower.*
2;1	fɔ:	floor.
2;2	fai	fly.
2;2	koufeik	cornflakes.
	f	**fr**
1;10	hʌfi	Humphrey.*
2;1	feʃ	fresh.
2;2	fɔgi	froggie.
2;3	fɔki	frockie.
2;3	fɔm	from.
2;3	faideg	fried-egg.
	t	**tr**
2;2	steit	straight.
2;2	tauzəz	trousers.
2;2	tein	train.
	t	**st**
2;0	touv	stove.
2;1	dautææə	downstairs.
2;2	tiki	sticky.
2;3	tiŋ	string.
2;3	ti:m	steam.
	t	**tʃ**
1;10	tææ	chair.
2;0	mætiz	matches.
2;0	ri:t	reach.
2;1	tææ	chamber.
	s	**st**
2;2	lasnait	last night.

Right panel

Age of Child.	Child's form.	Adult form.
	ʃ	**st**
1;11	touʃ	toast.
2;1	fə:ʃ	first.
2;1	lɔʃ	lost.
2;1	mʌʃ	must.
2;2	pouʃ	post.
	ʃ	**tʃ**
1;11	buʃə	butcher.
	d	**dr**
2;2	dɔ:ə	drawer.
2;3	desiŋgau	dressing-gown.
2;3	dein	drain.
2;3	dʌm	drum.
	d	**dʒ**
2;1	dʌst	just.
	n	**nj**
2;2	nu:	new.
	m	**mj**
1;11	muni	music.
	t	**sn**
2;3	tou	snow.
	k†	**tʃ**
2;2	kiki	chicken.
2;3	kɔki	chocolate.
2;3	hæŋkəki:k	handkerchief.
	k	**kl**
1;9	ki:	clean.
1;9	kou	close !
2;2	kælə	clever.
2;2	kouz	clothes.
2;3	kouz	close.
	b†	**kr**
1;6	biba	cream-pot.*
	k	**kr**
1;11	ki:	cream-pot.
	k	**sk**
1;8	ku:l	school.
1;10	biki	biscuit.
2;3	kru:	screw.
	g	**gl**
2;0	ga:ʃ	glass.
2;2	gisi	glycerine.
2;2	gʌbz	gloves.
	g	**gr**
1;7	gɑ	grannie.*
2;1	gei gei	Graham.
2;3	hʌŋgi	hungry.
2;3	gi:n	green.
	f	**sw**
2;3	fi:t	sweet.
	s	**sl**
1;9	si :	sleep.
	ʃ	**sl**
1;11	ʃi:ti	sleepy.
2;2	ʃitəz	slippers.

* = Compound attempted before the child can produce both sounds separately.
† With substitution.

ELISION: ANALYSIS OF CASES
HILDE STERN

Adult Compounds.	p	b	m	f	v	t	d	n	l	s	ʃ	k	g	Middle Cons.: Elided.	Middle Cons.: Retained.	Total.
Front and Middle — pl								1							1	1
ps(sp)	2								1					2	1	3
br		2						1						2	1	3
ʃm			2											2		2
fl				2										2		2
tr(rt)					1	3	2		1					6	1	7
st(ts)						1				3	1			1	4	5
ʃt						1								1		1
dr							2							2		2
Back and Middle — n								1						1		1
kl												1	1	2		2
kr												2		2		2
gl									1						1	1
gr									1						1	1
Total														**23**	**10**	**33**

w(v) Compounds	p	b	m	f	v	t	d	n	l	s	ʃ	k	g	Fronting.	Others.	Total.
ʃv				1										1		1
tsv				1				1			1			1	2	3
Total														**2**	**2**	**4**

Other compounds	p	b	m	f	v	t	d	n	l	s	ʃ	k	g	Elided	Retained	Total.
nk				1			2									3
ʃl								1								1
ʃr											2					2
pf	1			1												2
Total																**8**

DEVILLE'S DAUGHTER

Adult Compounds.	p	b	m	f	v	t	d	n	s	z	r	j	k	Middle Cons.: Elided.	Middle Cons.: Retained.	Total.
Front and Middle — pl	11	2		2	1									16		16
pr	8													8		8
pj	2													2		2
bl		3												3		3
br	1	9												10		10
bj					1									1		1
mj			1											1		1
fl	2		1	2										5		5
fr	2	2		4		1								9		9
vr					2									2		2

DEVILLE'S DAUGHTER (*continued*)

Adult compounds.	p	b	m	f	v	t	d	n	s	z	r	j	k	Middle Cons.: Elided	Middle Cons.: Retained	Total.
Front and Middle — tr						5								5	2	7
tj						1								1		1
dr							2							2		2
dj							1							1		1
sp	1													1		1
Back and Middle — sk						2			1	1				2	2	4
kl						6								6		6
kr	1	1				4					1		1	7	1	8
gl							1							1		1
gr							3							3		3
Total														**86**	**5**	**91**

Adult compounds.	p	b	m	f	v	t	d	n	s	z	r	j	k	Fronting.	Others.	Total.
w(ɥ) compounds — pw	5		1											6		6
pɥ	1													1		1
bw		3												3		3
mw			3											3		3
fw				1										1		1
vw		4			3	1								8		8
tw						2								2		2
trw						1								1		1
drw							1							1		1
nw								2						2		2
sw						1			1					1	1	2
sɥ				1										1		1
ʃw						1			1					1	1	2
zw										1					1	1
kɥ		1	1	1										3		3
krw				1										1		1
gɥ					1									1		1
Total														**36**	**3**	**39**

Adult compounds.	p	b	m	f	v	t	d	n	s	z	r	j	k			Total.
Others — lj												2				2
rj												1				1
sj						3			4							7
Total																**10**

K

Adult Compounds.	Child's sounds.												Middle Cons. :		Total.
	p	b	m	f	w	t	d	n	s	ʃ	k	g	Elided.	Retained.	
Front and Middle — pl	6												6		6
pr	3												3		3
pj	1												1		1
sp	3												3		3
bl		2											2		2
br		5											5		5
fl				4									4		4
fr				6									6		6
tr						3							3		3
st						5			1	5			5	6	11
ʃt(tʃ)						4				1		3	7	1	8
dr							4						4		4
dʒ							1						1		1
nj								1					1		1
mj			1										1		1
sn						1							1		1
Back and Middle — kl											5		5		5
kr		1									1		2		2
sk											3		3		3
gl												3	3		3
gr												4	4		4
Total													70	7	77

													Fronting	Others	
w(v) Compound sw				1									1	0	1
Total													1	0	1

Other compound sl								1	2						3
Total															3

7. SUBSTITUTION: HILDE STERN

Age	Child's form	Adult form	Substitution	Order of consonants — Replaced consonant						
				In child's repertory				Not in repertory		
				Substitution		Doubt-ful	Total	Substitution		Total
				By earlier cons.	By later cons.			By existing cons.	By new cons.	
0;10 to 1;6	didda	tiktack	d.t					1/11		
	dedda	Berta	d.t					1/11		
	muh	Kuh	m.k					5/11		
	mitze	Katze	m.k	5/11						
	ante	Hände	t.d		11/1					
	eischei	eins-zwei	ʃ.ts		19/7					
	schlüchel	Schlüssel	c.s					7/19		
	milss	Milch	s.c	7/18						
	nasse	Nase	s.z		8/7					
	bösche	Bürste	ʃ.s						8/9	
				2	3	0	5	4	1	5
1;7 to 1;9	nat	Knopf	t.p(f)			13/13				
	kaje	Kragen	j.g		11/2					
	ant	Hand	t.d		11/1					
	miesse	Gemüse	s.z	7/18						
	kuchel	Kuchen	l.n	9/13						
	kulle	Garnrolle	k.r	9/13						

					5	1	4	23	1
dalä	Taler	d.t	1/11						
beinene	Weihnachtsbaum	b.v	3/6						
atze	ritsche	s.ʃ	7/8						
dei	zwei	d.ts	1/9						
szoss	Schoss	s.ʃ	7/8						
slafe	schlafen	s.ʃ	7/8						
sette	Jette	s.j	6/13						
getsen	Gretchen	s.c	7/19						
pickel	Spiegel	k.g	11/13						
hing	Ring	h.r	3/13	13/9					
jeike	Zeitung	j.ts	11/13						
top	Knopf	t.n	11/13						
Total			16	6	1	23	4	1	5
1;10 onwards									
ssinken	trinken	s.r	7/13						
lief	Brief	l.r	9/13						
weppe	Treppe	v.r	6/13						
homm	komm	h.k	3/11						
hacker	Racker	h.r	3/13						
hein	herein	h.r	3/13						
hoss	horch	s.x	7/20						
Cumulative total			23	6	1	30	4	1	5

SUBSTITUTION : DEVILLE'S DAUGHTER [1]

0;11 to 1;6				
ato	encore	t.k	9/15	
bade	balai	d.l	9/15	
badon	ballon	d.l		
batin	bassin	t.s	5/7	5/20
bodo	bonhomme	d.n	9/4	

[1] See note, p. 262.

SUBSTITUTION: DEVILLE'S DAUGHTER *(continued)*

Age.	Child's form.	Adult form.	Substitution.	Replaced consonant. — In child's repertory. Substitution. By earlier cons.	By later cons.	Doubt-ful.	Total.	Not in repertory. Substitution. By existing cons.	By new cons.	Total.
0;11 to 1;6 *(contd.)*	boie	cuillère	b.k					6/20	7/8	
	chi	merci	ʃ.s	5/8						
	ia-ia	Suzanne	j.s	2/13	10/8					
	ia-io	Suzon	j.s	2/13	10/8					
	paton	poisson	t.s	2/13						
	pipu	fichu	p.f	5/7						
	poteu	fauteuil	p.f							
	peu	feu	p.f							
	ta	Charles	t.ʃ	5/8				5/20		
	tao	carotte	t.k	5/7				5/20		
	tata	canne	t.k							
	ta	sable	t.s							
	ta	chat	t.ʃ							
	tata	café	t.k	5/8				5/20		
	tata	caca	t.k	5/7				5/20		
	taté	caché	t.k	5/8				5/20		
	taté	saleté	t.s							
	té	chèvre	t.ʃ							
	té	sel	t.s							

			14	2	12	28	0	4	24
tété	sécher	t.s			5/20				5/8
tété	corset	t.k			5/20				5/8
ti	si	t.s			5/20				5/8
titi	quiqui	t.k							5/7
to	culotte	t.k							5/7
tô	seau	t.s							5/7
tô	chaud	t.ʃ							
ton	chausson	t.ʃ			5/20				5/8
ton	chiffon	t.ʃ							5/7
toti	coquille	t.k							
toti	saucisson	t.s							
toton	chausson	t.ʃ			5/20				
toutou	coucou	t.k		16/18				17/1	
vi	oui	v.w							
zou	jouer	z.ʒ							5/8
ate	assez	t.s							5/8
ati	assis	t.s							4/16
moni	musique	n.z							
Total . . .			14	2	12	28	0	4	24
1;7 botou	beaucoup	t.k			5/20				5/8
baté	bracelet	t.s			5/20				5/8
ta	carafe	t.k			5/20				5/7
taté	cassé	t.k							5/7
ti	cerise	t.s							5/8
até	chaise	t.ʃ							
toto	chaussette	t.ʃ			5/20				5/8
toto	ciseaux	t.s			5/20				
tato	corde	t.k							
tou	cou	t.k							
tan	descendre	t.s			5/20				5/8
tè	éclair	t.k							2/13
peté	ficelle	p.f / t.s							5/8

SUBSTITUTION : DEVILLE'S DAUGHTER (*continued*)

Age.	Child's form.	Adult form.	Substitution.	Order of consonants.						
				In child's repertory.				Replaced consonant. Not in repertory.		
				Substitution.		Doubt-ful.	Total.	Substitution.		Total.
				By earlier cons.	By later cons.			By existing cons.	By new cons.	
1;7 (*contd.*)	pi	fil	p.f	2/13						
	poté	fourchette	p.f, t.ʃ	2/13, 5/7						
	pon	front	p.f	2/13						
	taton	garçon	t.g	5/11						
	paté	marcher	p.m, t.ʃ	5/7						
	peteu	monsieur	p.m, t.s	5/8		2/2				
	pata	mouchoir	p.m, t.ʃ	5/7		2/2				
	poton	mouton	p.m, t.k			2/2				
	té	perroquet	b.p			2/2				
	bo-ion	pigeon	j.ʒ		6/2					
	teu	queue	t.k	10/18				5/20		
	jou	rouge	ʒ.r	18/12	18/12			5/20		

	child form	target word	phonetic	22	2	20	54	4	6	44
1;8	pé, ba-iè	sifflet, voilette	p.f, b.v, j.l							2/13, 6/17, 10/15
	Total . . .									44
	ane	aller	n.l							4/15
	boton	bouchon	t.ʃ							5/7
	tato	casserole	t.k			5/20				5/8
	mouni	chauve-souris	t.s, m.s							2/8, 4/12
	to	cloche	n.r			5/20				
	to	corne	t.k			5/20				
	tou	coudre	t.k			5/20				
	tou	courir	t.k			5/20				
	aba	cravate	b.v							6/17
	tin	crin	t.k			5/20				
	te	crochet	t.k			5/20				2/6
	apate	embrasser	p.b							6/17
	abo-ié	envoyer	b.v							6/13
	badu	fendu	b.f							2/13
	peté	fouetter	p.f							2/13
	pou	four	p.f							2/13
	pata	François	p.f							9/11
	da	grand	d.g							4/16
	ne	groseille	n.z							
	to	haricot	t.k			5/20				5/13
	ata	Lafargue	t.f						6/4	10/15
	ian	lampe	j.l							
	pato	marteau	p.m					2/2		5/8
	mati	merci	t.s					2/2		
	pata	moutarde	p.m							
	ba-io	noyau	b.n							
	paté	paquet	t.k			5/20				

SUBSTITUTION : DEVILLE'S DAUGHTER (*continued*)

Age.	Child's form.	Adult form.	Substitution.	Order of consonants. Replaced consonant. In child's repertory. Substitution. By earlier cons.	By later cons.	Doubt-ful.	Total.	Not in repertory. Substitution. By existing cons.	By new cons.	Total.
1;8 (*contd.*)	badu	pendule	b.p	10/16						
	ian	raisin	j.z	6/17						
	aba	revoir	b.v	5/8						
	ta	sac	t.s		6/2					
	fi	siffler	f.s	5/8						
	tin	singe	t.s	5/8	11/8					
	tou	sou	t.s	5/8						
	tu	sucre	b.v	6/17						
	ba-iin	vilain	j.l	10/15						
	batu	voiture	b.v	6/17						
	ta	chocolat	t.l	5/15						
	Total . .			71	9	6	86	29	2	31
1;9	até	acheter	t.ʃ	5/7						
	peté	bifteck	p.b	2/6						
	ta	cave	t.k					5/20		
	taté	chercher	t.ʃ	5/7						

child form	French	code	36	11	81				
						38	2	98	6
tou	clou	t.k	5/20						
toum	clown	t.k	5/20						
toton	cochon	t.k	5/20						
totim	coquine	t.k	5/20						
da	courant	d.r	5/20		9/12				
zan	Jean	z.3			16/18				
etou	écouter	t.k	5/20	9/5					
adin	éteindre	d.t		9/5					
adadu	éteint	d.t							
pata	placard	t.k							
abodi	refroidir	b.f			6/13				
apaté	repasser	t.s			5/8				
iin	rien	j.r			10/13				
ta	sage	t.s			5/8				
abeié	travailler	b.v			6/17				
Total .			**36**	**11**	**81**	**38**	**2**	**98**	**6**
1;10									
vose	fourchette	v.f		17/13					
		s.ʃ		8/7					
tou	couche	t.k	5/20						
atosé	accrocher	t.k	5/20						
		s.ʃ		8/7					
tae	carré	t.k	5/20						
son	citron	s.t		8/5					
potu	confiture	p.k			2/20				
to	coq	t.k	5/20						
totodi	crocodile	t.k	5/20						
		f.k	13/20						
fi	cuisse	b.m							
abadé	demander	t.k		6/2					
ti	écrire	b.f			6/13				
baza	fondu	z.d	5/20	17/9					
do	gauche	d.g			9/11				
da	glâce	d.g			9/11				

SUBSTITUTION : DEVILLE'S DAUGHTER (continued)

Age.	Child's form.	Adult form.	Substitution.	Order of consonants. Replaced consonant. In child's repertory. Substitution. By earlier cons.	By later cons.	Doubt-ful.	Total.	Not in repertory. Substitution. By existing cons.	By new cons.	Total.
1;10 (contd.)	dognou	grenouille	d.g	9/11	13/2					
	ii	lit	j.l	10/11	8/7					
	fosa	mouchoir	f.m		6/2					
			s.ʃ		6/1					
	boton	mouton	b.m							
	bazo	oiseau	b.w							
	paté	passer	t.s	5/8						
	fè	pêche	f.p		13/2					
	apase	ramasser	p.m		17/12					
	voi	tiroir	v.r	6/17				5/20		
	bezé	verser	b.v			2/2				
	sa	chat	s.ʃ		8/7					
	tasé	corset	t.k							
	Total . .			89	24	7	120	44	2	46
1;11	amuié	amuser	j.z	10/16	8/7					
	aposé	approcher	s.ʃ		8/7					
	atasé	attacher	s.ʃ							

		Transcription		
botim	bottine	m.n	2/4	8/7
tabiné	cabinet	t.k	5/20	8/7
tao	carreau	t.k	5/20	8/7
sam	chante	s.J		
siïn	chien	s.J		
sa	chocolat	d.g		
sida	cigare	t.k		
tè	clair	t.k		
togné	cogné	b.k	9/11	8/5
to	col	s.t	5/20	
bosu	confiture	t.k	5/20	
tou	coup	t.k	6/20	8/7
touvé	couvercle	s.J	5/20	
tem	crème	m.n	5/20	
sasé	crochet	m.n	5/20	
diam	Diane	t.k	2/4	8/5
dom	donne	s.t	2/4	16/11
taié	escalier	z.g	5/20	13/2
fôseu	fauteuil	f.p		
zo	gauche	m.n		
fon	jupon	s.J		
lem	laine	s.J		
masé	marcher	n.z	2/4	8/7
mosé	moucher	f.p		8/7
ané	oseille	f.p		
fa	place	v.p	4/17	
fam	planche	t.k		
veian	pliant	m.ɲ		13/2
toua	quoi	m.n		13/2
sem	saigne	z.r	5/20	17/2
sem	Seine	m.n	2/19	
zo	sirop	t.s	2/4	16/12
som	sonne		2/4	
tu	sur		5/8	

SUBSTITUTION: DEVILLE'S DAUGHTER (*continued*)

Age.	Child's form.	Adult form.	Substitution.	Order of consonants.						
				Replaced consonant.						
				In child's repertory.				Not in repertory.		
				Substitution.		Doubt-ful.	Total.	Substitution.		Total.
				By earlier cons.	By later cons.			By existing cons.	By new cons.	
1;11 (*contd.*)	zazam	Suzanne	m.n	2/4						
	sa	tasse	s.t	2/4	8/5					
	toum	tourne	m.n	2/4						
	vazim	vaseline	m.n	5/20						
	tam	canne	t.k	2/4						
			m.n							
		Cumulative total	.	116	41	7	164	44	2	46

SUBSTITUTION: K

Age.	Child's form.	Adult form.	Substitution.	By earlier cons.	By later cons.	Doubt-ful.	Total.	By existing cons.	By new cons.	Total.
0;9 to 1;6	biba	cream-pot	b.p	0	3/2	0	1	3/16 5/10	0	2
	eba	ever	b.v							
	da	again	d.g							
	Total .	.		0	1	0	1	2	0	2

				3	3	0	6	4	1
					3/2 16/8			8/18 8/21	16/18
I.S.									
1;7 to 1;9									
be	pen	b.p							
fɔtʃi	water	f.w							
vrɔki	frock	v.f							
vɔki	walk	v.w							
baːti	bathie	t.θ	11/14					
pijou	pillow	j.l	10/14					
aigu	Eileen	g.l	13/15					
ʃiː	sea	ʃ.s						
Total .			**3**	3					
1;10 to 2;0									
friː	three	f.θ	16/18					
fænku	thank-you	f.θ					8/21	
vata	water	v.w	13/15				8/21	
badi	bunny	d.n	9/21					
ʃʌti	supper	t.p	11/14	5/3				
maːti	mouth	t.θ	11/17	9/2				
dɔji	dolly	j.l	11/17					
jeidi	lady	j.l	11/17					
djiɲki	drink	j.r						
djes	dress	j.r						
ʃiːti	sleepy	t.p	13/15	9/2				
gɑːʃ	glass	ʃ.s	13/15					
hɔʃ	horse	ʃ.s	13/15					
kjɔʃ	cross	j.r	11/17					
haiʃiːk	hide-seek	ʃ.s	13/15					
naiʃ	nice	ʃ.s	13/15					
puʃi	pussy	ʃ.s	13/15					
peiʃi	Pacey	ʃ.s	13/15					
pɔʃul	parcel	ʃ.s	13/15					
ʃʌn	sun	ʃ.s	13/15					

U

SUBSTITUTION : K (*continued*)

Age.	Child's form.	Adult form.	Substitution.	In child's repertory. By earlier cons.	In child's repertory. By later cons.	Doubtful.	Total.	Not in repertory. By existing cons.	Not in repertory. By new cons.	Total.
1;10 to 2;0 (*contd.*)	ʃiʒiʒ	scissors	ʃ.s	13/15						
			ʒ.z	18/20						
	ʃoup	soap	ʃ.s	13/15						
	touʃ	toast	ʃ.s	13/15						
	tiːʃ	teeth	ʃ.θ					13/21		
	laiki	light	k.t	6/9						
	aiʒ	eyes	ʒ.z	19/20						
	biːdʒ	beads	ʒ.z					18/21		
	nouʒ	nose	ʒ.z	19/20						
	piːʒ	please	ʒ.z	19/20						
		Total . .		29	6	0	35	8	1	9
2;1 to 2;3	ʌbʌn	oven	b.v	3/16						
	gʌbz	gloves	b.v	3/16						
	faim	Thymol	f.θ	8/21						
	fiŋ	thing	f.θ	8/21						
	fruː	through	f.θ	8/21						
	vaid	ride	v.r	16/17						

Phonetic	English	Symbol			
vʌn	one	v.w	16/18		16/22
vindou	window	v.w	16/18		16/22
væt	that	v.ð			
wiv	with	v.ð			
dɑːjin	darling	n.ŋ	2/12		5/22
ʃɒkin	shocking	n.ŋ	3/12		5/22
edə	ever	d.v	5/15		
vedi	very	d.r	5/17		
hʌdi	hurry	d.r	5/17		
dis	this	d.ð			
douz	those	d.ð			
ʃitəz	slippers	t.p		9/2	
tou	snow	t.n		9/3	
dɑːjin	darling	j.l	11/14		
hʌjou	hullo	j.l	11/14		
jaiti	light	j.l	11/14		
jetis	lettuce	j.l	11/14		
jiv	live	j.l	11/14		
jift	lift	j.l	11/14		
jegiz	leggings	j.l	11/14		
jʊk	look	j.l	11/14		
jidi	lid	j.l	11/17		
jaik	like	j.l	11/17		
djɑːft	draught	j.r	11/17		
gjeit	great	j.r	11/17		
hɒjid	horrid	j.r	11/17		
jedi	ready	j.r	11/17		
joud	road	j.r	11/17		
kjiːmi	creamy	j.r			
mæeji	Mary	j.r			
sigijæt	cigarette	j.r			
ɔjinʒ	orange	j.r			
ja	there	j.r			11/22
jæts	that's	j.ð			11/22
hauʃ	house	ʃ.s	13/15		

SUBSTITUTION : K (*continued*)

Age.	Child's form.	Adult form.	Substitution.	In child's repertory. Substitution. By earlier cons.	By later cons.	Doubt-ful.	Total.	Not in repertory. Substitution. By existing cons.	By new cons.	Total.
2;1 to 2;3 (*contd.*)	loʃ	lost	ʃ.s	13/15						
	mæŋkupiːʃ	mantlepiece	ʃ.s	13/15						
	mʌʃ	must	ʃ.s	13/15						
	pouʃ	post	ʃ.s	13/15						
	piːʃ	piece	ʃ.s	13/15						
	penʃəl	pencil	ʃ.s	13/15						
	ʃɔː	saw	ʃ.s	13/15						
	ʃtææʒ	stairs	ʃ.ʒ	13/15						
	ʃei	say	ʃ.s	13/15						
	ʃitəz	slippers	ʃ.s	13/15						
	ʃeti	settee	ʃ.s	13/15						
	ʃolʃ	self	ʃ.s	13/15						
	ʃæm	Sam	ʃ.s	13/15						
	ʃuːn	soon	ʃ.s	13/15						
	ʃoːʃə	saucer	ʃ.s	13/15						
	ʃævil	Saville	ʃ.s	13/15						
	jæʃtədei	yesterday	ʃ.s	13/15						
	fəːʃ	first	ʃ.s	13/15						
	ʃtææʒ	stairs	ʒ.z	19/20						

				19/22		
bu:ʒ	Booth	ʒ.ð	6/9			
bokl	bottle	k.t	6/9			
likl	little	k.t	6/9			
mæŋkupi:ʃ	mantlepiece		10/3			
gʌgi	another	g.n				
Cumulative Total		85	9	0	94	15	1	16

ANALYSIS OF SUBSTITUTIONS

	Front for front.	Middle for middle.	t or d with k or g.	t, d, ts, ð or θ with s, z, ʃ, or ʒ.	Others.	Total
Hilde Stern . .	b.v 1 d.t 3 d.ts 1 t.d 2 t.p 1 t.n 1	l.r 1 ʃ.s 1 s.z 2 s.ʃ 3 s.j 1 s.r 1 s.c 2 c.s 1		ʃ.ts 1	m.k 2 v.r 1 l.n 1 j.g 1 j.ts 1 s.x 1 k.r 1 h.r 3 h.k 1 k.g 1	
Total . . .	9	12	0	1	13	35
Deville's daughter	p.f 12 p.m 7 p.b 2 b.p 2 b.v 8 b.f 3 b.n 1 b.m 2 b.w 1 f.p 4 v.f 1 v.p 1 v.w 1 m.n(ŋ) 11 t.f 1 d.t 2 d.n 1	j.z 3 j.ʒ 1 j.l 4 j.r 1 j.s 2 s.ʃ 12 ʃ.s 1 z.r 1 z.ʒ 2 ʒ.r 1	t.g 1 t.k 54 d.g 5 d.k 1	t.s 26 t.ʃ 16 s.t 4 z.d 1	b.k 1 f.s 1 f.k 1 f.m 1 v.r 1 m.s 1 d.l 2 h.l 1 n.r 1 n.z 3 z.g 1	
Total . . .	60	28	61	47	14	210
K.	b.p 2 b.v 3 f.w 1 f.θ 5 v.f 1 v.w 4 v.ð 2 d.n 1 d.v 1 d.ð 2 t.p 3 t.n 1 t.θ 2	j.l 13 j.r 12 ʃ.s 35 ʒ.z 4	d.g 1 k.t 4	ʃ.θ 1 ʒ.ð 1	v.r 1 m.ŋ 2 g.n 1 d.r 2 j.ð 2 g.l 1 n.d 1 ŋ.z 1	
Total . . .	28	64	5	2	11	110

8. REDUPLICATION : DEVILLE'S DAUGHTER

Child's form.[1]	Adult form.	Child's form.	Adult form.
bébé	bébé.	*sasé	cassé.
kaka	caca.	sèsô	cerceau.
*nanu	canule.	*fôfé	chauffer.
*tati-n	Catherine.	tatam	content.
*papo	chapeau.	toutou	coucou.
*sôsé	chaussette.	*totodi	crocodile.
chèché	chercher.	dedon	édredon.
*tôté	côté.	*fifu	fichu.
*papô	crapaud.	*tatò	gâteau.
dodo	dodo.	gugu	Gugusse.
*taté	étrangler.	mimi	mimi.
*sason	garçon.	apapi	parapluie.
*tati	gentil.	*momonè	porte-monnaie.
lolo	lolo.	*tat	quatre.
papa	papa.	*vavon	savon.
*fouf	pouf.	*tuté	sucré.
*sasé	saleté.	tété	téter.
*vavè	serviette.	*vouv	Louvre.
tatim	tartine.	babo	barboter.
*mamoné	tramway.	bobo	bobo.
bibi	bibi.	*nana	canard.
*chaché	cacher.	*saso	casserole
*taton	carton.	*mamo	chameau.
sasu	celui-ci.	*chôché	chausser.
*babon	charbon.	*fafé	chemin-de-fer.
*chôchon	chausson.	*aleli	Cornelie.
*popo	compôte.	*toto	couteau.
*toton	coton.	*sason	croissant.
*sasé	crochet.	*nanu	éternue.
dedan	dedans.	*amim	gamine.
*mamé	fermer.	*taté	gâté.
*dadé	garder.	popotam	hippopotame.
*touté	goûter.	*tamatiin	pharmacien.
maman	maman.	*dadé	regarder.
papié	papier.	*chéché	sécher.
pipi	pipi.	*zazam	Suzanne.
poupé	poupée.	tomomé	thermomètre.
*toté	sauter.	bonbon	bonbon.
*foif	soif.	*mam	manche.
tatu	teinture.	mama-ié	mademoiselle.
*sosé	retrousser.	babouillon	barbouillon.
*apapé	attraper.	kokim	coquine.
bobè	bobèche.	*bibu	omnibus.
*fafé	café.	babeion	papillon.

* = Absence of reduplication in adult form   [1] See note, p. 262.

REDUPLICATION : K

Child's form.	Adult form.	Child's form.	Adult form.
*biba	cream-pot.	pʌpʌ	puff-puff.
dada	dada.	*gaːgi	girlie.
*dədə	Dempy.	*gɔgi	doggie.
*gɔga	chocolate.	*neini	navel.
kæke	cakie.	*papa	grandpa.
mama	mama.	kuku	cuckoo.
nana	nana.	*tætoun	telephone.
papa	papa.	ʍiːwiː	wee-wee.
titta	tick-tick.	*geigei	Graham.
bibi	bib.	*nuːni	balloon.
bæba	baby.	*kiki	chicken.
*dindin	dinner.	*kɔki	chocolate.
*nini	Winnie.	pæpə	paper.
pʌpʌ	powder-puff.	ʃɔːʃə	saucer.
tæta	tatta.	*gʌgi	another.
tæti	potato.	tiːtɔt	tittot.

9. ASSIMILATION : HILDE STERN

Child's form.	Adult form.	Sounds.	Assimilation		
			of later to earlier.	of earlier to later.	Doubt-ful.
dedda	Berta	d.b†	1/3		
mamau	Baum	m.b		5/3	
mammel	Semmel	m.z	5/18		
luppel	nuppeln	l.n	9/13		
Schlell	Schnell	l.n	9/13		
fofa	Sofa	f.z	17/18		
hoppeheite . . .	Hoppereiter	h.r	3/13		
beinene	Weihnachtsbaum	n.b		13/3	
hinnehofen . . .	hingeworfen	h.v	3/6		
ssoss	Schoss	s.ʃ	7/8		
ging ging . . .	Klingling	g.k		13/11	
Total . .			8	3	0

DEVILLE'S DAUGHTER[1]

			of later to earlier.	of earlier to later.	Doubt-ful.
baba	balle	b.l	6/15		
dade	regarder	d.g	9/11		
moni	musique	m.z	2/16		
tété	laitier	t.l	5/15		
tété	côtelette	t.k	5/20		
toto	couteau	t.k	5/20		
babo	bravo	b.v	6/17		
dadi	radis	d.r	9/12		
nana	canard	n.k	2/20		
pipu	fichu	p.ʃ	2/7		
tata	tasse	t.s	5/8		
tété	sécher	t.ʃ	5/7		
toti	coquille	t.k	5/20		
bibu	omnibus	b.m		6/2	
niénié	panier	n.p		4/2	
popo	chapeau	p.ʃ	2/7		
toton	torchon	t.ʃ	5/7		
taté	cassé	t.s*	5/8		
toté	chaussette	t.s*	5/8		
tôtô	ciseaux	t.z	5/16		
taton	garçon	t.s*	5/8		
tato	casserole	t.s*	5/8		
daté	danser	d.s		9/8	
papo	drapeau	p.d	2/9		
omené	omelette	m.l	2/15		

* = With substitution   † Read : **d** dominates **b.**
[1] See note, p. 262.

ASSIMILATION : DEVILLE'S DAUGHTER (*continued*)

Child's form.	Adult form.	Sounds.	Assimilation		
			of later to earlier.	of earlier to later.	Doubt-ful.
tatô	rateau	t.r	5/12		
taté	cacher	t.ʃ*	5/7		
taté	chanter	t.ʃ	5/7		
tati	sentir	t.s	5/8		
menu	venu	n.v	4/17		
achoché	accrocher	ʃ.k	7/20		
nanu	canule	n.k	4/20		
tatin	Catherine	t.k	5/20		
sôsé	chaussette	s.ʃ		8/7	
tôté	côté	t.k	5/20		
papô	crapaud	p.k	2/20		
taté	étrangler	t.g	5/11		
sason	garçon	s.g	8/11		
tati	gentil	t.ʒ	5/18		
sasé	saleté	s.t		8/5	
vavé	serviette	v.s		17/8	
mamoué	tramway	m.t	2/5		
chaché	cacher	ʃ.k	7/20		
taton	carton	t.k	5/20		
babon	charbon	b.ʃ	6/7		
chochon	chausson	ʃ.s	7/8		
popo	compôte	p.k	2/20		
mamé	fermer	m.f	2/13		
dade	garder	d.g	9/11		
touté	goûter	t.g	5/11		
toté	sauter	t.s	5/8		
foif	soif	f.s		13/8	
sosé	retrousser	s.t		8/5	
apapé	attraper	p.t	2/5		
fafé	café	f.k	13/20		
sasé	cassé	s.k	8/20		
fôfé	chauffer	f.ʃ		13/7	
tatam	content	t.k	5/20		
totodi	crocodile	t.k	5/20		
fifu	fichu	f.ʃ		13/7	
tatô	gâteau	t.g	5/11		
mamoné	portemonnaie	m.p			2/2
tat	quatre	t.k	5/20		
vavon	savon	v.s		17/8	
tuté	sucré	t.s*	5/8		
moné	bonnet	n.b*	4/6		
sasu	ceinture	s.t		8/5	
dodo	rideaux	d.r	9/12		
vouv	louvre	v.l		17/15	
saso	casserole	s.k	7/20		
mamo	chameau	m.ʃ	2/7		
chôché	chausser	ʃ.s	7/8		

ASSIMILATION : DEVILLE'S DAUGHTER (continued)

Child's form.	Adult form.	Sounds.	Assimilation		
			of later to earlier.	of earlier to later.	Doubt-ful.
aleli	Cornelie	l.n		15/4	
sason	croissant	s.k	8/20		
nanu	éternue	n.t	4/5		
amim	gamine	m.n	2/4		
taté	gâté	t.g	5/11		
chéché	sécher	ʃ.s	7/8		
fouf	pouf	f.p		13/2	
toton	coton	t.k	5/20		
sasé	crochet	s.k*	8/20		
zazam	Suzanne	z.s		16/8	
Total			65	16	1

K

lædəti	lavatory	t.v	9/16		
nini	Winnie	n.w	3/18		
tætoun	telephone	t.f		9/8	
tʃiti	chippy	tʃ.p		13/2	
neini	navel	n.v	3/15		
gɑːki	Gertie	g.t		10/9	
gaːgi	girlie	g.l	10/13		
gɔgi	doggie	g.d		10/5	
muɲi	music	m.z	1/20		
meɲit	mend-it	m.d	1/5		
taːnt	can't	t.k		9/6	
maːni	Marjorie	m.dʒ	1/19		
nuːni	balloon	n.l	3/14		
kouk	coat	k.t	6/9		
kiki	chicken	k.tʃ	6/13		
kæŋkəreitə	camphorated	k.f	6/8		
kɔki	chocolate	k.tʃ	6/13		
kikl	tickle	k.t	6/9		
mɔkəkaː	motor-car	k.t	6/9		
hæŋkəkiːk	handkerchief	k.tʃ	6/13		
gɑːk	dark	k.d		6/5	
kæŋgik	candlestick	k.t	6/9		
nemənout	envelope	n.v n.l	3/16 3/14		
biba	cream-pot	b.k*	3/6		
gɔga	chocolate	g.tʃ	10/13		
papa	grandpa	p.g	2/10		
kæg	Tagg	g.t		10/9	
ʃɔlʃ	self	ʃ.f*		13/8	
Total			21	8	0

RESPONSE AND UTTERANCE

(C = Child ; M = Mother ; F = Father ; A = Adult)

1. RESPONSE TO LANGUAGE BY K

Age.	Form.	Circumstances and response.
0;8,20	*Cuckoo, Cuckoo*	When M sings this in special tone of voice, C turns towards her and smiles.
0;8,24	*nan nan*	When M says this, C turns towards maid (doubtful).
0;9,5	*No !*	C sitting in " play-pen " ; about to put piece of newspaper in his mouth. When F says this in a loud voice, C desists from act.
0;9,6	*Say Good-bye*	C's parents leaving the house : C being held up at window by maid, who says this. C waves his hand.
0;9,14	*Baby, where is the ballie ?*	C in play-pen, with eiderdown, cushion, silver bell, rattle, toy dog and small white ball, which he has had a fortnight. M says this. C slowly turns and touches ball. This repeated successfully three times. No response at 5th, 6th, 7th times.
1;0,10	*Give mummy crustie* *Give daddy crustie*	M and F having tea with C, who is munching a crust. M says this. C puts crust into her hand. Repeated twice more with same effect. M then says this. No response from C.
1;0,12	*Give mummy teddy* *Give auntie teddy*	M and " auntie " out with C who is hugging his toy teddy bear. M says this. C holds it out to her. Then M says this. No response from C. M repeats it three times more ; at fourth time, C gives it to *M.*
1;0,15	*Come out, Baby !*	C lying in bath, which he enjoys. M says this, without making any movement. C crawls to further end of bath.

Age.	Form.	Circumstances and response.
1;0,27	Baby, where's shoe-shoe ?	C in play-pen. One shoe lying outside, beyond his reach. M says this. C immediately crawls towards shoe, and tries to reach it.
1;0,29	Mamma not speaking to you	C refuses to lie down in baby-carriage, in spite of M's efforts. Finally she says this, in tone of annoyance. Immediately C flings himself backwards in rage, and screams.
1;3,0	Where's choc ?	M has recently given him, on two or three occasions, a small piece of chocolate, which she keeps in a certain drawer. On her saying this, C looks towards the drawer.
1;3,1	Where's cream-pot ?	C is fond of playing with pot containing face-cream. On this occasion the pot is standing on a chair near him. When M says this he leans over it and seizes it.
	Honey, baby !	At breakfast-time he regularly has honey. On this occasion, when the honey has not yet been removed from the cupboard in which it is kept, M says this, whereupon C waves his hand towards the closed cupboard door.
	Have some porridge !	There is porridge on the breakfast table. When M says this, C stretches out towards it.
1;3,2	Where's the cream-pot ?	Under similar conditions to those in entry of previous day, with same effect.
	Have some honey !	At breakfast-time. The honey is still in the cupboard. When M says this, C dances gleefully in his chair.
1;3,3	Baby hold spoonie !	C will not take his orange juice. Turns his back on M, who is trying to feed him. When she says this he immediately turns round, takes the spoon and tries to feed himself.
	Baby, have honey !	At the end of his breakfast ; C has not yet had his honey. When M says this, he turns to the cupboard where it is kept, in great glee.
1;3,5	Where's apple ?	He has been nibbling an apple, while crawling about on the floor, and has thrown it into a corner. M does not know this, and asks the question, whereupon C crawls straight towards the apple and brings it to her.

2. MEANINGFUL UTTERANCE BY K IN HIS 11TH, 14TH AND 17TH MONTHS

Age.	Form.	Circumstances.
0;10,4	a a a a	In apparent glee, when children pass by his baby-carriage.
0;10,26	næ næ	Looking up at maid, while being held in her arms (doubtful).
0;10,28	a a a	C sitting on M's lap, playing with toy dog. He drops this, and makes strenuous efforts to reach it, without success. Puts his hand on her, then looks at dog. No response from M. C turns over on her lap, face downwards, then in great excitement cries out.
	a	Utters this in tone of rage, on being reprimanded.
1;1,8	ɛbɔ	Utters this (when M says *Peep bo*) and covers his head with his eiderdown. Repeats word and action six times without further stimulus from M.
	nana nana mama mama	When maid enters room, C says this several times, waving his hand. M is walking by C's baby-carriage. He says this repeatedly to himself, occasionally glancing up at her with a smile.
1;1,9	ɛbɔ	F and M with C. M puts napkin over F's face. C pulls it away saying this.
	ɛbɔ	M has laid a woolly shawl at lower edge of door to keep out draughts. C crawls over to it, puts it on his head, and says this.
1;1,15	dáda dáda	When M says *Where's Daddy?* C turns towards F and says this.
	a a a a a	A plaything is out of C's reach. He tries to reach it, unsuccessfully. At length, he turns to M, and looks alternately at her and at plaything, saying this. Is overjoyed when she gives it to him.
1;1,20	iːpba	F puts cloth over C's head. He pulls it off and says this.
1;1,24	a a a a a	Is given an apple, receives it with expression of joy and says this in a chuckling gleeful manner.
1;1,26	ɛ ɛ ɛ ɛ	While being fed, stretches out his hand towards milk or water according as he wants either. When it is not immediately forthcoming, says this in a querulous tone.

MEANINGFUL UTTERANCE BY K (continued)

Age.	Form.	Circumstances.
1;1,27	**a a a a**	On being allowed to grasp the end of a stick in play, says this in a gleeful manner. When stick is removed beyond his grasp he reaches for it and makes same sounds in a querulous manner.
1;4,0	**kæke**	M offering him cake says *Cakie, Baby ?* C says this softly, and with a smile ; repeats this each time he is offered a piece of cake, and also occasionally while eating it.
1;4,1	**ɛ ɛ ɛ**	On seeing cake at teatime, reaches out for it. When it is kept beyond his reach, says this with growing impatience.
	ka ka	M says *Cakie*, whereupon C says this and is given cake.
	kæke	C says this while eating the cake.
1;4,2	**ɛ ɛ ɛ**	Says this impatiently while trying to reach his toy rabbit, which is beyond his grasp.
1;4,6	**bɑ**	Seeing nursery table, at bath-time, with toilet things on it, including bath-towel.
	bɑ	On being taken into bathroom, where water is running into his bath, says with this great joy.
1;4,7	**ɛ ɛ ɛ**	Says this in gleeful manner on passing the house where a friend lives.
1;4,8	**ahaaa**	On being given a handkerchief scented with lavender by M who says : *Smell handkerchief*, C puts it to his nose, sniffs it, and says this.
1;4,12	**a a a**	Says this on being offered flowers by M, who says : *Smell the pretty flowers.*
1;4,15	**da da**	On M saying, *Play game of up-and-down* (a game of which he is very fond), says this, heaving himself backward in the accustomed manner.
1;4,16	**ba**	Says this in response to maid, on her saying *Good-bye* to him at bedtime.
1;4,17	**ha**	Says this at breakfast-time, turning towards the sideboard cupboard where the honey, which he generally has at breakfast, is kept.
	ba	Says this on hearing M, who is speaking on telephone, say *Good-bye.*
	ba ba	Says this on pointing to button on M's jacket.
1;4,18	**bai**	When F says *Good-bye* on leaving house, C says this and waves his hand.
	a a	When he needs the chamber-pot.
	ba	While fingering the buttons on his coat.

3. K'S RESPONSE TO " BALLIE "

Age.	Form.	Circumstances.
0;9,14	*Baby, where's the ballie ?*	C in play-pen, with eiderdown, cushion, silver bell rattle, toy dog and small white ball, which he has had a fortnight. M speaks. C slowly turns and touches ball. This repeated successfully three times. No reponse at 5th, 6th, 7th times.
0;9,15	*Baby, where is the ballie ?*	C as above. Correct response twice out of five trials. On one of these successful occasions the ball is well out of his line of sight ; C turns until he sees it.
0;9,16	*Baby, where is the ballie ?*	C as above. Correct response once out of four trials.
0;9,29	*Baby, where is the ballie ?*	C in play-pen with ball and other articles. Invariably reaches for ball when A speaks.
0;10,12	*Where's the ballie ?*	C finds the ball when A says this.
0;10,21	*Where's the ballie ?*	C in play-pen with two balls ; a large coloured one in addition to the original small white one. F speaks. C touches small ball, never large one.
0;10,26	*Where's the ballie ?*	C in play-pen with large ball only. F speaks. No response from C.
0;10,27	*Doggie !*	C in play-pen with brown toy dog, blue toy rabbit. eiderdown, large coloured ball. M holds up dog and repeats this several times. No response from C.
	Where's ballie ? *Where's doggie ?*	Ten minutes later, F speaks. C holds up ball. F speaks again. C holds up dog. This repeated in irregular alternation three or four times, with correct results.
	Where's ballie ?	Then small white ball put into play-pen. C plays with it for a time. Then F speaks. C holds up small white ball. On second occasion, responds similarly. On third occasion, holds up *large* ball.
0;10,29	*Ballie !*	C in play-pen with large ball, and teddy bear, lying together. F speaks. After some delay, C crawls towards both articles, but does not touch either of them. F repeats word, but with no further effect.
1;1,5	*Baby, where's ballie ?*	C playing with toy ; has not played with large coloured ball all day ; at this moment it is lying in corner of room, in shadow. M speaks. C turns round and crawls towards ball. On the way, he halts at the coal-box, a favourite plaything. When M repeats phrase, C resumes journey, seizes ball, and looks at M.

4. K: USE OF **aa, ɛɛ** AND VARIANTS

Age.	Circumstances.	Sound used.
0;9,16	On seeing a person of whom he is fond ; or hearing footsteps of familiar person : in a tone of delight.	**a a a**
	On seeing his bottle of " gripe-water," of which he is fond. In a delighted tone.	**a a a**
0;10,4	On being wheeled past children in the street. Calls out in great glee.	**a a a**
0;10,28	Sitting on M's lap, drops his toy dog. Makes effort to reach it, but is unsuccessful. Calls out rather excitedly.	**a a a**
	Seizing something that is forbidden, he is reprimanded by the maid, who wags her finger at him, saying *Now, Sir !* He replies in a tone of rage.	**a**
0;10,29	Is playfully reprimanded as on previous day and replies in a tone of rage.	**a**
1;0,15	Drops one of his playthings, tries to reach it, but unsuccessfully ; calls out excitedly.	ɛ ɛ ɛ
1;1,15	Tries to reach a box of chessmen, one of his favourite toys ; failing, he looks towards M and calls out, in series of sharp cries.	**a a a**
1;1,24	Being given an apple, says this in chuckling, gleeful manner.	**a a a**
1;1,26	During a meal, stretches out hand towards drink ; when this is not immediately handed to him, says querulously :	ɛ ɛ ɛ
1;1,27	F playing with him, allows him to seize knob of walking-stick. C says this in contented tone : When knob is withdrawn out of his reach, says this in querulous tone :	**a a a** **a a a**
1;2,0	Turning over leaves of picture book, comes upon drawing of a doll. Points to this and speaks in chuckling gleeful manner. (*Note.*—C has no doll, and no toy resembling a doll.)	**ha ha ha**
1;2,21	On seeing chamber-pot.	**aa aa**
1;3,26	The sound is still being commonly used as an indication that something is desired.	**a a a**
1;4,1	On the previous day, he had been told the word *cakie* on being given a piece of cake at tea, and had repeated the word **kæke.** To-day, on seeing similar cake at tea, stretches out this hand and says this :	ɛ ɛ ɛ

K : USE OF **aa,** **εε** AND VARIANTS (*continued*)

Age.	Circumstances.	Sounds used.
1;4,2	Trying to reach his toy-rabbit, which is just beyond his play-pen.	ε ε ε
1;4,7	The sounds occur in the course of apparently meaningless babbling.	ε ε ε hə hə hə
1;4,8	On being wheeled by the house of friends, makes signs of glee and cries out joyfully, stretching his hand out in direction of the house.	ε ε ε
	M gives him a handkerchief scented with lavender, saying *Smell handkerchief.* C holds it to his nose and sniffs, saying this in tone of satisfaction.	ahaaa
1;4,12	M brings C near to some jonquils growing in a bowl ; he bends over and smells them, saying this.	a a a
1;4,17	As an indication that he needs the chamber-pot.	aa, aa
1;5,10	M dressing C in front of fire ; he points to this and calls out in tone of satisfaction ; soon afterwards he says f f f, then fa.	ahaaa
1;5,30	Turning over leaves of picture book, comes upon drawing of a doll, upside-down. Lays his head on the picture, and says this, just as when he is told *Love* (*so-and-so*).	a a a
1;6,3	Looking at picture book, comes upon drawing of a horse. Looks up at his mother inquiringly ; she says *horse.* Comes next to picture of a jug, points to it and looks at her ; when she does not reply, repeats these sounds urgently.	ε ε ε
1;6,24	Reaching towards half an apple.	ɑ ɑ
1;6,25	While C is playing on floor, M says *Apple, Baby ?* C says ɑ ɑ, crawls quickly towards door and begins to rattle the knob. M takes him into next room, where fruit is kept ; she lifts him up to the fruit-dish and he takes an orange. M says *Take an apple.* C drops orange and picks up an apple.	ɑ ɑ

K : USE OF aa, εε AND VARIANTS (*continued*)

Age.	Circumstances.	Sounds used.
1;6,25	C watching M darning. M says, *Baby, where's my darner ? Mummie wants her darner.* C puts his hand under a chair, brings out darner, and says :	ε ε ε
1;7,1	When he desires his eiderdown (**aidi**) says :	a
1;8,10	On being given new shoes, says ʃ ʃ ε ε.	ε ε
	In the garden with M ; C suddenly points and looks upwards, saying ε ε ε. It is an aeroplane.	ε ε ε
1;8,16	Until now, when he wishes for toast and butter at breakfast, has said ε ε pointing. To-day for the first time says **bʌti.**	ε ε
1;9,12	In M's room are two small cupboards side by side, one of which he is forbidden to open. To-day C points to forbidden cupboard and says ε ε interrogatively. When M says *No !* C points to other cupboard, saying ε ε as before. M replies *Yes !* C repeats this as a sort of game about a dozen times.	ε ε
1;9,13	C has spots on his skin, which M treats with calamine. To-day, while dressing him, she has omitted the treatment ; C points to spots, saying :	ε ε
1;9,15	On seeing aeroplanes through the window.	ε ε
1;9,21	Says this repeatedly, trying to attract M's attention.	ε ε
1;9,22	Used interrogatively. M finds him playing with forbidden object, says *No !* and he desists. C then picks up a box with which he often plays and says ε ε. M replies *Yes.* C then points again to forbidden object, saying ε ε. M replies *No !* All this is repeated several times.	ε ε
1;9,27	Sees aeroplane ; instead of usual sound now says **pei pei.**	
1;9,28	On seeing a kite, points to it and says **pei.**	
1;10,2	Dialogue between M and C. C : **dædi ?** M : *Gone ta-ta. Where's mummie ?* C (pointing) : ε ε ε.	ε ε ε
2;0,6	Still uses this in game of " loving " a person ; i.e. leans his head against someone and says this caressingly.	a a a

5. USE OF mama (AND ITS VARIANTS) BY K
A SUMMARY OF EVERY NEW USE AS IT OCCURRED.

Age.	Response to language. Circumstances.	Form.	Utterance. Form.	Circumstances.
0;5,11			m m m m	During a chain of babbling, after a feed.
0;8,20			mammam	When he is mildly lacking something; e.g. when he is alone and " wishes for company " (i.e. the cry ceases when someone appears), or when he is reaching for a plaything.
0;8,26			mæm mæm mʌmmi	When very uncomfortable; in the course of struggling and crying.
0;9,6			mæmmæm	Uttered in very contented tone, while lying in M's arms and looking up at her.
0;9,8			mama, əmám	Uttered once or twice (no chain of babbling) when playing contentedly by himself.
0;9,29			mamama	Sitting alone in his play-pen. His ball rolls out of his reach. He stretches towards it, but unsuccessfully. After several efforts he begins to say this while reaching for the ball.
1;0,6	C gnawing at crust. M sitting near by says this: C holds up crust and whimpers a	*Baby, give mama crustie*		

USE OF **mama** BY K (*continued*)

| Age. | Response to language. | | Utterance. | |
	Circumstances.	Form.	Form.	Circumstances.
	little. (M had tried this on several occasions in past three weeks, but with no effect.)			
	C in play-pen. Toy musical box (which he has had about one week) lying within his reach. M says: No response from C. An hour later, similar conditions. M speaks as before. C immediately holds musical box out towards her.	*Give mummy tinkle box.*		
1;0,28			m m m m	C sitting with M, stretches out his hand, touches her sleeve, saying this.
			mʌmmʌ mʌmmʌ be be	C lying on M's lap after his bath. Puts up his hands on either side of her chin, saying this.
1;1,6	F and M with C who is gnawing a crust. M says: C offers it to *M*. M repeats phrase, with same effect. M says: C offers it to F	*Give daddy crustie* *Give mummy crustie*		
1;1,8			mama, mama	C in baby-carriage, M walking beside him. Much of the time he says this, as if to himself, but every now and then he glances up at M with a smile.

USE OF **mama** BY K (*continued*)

Age.	Response to language.		Utterance.	
	Circumstances.	Form.	Form.	Circumstances.
1;1,15	F and M with C. M says : C nestles head in her neck M says : C nestles head in F's neck. But after this, whichever of the two M says, C nestles only to *M*	*Love mummy* *Love daddy*		
1;2,1			**máma** (or **mamá, míma, mimá**)	C utters this on the following occasions : (1) In his baby-carriage, being wheeled by M, says this many times in a babbling manner. (2) Having dropped the cream-pot (a favourite plaything) searches for it unsuccessfully, then looking at M, says this. (3) He is asked to find an object which is in the room, but which he cannot see. Looking round for it, says this. (4) Seeing a visitor for the first time, he picks up several of his playthings, brings them to her, and says this each time. (5) Very often this is his first remark on waking up in the morning.
1;4,2	If M says this, C responds according to circumstances. If he is tired, or needs	*Come to mummy*		

USE OF **mama** BY K (*continued*)

Age.	Response to language.		Utterance.	
	Circumstances.	Form.	Form.	Circumstances.
	help, he comes at once. Sometimes however he will scuttle away in play, hide his face and then look up roguishly.			
1;5,8	C and M in front of mirror. C points to reflection of self when M says : But he makes no response at all, when she says : (The whole of this was repeated four times, with the same result.)	*Where's Baby ?* *Where's mummy ?*		
1;6,2	C playing in a corner of room. M says : C crawls over to her chair where the newspaper is, and takes it up in his hands, then puts it down again. M then says : C takes it up again and hands it to her.	*Baby, where's the news-paper ?* *Give mummy news-paper.*		
1;6,13	M says : M says : M says :	*Where's auntie ?* *Where's Dempy ?* *Where's mummy ?*	**a:ti** **de de**	In reply, C points in right direction, and says this. C points in right direction, saying this. C points in right direction, but remains silent.
1;6,15			**mama mama**	From his baby-carriage he catches sight of a poster on a hoarding—a picture of a smiling woman. Immediately, he says this.

6. USE OF tik tik (AND ITS VARIANTS) BY K

Age.	Form.	Circumstances.
		For some days past C has listened to F's watch ; F has often said **tik tik tik** in rhythm of ticking.
1;5,22	tik tik	F sitting down. C spontaneously comes over to him, seizes lapels of coat and tries to push them apart.
1;5,23	tik tik	Exact repetition of what occurred on previous day.
1;5,24		A number of articles, including a brightly coloured watch, are depicted on the same page of a book which he has just been given. When F says *Find* **tik tik,** C points to picture of watch.
1;5,30	tit tit	C looking at picture-book, upside down. When he comes to picture of watch, puts finger on it, and says this.
1;6,9	tit tit	F sitting down. C comes over to him, seizes lapels of coat and says this rapidly in a whisper until F shows him his watch.
1;6,11	tita tita	C in chair finishing his dinner. Suddenly he points and says this. M looks up and discovers he is pointing to picture of watch in opened book.
1;6,15	tit tit	After trying in vain to obtain chocolate from M, C comes over to F and says **tit tit tit** rapidly until he is shown the watch.
1;7,18	titta	C happens to come upon a bowl which has been out of his reach for some months. Among the odds-and-ends which it contains he sees a small clock lying on its face. Immediately he says this.
1;8,28	tittit	The church clock strikes the quarter. C looks up at the clock and says this.

7. USE OF goga BY K

Age.	Form.	Circumstances.
1;3,0		On two or three occasions recently M has given him a piece of chocolate which she keeps in a certain drawer. When now she says *Where's choc ?* he looks towards drawer.
1;6,9	goga goga	M says, standing by bureau in which chocolate is kept : *I've got something nice for you.* C says this.
	goga goga	C crawls over to bureau, reaches up to handle of drawer and says this.
1;6,13	goga goga	At dinner, C is offered a banana. He waves this away and says this.
1;6,14	goga goga	M takes him into a shop and asks for chocolate. C keeps on repeating this in a whisper.
	goga goga	When bag is put into baby-carriage, C tries to open it, saying this.
	goga	When M says *What would Baby like ?* C replies :
1;6,15	goga goga	When M says *What have I got ?* in a certain tone of voice, C almost invariably replies :
	goga goga	C goes over to drawer where chocolate is kept. M asks, *What do you want ?* C says this in reply. As no chocolate is forthcoming he stands there repeating this many times until at last he desists.
1;6,23	goga	M stops with C outside sweet shop. He looks in at the window and says this. On being handed the packet he says this again.
1;7,28	goga	C picks up a crust of brown bread ; says this, bites into it, then drops it hastily.
1;8,18	goga	C opens M's hatbox, takes out her hat and says this. *Note.*—On putting on her hat before setting out M sometimes says, *I shall buy you* **goga.**

THE APPROACH TO CONVENTIONAL USAGE

AMENT'S NIECE

Use of word *mämmämm* (*mómi*, *máma*)

Age.	Circumstances.
days 206	In the course of babbling.
354	With reference (a) to food, particularly bread ; (b) to her sister, who often fed her.
513	With reference to any food or drink.
517	She drops a toy ; her sister tries to pick it up ; she protests *mämmämm*
528	To indicate that she desires her supper.
537	Still with reference to various kinds of food and drink.
571	With reference to her mother : *mómi*
592	Still with reference to various kinds of food and drink.
597	With reference to her mother : *mama.*
602	Particularly with reference to chocolate.
603	In the course of babbling (*m, mm, monné, mimi*).
615	With reference (a) to her aunt ; (b) to an egg. (*mama* in each case.)
685	Apparently with reference to her mother : *mama.*

Use of word *mimi* (also *minni*)

days 578	With reference to the cat.
593	With reference to a dead rat seen in the street.
594	With reference to a rabbit.
597	With reference to pictures of various animals and birds.
608	In the course of babbling.
609	With reference to milk ; uses the learnt word *mimi.*
610	With reference to picture of a cat.
653	With reference to a milk bottle.
662	With reference to a champagne bottle.
672	With reference to a cup of chocolate.
689	Again with reference to milk.
743	Wakes up in a fright saying *minni* ; it is evident from the circumstances that she has been dreaming of a cat.
744	As in the previous entry ; uses *minni* with reference to dream of a cat.
745	Again with reference to cat.
754	Again with reference to cat.

Use of word *mĕdi* (from *mädchen*)

days 578	Uses the word in imitation of *mädchen.*
594	In calling her sister's attention to picture of girls in a book.
597	With reference to picture of elephants.
621	In addressing two of her sisters (Irma and Sophie) ; her sister Daisy she has called *dĕsi* since 571st day.
623	With reference to picture of frog walking upright and reading.
626	With reference to various pictures of people.
662	With reference to chocolate figure of Santa Claus.
773	With reference (a) to pictures of various animals ; (b) to her three sisters who are together in a group.

IDELBERGER'S SON

Use of word *a a*

Age.	Circumstances.
days 258	While playing with his father, strokes his hair and says *a a*.
260	With reference to various objects, including dog, bird, horse, carriage.
372	With reference to urine ; also referring to spilt milk.
373	As expressing his need to urinate.
375	Again with reference to spilt milk.
376	With reference to chamber-pot. Also while looking at his soiled hands after a meal.

Use of word *dada* (also *deide*)

days 320	While rumpling his mother's hair ; spoken with smile and happy intonation.
331	While pulling his father's hair or beard.
337	While putting his arms round his mother's neck and laying his head against her.
430	Still used while rumpling his mother's or father's hair.
473	With reference to horse seen in the street. (*Note.*—For some time past he has referred to his rocking-horse as *dudu*.)
484	With reference to his rocking-horse.

Use of word *baba*

days 331	In the course of crying.
394	On seeing his father. (*Note.*—For some time past has responded correctly to *papa*.)
403	On seeing his mother.
409	With reference to pictures of men in a tailor's catalogue.
411	When he wished to be lifted on to his father's lap.
414	As expressing his desire to eat out of his father's plate.
448	With reference to his father's trousers hanging on a hook.
451	On seeing a portrait of his father.
465	On hearing the bell of a vehicle in the street. (*Note.*—Some little time previously his father had mended the electric bell in the house.)
473	On seeing various pieces of writing.

Use of word *wauwau*

days 251	On seeing the figure of a dog in porcelain.
257	Again on seeing the porcelain dog.
302	On seeing the picture of a sewing-table.
307	On hearing the barking of a dog (which he could not see) ; also on looking at a hobby-horse ; on looking at a picture of his grandfather ; on looking at a clock on the wall.
314	Again with reference to the porcelain dog.
331	With reference to a lady's fur collar with head of a dog ; also to another fur collar without any head.
334	With reference to a sqeaking rubber doll.
337	With reference to buttons on a coat.
398–428	With reference to various objects : (*a*) buttons, (*b*) dogs, (*c*) toy dog, (*d*) bathroom thermometer.
454	On seeing his brown slippers. (*Note.*—His toy dog is brown.)
466	Being shown his new-born brother, says *wauwau*, smiling and pointing.
577	With reference to various animals (feline and canine) seen in the Zoological Gardens.

K : USE OF **da** AND **da** (DOWN)

Age.	Circumstances.	Spoken to child.	Child's behaviour.	Spoken by child.
1;4,15	C is accustomed to throw himself backwards on hearing word *down*. This day, while he is sitting in his cot, M speaks to him :	*Play the game of up and down.*	C throws himself backward and says :	**da da**
1;6,8	C sitting on his mother's knee.		Says this, then scrambles off :	**da**
1;6,9	C is fond of cod-liver oil. At this moment is sucking washing-flannel, which his mother wishes him to release. She speaks to him :	*Put down your flan-tie, and I'll give you cod-liver.*	C throws flannel vigorously on to floor, and says :	**da**
1;6,16	C has developed a passion for climbing up and down stairs.		To-day, on seeing the foot of the stairs, screams in excitement :	**da da da**
1;6,26			On being brought to foot of the stairs indicates (that he wants to climb) them by saying :	**da da**
1;7,6	C is building blocks into a high column. M speaks to him :	*Baby, da*	C immediately knocks down the column.	

æg (EGG)

1;5,24	C looking at picture book.	*Find eggie.*	Points to picture of an egg.	
1;5,30	C busy playing with his toys.	*Find eggie.*	C crawls over to picture book on hearing word, turns over several pages, fails to find picture of egg, then crawls back to his toys.	
1;6,3	C looking at picture book.	*Where's eggie ?*	Points to picture of an egg.	

æg (EGG) *(continued)*

Age.	Circumstances.	Spoken to child.	Child's behaviour.	Spoken by child.
1;7,9	C is brought down to breakfast, sees empty eggshell, and says :			æg
1;7,28	At breakfast-table C sees an empty eggshell, says :			æg
1;7,29	C is in the room where breakfast is usually served ; *before* the table is laid, he says :			æg
1;7,30	C is with M to whom early morning tea is brought on a tray (which sometimes is used for C's own teatime meal, including an egg).		On seeing the tray, C says :	æg
1;11,9	M speaking to C before breakfast.	*What is Baby going to have for breakfast this morning ?*	C replies :	agu

fa (FLOWER)

Age.	Circumstances.	Spoken to child.	Child's behaviour.	Spoken by child.
1;4,12	M brings C near to some jonquils growing in a bowl.	*Smell the pretty flowers.*	C bends over and smells them, says :	a a a
1;4,13	As above.	*Smell flowers. Smell pretty flowers.*	As above ; says :	a a a
	C crawling about room.	*Where are the flowers ?*	C crawls towards flowers and holds out his hand towards them.	
1;4,16	There are pink tulips in a bowl in a room different from that concerned in the previous entries. M speaks :	*Baby, where's flowers ?*	C points to tulips.	

fa (FLOWER) *(continued)*

Age.	Circumstances.	Spoken to child.	Child's behaviour.	Spoken by child.
1;5,24	Two pictures of flowers in a book put before C. M speaks :	*Where's flowers ?*	No response from C.	
1;6,14	M holding C by window, through which he can see hyacinths in a bowl in the room.		C puts his hand on the window-pane, and speaks :	**fa fa**
	Later. Again he is being held up to window.		C stretches out towards the window, and speaks :	**fa fa**
1;6,15	M wheels C's carriage towards bed of tulips, and speaks.	*Where are the flowers ?*	C repeats this many times.	**fa fa**
1;6,21	M takes C into a room where there is a bowl of irises, and speaks :	*Where are the flowers ?*	C stretches out hand towards flowers.	**fa fa**
1;6,27	C being wheeled, is brought beneath branches of a flowering cherry.		C looks up towards blossoms, and says :	**fa fa**
1;7,27	C playing in garden. M speaks :	*Pick a flower and give it to daddy.*	C picks a flower (probably Virginia Stock) and brings it to his father.	
	As above.	*Pick a flower and give it to mummy.*	C picks and brings flower to his mother.	
1;10,26	C has a biscuit with a tiny sugar flower.		As soon as he gets it, C says :	**fa fa**
	C has slippers with embroidered flowers.		Points with signs of joy, and says :	**fa fa**

ʃi: (SEA)

Age.	Circumstances.	Spoken to child.	Child's behaviour.	Spoken by child.
1;9,23	At the seaside. M has taken C for a few minutes' walk by the sea, in the course of which she has said *sea* several times to him. Later on, out of sight of the water, she asks him the question :	*Where's the sea ?*	C points in right direction.	
1;9,27			Says this, apparently when he wishes to be taken up over the sandhills to the sea :	ʌpi (up)
1;9,28	When C is is bed, a thunderstorm. C cries and M goes to him. He is standing up in his cot.		C points in direction of the sea, and says :	ʃi: ʃi:
1;9,29	M takes C for a walk on the land side of the sandhills, beyond which is the sea.		C tugs towards the sea, saying :	ʃi: ʃi :
	M says :	*Where's the sea ?*	C points in right direction.	
	Later, C playing in garden.		Tugs at M's sleeve, and says :	ʃi: ʃi:
	M asks :	*Where ?*	C points in right direction.	
1;10,27	C is being taken for a walk (near his home in an inland town). He is taken across a railway bridge.		C says :	ʃi: ʃi:
1;11,2	C during a walk is brought near a grassy bank (something like the sandhills seen by the sea).		C says :	ʌpi ʃi: ʃi:

WORDS USED TO REFER TO ANIMALS

Age.	Circumstances.	Spoken to child.	Spoken by child.
	For some time past on seeing cat, Timmy.		ti:
1;9,11	On seeing the dog Scamp, newly acquired by the family.		ti:
	The same day, on seeing a dog in the street.		ti:
1;10,18	Looking through window of train, at sight of cows :		ti:
	On seeing sheep through the window.		ti:
1;11,1	On seeing his own toy dog (imitation of *doggie*) :		gɔgi
1;11,2	With reference to a dog he has seen :		gɔgi
1;11,24	On seeing a horse in the street, says : F then says :	*horse*	ti:
1;11,25	Out in the street with M who, pointing to rider, says :	*There's a little girl riding on a ——*	
	C adds : M repeats her remark, with same response from the child.		hɔʃ
1;11,26	On seeing a horse in the street : Hearing this, F says : C repeats :	*horse*	ti: hɔʃ
1;11,27	Looking at book, sees picture of a cat ; says : For pictures of other animals, and of birds, says :		puʃi gɔgi
2;0,10	In the street, seeing large St. Bernard dog, says :		hɔʃ
2;0,20	Again, on seeing large St. Bernard, says :		bigi gɔgi

USE OF bɔ (BOX) AND SUBSTITUTES

1;6,23	For some time past, on seeing a wooden box, 4 by 6 inches and 4 inches deep, brightly coloured :		bɔ
	Takes from cupboard a flat cardboard box, 5 by 2 inches and 1 inch deep, containing a bottle, holds it up and says :		bɔ
	F shows C small tin box containing tobacco, about 3 by 1½ inches and ½ inch deep. C says :		bɔ

APPENDIX V

USE OF **bɔ** (BOX) AND SUBSTITUTES (*continued*)

Age.	Circumstances.	Spoken to child.	Spoken by child.
1;7,8	Playing with box of bricks. Having hidden the box he wants some of the bricks which are out of his reach. Stretches towards them, saying :		bɔ bɔ bɔ
	F, as a test, says : Whereupon C hands him a brick.	*Give daddy* **bɔ**	
1;7,10	C has been playing with bricks ; M says: C searches in drawer and produces a brick.	*Give mummy bricks.*	
1;7,11	M says : Whereupon C produces them.	*Get out the bricks.*	
1;7,15	C has emptied tablets of soap from tin box where they are kept. M says : C does so.	*Put all the soap back into the box.*	
1;10,4	Away from home ; has not seen his bricks for a fortnight. M says : C repeats eagerly	*Baby, come and buy some bricks.*	biki biki
1;10,22	Goes to his drawer where bricks are kept, says many times : M says : C goes into the kitchen and says : He receives his bricks with signs of joy.	*Go and ask Carrie.*	biki biki biki
1;11,2	At the shoe-shop, calls out : Ceases only when he is given a shoe-box.		bɔ bɔ
2;1,5	In the early morning is accustomed to have *stove* lit, to be propped up with a *pillow*, and allowed to play with his *doggie* and his *box* of *bricks*. This morning says :		tɔuv— pidɔu— gogi— bɔkiʃ— bikiʃ

SCHÄFER'S SON

Age.	Circumstances.
0;9,7	F brought C's hands together, saying *Mache bitte bitte* with exaggerated intonation and in a definite rhythm ($\diagdown$x$\diagup$x$\diagdown$x) corresponding to rhythm of clapping. In a few days, C would imitate movement, on seeing it performed, but not in response to phrase alone.
0;9,19	C responded correctly to phrase when this was unaccompanied by any movement of F, but only when uttered in special tone and rhythm.
0;10,0	C responded correctly to *bitte bitte* uttered in ordinary tone of voice.
0;10,9	C responded correctly to *kippe kippe* in " Ammenton " and special rhythm. No response to *lalalala*, although uttered in " Ammenton " and special rhythm.
0;10,14	F began to say *bitte bitte* to C on occasions when latter was reaching out for food ; as soon as he had made the clapping-movement he was given the desired object.
0;10,24	When C wanted cake, F said usual phrase ; no response from C. On being given cake, C made clapping-movement.
0;10,27	C made clapping-movement on merely seeing cake. In the following days he made the movement on seeing different varieties of cake. On every such occasion the response was reinforced by the award of cake.
0;11,0	F holding a letter in front of C said *Ei ei ei, du schöne Brief.* C immediately made the clapping movement, and was given the letter.
0;11,3	C showed that he desired a certain box ; this was given to him and he then made the clapping-movement. The same thing happened when he wished to be given a piece of string.
0;11,4	While F was reading, C made the clapping-movement and was given the book.
0;11,11	By this date, C was making the movement on a large variety of occasions when he desired some object or activity (such as being taken up into someone's arms), and even at times when, as far as he knew, nobody else was present to give him what he wanted.

REFERENCES

ALEXANDER   BV   Alexander, S. *Beauty and other Forms of Value.* 1933.

ALEXANDER   CP   Alexander, S. Creative Process in the Artist's Mind. *B.J.P.*, XVII, 1927.

ALLPORT   SP   Allport, F. H. *Social Psychology.* 1924.

AMENT   SD   Ament, W. *Die Entwicklung von Sprechen und Denken beim Kinde.* 1899.

BALDWIN   MD   Baldwin, J. M. *Mental Development.* 3rd edn., 1906.

BARTLETT   R   Bartlett, F. C. *Remembering.* 1932.

BATEMAN   LD   Bateman, W. G. A Child's Progress in Speech, *J. Educ. Psych.*, V, 1914.

BEAN   PL   Bean, C. H. An Unusual Opportunity to investigate the Psychology of Language. *J. Genet. Psych.*, XL, 1932.

BEKHTEREV   ER   Bekhterev, W. M. Emotions as Somatomimetic Reflexes, *in* Reymert, M. L. *Wittenberg Symposium on Feelings and Emotions.* 1928.

BEKHTEREV   PO   Bekhterev, W. M. *La Psychologie Objective.* 1913.

BELL   AE   Bell, C. *The Anatomy of Expression.* 7th edn., 1877.

BERNFELD   PI   Bernfeld, S. *The Psychology of the Infant.* 1929.

BLANTON   BI   Blanton, M. G. Behaviour of the Human Infant. *Psych. Rev.*, XXIV, 1924.

BRIDGES   GT   Bridges, K. M. B. A Genetic Theory of the Emotions. *J. Genet. Psych.*, XXXVII, 1930.

BÜHLER   GEK   Buhler, K. *Gie geistige Entwicklung des Kindes.* 3te Aufl., 1922.

BÜHLER   FY   Bühler, C. *The First Year of Life.* 1930.

BÜHLER   KJ   Bühler, C. *Kindheit und Jugend.* 3te Aufl., Leipzig, 1931.

BÜHLER   KP   Bühler, K. *Die Krise der Psychologie.* 1929.

BÜHLER   LE   Bühler, K. Les Lois génerales d'Evolution dans le langage de l'Enfant. *J. de Psych.*, XXIII, 1926.

BÜHLER   MDC   Bühler, K. *The Mental Development of the Child.* 1930.

BÜHLER   VA   Bühler, C., and Hetzer, H. Das erste Verständnis für Ausdruck im ersten Lebensjahr. *Z. für Psych.*, CXCVII, 1928.

BÜHLER   TS   Bühler, K. Kritische Musterung der neuern Theorien des Satzes. *Indo-Germ. Jahrbuch.* VI, 1920.

323

CANNON BC Cannon, W. B. *Bodily Changes in Pain, Hunger,* etc. 1925.

CASSIRER CS Cassirer, E. Étude sur la pathologie de la conscience symbolique. *J. de Psych.,* XXVI, 1929.

CHAMBERLAIN SC Chamberlain, A. F., and I. C. Studies of a Child. I. *Ped. Sem.,* XI, 1904.

CLAPARÈDE EP Claparède, E. *Experimental Pedagogy.* Eng. tr., 1911.

CROCE A Croce, B. *Æsthetic.* Tr. D. Ainslie. 2nd edn., 1922.

CURTI CP Curti, M. W. *Child Psychology.* 1930.

DARWIN BI Darwin, C. The Biography of an Infant. *Mind,* II, 1877.

DARWIN EE Darwin, C. *The Expression of the Emotions.* 1873.

DELACROIX LP Delacroix, H. *Le Langage et la Pensée.* 2me ed., 1930.

DE LAGUNA S De Laguna, G. A. *Speech.* 1927.

DEMPE WS Dempe, H. *Was ist Sprache?* 1930.

DE SAUSSURE LG De Saussure, F. *Cours de Linguistique générale.* 1916.

DESCOEUDRES DE Descoeudres, A. *Le Développement de l'Enfant.* 1927.

DEVILLE DL Deville, G. Notes sur le développement du langage. *Rev. de Ling.,* XXIII, 1890 ; XXIV, 1891.

DEWEY CT Dewey, J. Context and Thought. Univ. of Calif. *Pubns. in Philos.,* XII, 3, 1931.

DEWEY PI Dewey, J. Psychology of Infant Language. *Psych. Rev.,* I, 1894.

DREVER IM Drever, J. *Instinct in Man.* 2nd edn., 1921.

ENGELHARDT VT Engelhardt, V., und Gehrcke, E. Über die abhängigkeit der Vokale von der absoluten Tonhöhe. *Z. für Psych.,* CXV, 1930.

FOX MB Fox, C. *The Mind and its Body.* 1931.

FREUD PP Freud, S. *Beyond the Pleasure Principle.* 1922.

GARDINER SL Gardiner, A. H. *The Theory of Speech and Language.* 1932.

GESELL IG Gesell, A. *Infancy and Human Growth.* 1929.

GHEORGOV AA Gheorgov, I. A. *Die ersten Anfänge des Sprachlichen Ausdrucks für des Selbstbewusstseins bei Kindern.* 1905.

GRAMMONT PP Grammont, M. Observations sur le Langage des Enfants, in *Mélanges . . . offerts à A. Meillet.* 1902.

GRÉGOIRE AP Grégoire, A. L'apprentissage de la parole pendant les deux premières années de l'enfance. *J. de Psych.,* XXX, 1933.

GROOS PM Groos, K. *The Play of Man.* Eng. tr., 1901.

GROOS SM Groos, K. *Die Spiele der Menschen.* 1899.

GUERNSEY SN Guernsey, M. Eine genetische Studie über Nachahmung. *Z. für Psych.*, CVII, 1928.

GUILLAUME DP Guillaume, P. Les débuts de la phrase chez l'Enfant. *J. de Psych.*, XXIV, 1927.

GUILLAUME IE Guillaume, P. *L'Imitation chez l'Enfant.* 1925.

GUTZMANN SK Gutzmann, H. Die Sprachlaute des Kindes. *Z. für Päd. Psych.*, I, 1899.

HEAD A Head, H. *Aphasia and Kindred Disorders of Speech.* 2 vols., 1926. (References to Vol. I.)

HETZER SM Hetzer, H., und Reindorf, B. Sprachentwicklung und Soziales Milieu. *Z. für Angew. Psych.*, XXIX, 1928.

HOCART PL Hocart, A. M. The Psychological Interpretation of Language. *B.J.P.*, V, 1912.

HOYER LK Hoyer, A., und Hoyer, G. Über die Lallsprache eines Kindes. *Z. für Angew. Psych.*, XXIV, 1924.

IDELBERGER KS Idelberger, H. Hauptproblemen der kindlichen Sprachentwicklung. *Z. für päd. Psych.*, 1903.

JACKSON B Jackson, Hughlings. Aphasia. *Brain*, XXXVIII, 1915.

JESPERSEN ND Jespersen, O. *Language, its Nature, etc.* 1922.

JONES ER Jones, H. E. The Retention of Conditioned Emotional Reactions in Infancy. *J. Genet. Psych.*, XXXVII, 1930.

JONES PE Jones, D. *The Pronunciation of English.* 2nd edn., 1927.

KAMPIK LT Kampik, A. Das Lallen beim taubgeborenen Kinde. *Bl. für Taubst.bldg.* 1930.

KELLER SL Keller, H. *The Story of my Life.* 1904.

KENYERES PM Kenyeres, E. Les premiers mots de l'enfant. *Arch. de Psych.*, XX, 1927.

KERN AS Kern, E. Vergleichende Analyse des Sprachwerdens beim vollsinnigen und taubstummen Kinde. *Bl. für Taubst.bldg.* 1930.

KOFFKA GM Koffka, K. *The Growth of the Mind.* 2nd edn., 1928.

LAMSON LB Lamson, M. S. *Life of Laura Bridgman.* 1878.

LANDIS EE Landis, C. The Expression of Emotion *in* Murchison, C. *Foundations of Exper. Psych.*, 1930.

LE DANTEC MI Le Dantec, F. Le Mecanisme de l'Imitation. *Rev. Philos.*, X, 1899.

LIEBER LB Lieber, F. On the vocal sounds of Laura Bridgman. *Smithsonian Cont. to Knowledge*, II, 1851.

LINDNER B Lindner, G. Beobachtungen. *Kosmos*, VI, 1882.

LORIMER GR Lorimer, F. *The Growth of Reason.* 1928.

LÖWENFELD RS Löwenfeld, B. Reaktionen der Säuglinge auf Klänge und Geräusche. *Z. für Psych.*, CIV, 1927.

MAJOR	FS	Major, D. R. *First Steps in Mental Growth.* 1906.
MALINOWSKI	MM	Malinowski, B. Appendix to Ogden and Richards : *The Meaning of Meaning.* 2nd edn., 1927.
MARICHELLE	RA	Marichelle, H. Le Réeducation Auditive chez les Sourds-muets. *J. de Psych.,* 1922.
MARKEY	SP	Markey, J. F. *The Symbolic Process.* 1928.
MCDOUGALL	OP	McDougall, W. *An Outline of Psychology.* 5th edn., 1931.
MCDOUGALL	SP	McDougall, W. *An Introduction to Social Psychology.* 21st edn., 1931.
MERINGER	LS	Meringer, R. *Aus dem Leben der Sprache.* 1908.
MEUMANN	EK	Meumann, E. Die Enstehung der ersten Wortbedeutungen beim Kinde. Wundt's *Philos. Stud.,* XX, Leipzig, 1902.
MEUMANN	SK	Meumann, E. *Die Sprache des Kindes.* 1903.
MÜLLER	ST	Müller, M. Identity of Language and Thought, in *Three Lectures,* 1887.
NICE	CT	Nice, M. M. A Child who would not talk. *Ped. Sem.,* XXXII, 1925.
OGDEN	MM	Ogden, C. K., and Richards, I. A. *The Meaning of Meaning.* 2nd ed., 1927.
OLTUSCEWSKI	GE	Oltuscewski, W. *Die geistige und Sprachliche Entwicklung des Kindes.* 1897.
O'SHEA	LD	O'Shea, M. V. *Linguistic Development and Education.* 1907.
PAGET	HS	Paget, R. *Human Speech.* 1930.
PALMER	EI	Palmer, H. E. *English Intonation.* 1922.
PAVLOVITCH	LE	Pavlovitch, H. *Le Langage enfantin.* 1920.
PELSMA	CV	Pelsma, J. P. A Child's Vocabulary and its development. *Ped. Sem.,* 1910, XVII.
PIAGET	LP	Piaget, J. *Le langage et la Pensée chez l'Enfant.* 1923.
PREYER	MC	Preyer, W. *The Mind of the Child,* Vol. II.
RONJAT	DL	Ronjat, J. *Le Développement du langage observé chez un enfant bilingue.* 1913.
SAPIR	L	Sapir, E. *Language.* 1921.
SCHÄFER	BV	Schäfer, P. Beobachtungen und Versuche an einem Kinde. *Z. f. Päd. Psych.,* XXIII, 1922.
SCHÄFER	RS	Schäfer, P. Die Kindliche Entwicklungsperiode des reinen Sprachverständnisses nach ihrer Abgrenzung. *Z. f. Päd. Psych.,* XXII, 1921.
SHINN	BB	Shinn, M. W. *The Biography of a Baby.* 1905.
SIGISMUND	KW	Sigismund, B. *Kind und Welt.* 1856.
SPEARMAN	NI	Spearman, C. *The Nature of Intelligence.* 1923.
STERN	KSp	Stern, C., und W. *Die Kindersprache.* 4te. Aufl., 1928.
STOUT	AP	Stout, G. F. *Analytic Psychology.* 1906.
STOUT	MP	Stout, G. F. *Manual of Psychology.* 4th edn., 1929.

STUMPF EE Stumpf, C. Eigenartige sprachliche entwicklung eines Kindes. *Z. f. päd. Psych.*, II, 1900.

SULLY OP Sully, J. *Outlines of Psychology.* 1899.

SULLY SC Sully, J. *Studies of Childhood.* 1896.

TAINE AL Taine, H. Acquisition of Language by Children. *Mind*, II, 1877.

TRACY LC Tracy, F. The Language of Childhood. *Amer. J. Psych.*, 1893.

VALENTINE PA Valentine, C. W. Presidential Address. Brit. Assoc., 1930.

VALENTINE PI Valentine, C. W. The Psychology of Imitation. *B.J.P.*, 1930.

WALLON IE L'interrogation chez l'Enfant. *J. de Psych.*, 1924.

WARD PP Ward, J. *Psychological Principles.* 1918.

WATSON PB Watson, J. B. *Psychology from the Standpoint of a Behaviorist.* 2nd edn., 1924.

WERNER EP Werner, H. *Einführung in die Entwicklungspsychologie.* 1926.

WHITNEY LG Whitney, W. D. *The Life and Growth of Language.* 1895.

WHITNEY MM Whitney, W. D. Max Müller's *Science of Language.* 1892.

WHITNEY SL Whitney, W. D. *Language and the Study of Language.* 1867.

WUNDT VP Wundt, W. *Völkerpsychologie.* 4te Aufl., Bd. I, 1924.

INDEX

Adult, function of, in growth of speech, 79, 87–8, 137, 162, 194, 212–13, 218–19, 221–2 ; speech, see Words, conventional

Æsthetic emotion, 67–8

Affect, in child's speech, 136, 143, 148, 151, 153, 154, 156–7, 160, 162, 192, 194, 196, 205–6, 211, 219, 230 ; in language, 17 ; response to, 43, 46, 48, 118–20, 146, 155, 191, 211–12, 217

Affective discrimination, see Discrimination ; inhibition, 155, 161, 212 ; similarity, see Similarity

Alexander, S., æsthetic emotion, 67–8

Allport, F. H., Circular Reaction, 79, 81 ; imitation of unfamiliar acts, 99 ; origin of repetition, 59

Ament, W., expansion of word's use, 208, 213–15, 219–20, 228, 314

Ammensprache, 113–14

Anticipatory movements in sucking, 34

Aphasia, verbal, 184–8

Art, and babbling, 66–9

Assimilation, in form of words, 177, 181–3, 184, 187, 297–9

Attention in imitation, 74

Babbling, and art, 66–9 ; and deafness, 60 ; and expression, 55, 65, 135 ; and imitation, 99, 140 ; and meaning, 135, 140 ; and play, 60–3 ; and repetition, 58 ; definition of, 55 ; development of, 55 ; incentive in, 63–6 ; intervention of adult in, 79, 87–8, 137 ; isolated sounds, 58 ; kinæsthetic sensation, 59–60 ; patterns in, 65 ; preparatory function of, 93 ; repetitive chains in, 56 ; transformation of discomfort cries, 57, 64

Back-consonants, see Consonants, back

Baldwin, J. M., Circular Reaction, 79 ; origin of repetition, 59

Bartlett, F. C., schema, 187–8

Bateman, W. G., conventional words ; earliest occurrence, 124

Bean, C. H., front-consonants in a blind child, 35

Behaviour and the child's speech, 144–5, 147, 149

Bekhterev, W. M., Circular Reaction, 79 ; differentiation of expression, 21 ; repetition of unpleasant experience, 64

Bell, C., expression, 12

Blind child, front-consonants in, 35

Bridges, K. M. B., differentiation of expression, 22

Bridgman, L., back comfort-sounds, 32

Bühler, C., babbling in isolated sounds, 58 ; expression of satisfaction, 33 ; hunger cry, 22 ; intention in play, 63 ; intonational form in imitation, 75 ; mastery in play, 65 ; phonetic form in imitation, 75 ; purposive movements, 111–12 ; repetitive babbling, 56 ; vocal response to voice, 41 ; and *Hetzer, H.*, gestures, rôle of, 117 ; — occurrence of earliest words, 124 ; — response to intonation, 44 ; — response to speech, 39, 46 ; — sucking movements, 34

Bühler, K., babbling and expression, 56 ; babbling in isolated sounds, 58 ; continuity of development, 191 ; *Dempe, H.*, on, 14 ; expression, 12 ; intention in play, 63 ; repetition and babbling, 58

Cannon, W. B., expression, 12

Cassirer, E., symbolisation, 15

" Centrifugal " and " centripetal " consonants, 128–30, 133

Chains of babbling, 56

Chamberlain, A. F., expansion of word's use, 189–90

Chimpanzees, *Köhler's*, 202

Circular reaction, 79–81

Claparède, E., " instinct to conform ", 100

329

Comfort-sounds, phonetic analysis, 30 ; and satiety, 32
Communication in language, 15, 222
Compounds, consonant, see Consonant-compounds
Comprehension, and metalalia, 97 ; of conventional words, 47–8, 105 ; relation to meaningful utterance, 105 ; training in, 110, 116, 118, 138–40, 160 ; see also Meaning
Conational factors in speech, 143, 154, 156–7, 160, 162, 196, 212, 217
Conceptual thinking, growth of, 210, 225–30 ; —, nature of, 223–5
Confusion, 227–30
Consonant-compounds, 171–7, 183–4
Consonants, and vowels, distinction between, 26 ; back, 30–2, 170, 175–6, 178 ; " centrifugal " and " centripetal ", 128–30, 133 ; classification of, 259 ; early, in crying, 29 ; order of appearance, 25, 177–9 ; " strong " and " weak ", 128, 133 ; front, and imitation, 35 ; — and onomatopœia, 141–2 ; — and sucking-movements, 33, 127–35 ; — in a blind child, 35 ; — in crying, 26 ; — in earliest conventional words, 125, 137, 169–71, 175–80, 184, 257–8 ; middle, 170, 175–6, 178–80, 184 ; nasal, see Nasals
Conventional patterns of speech, 118, 260–9 ; words, see Words
Cries, discomfort, see Discomfort ; expressive, 17 ; response to, by child, 39
Croce, B., expression, 11
Curti, M. W., sucking-movements, 34

Darwin, C., beginning of imitation, 72 ; discomfort cries, 27 ; expansion of word's use, 189 ; expression, 11–12 ; imitation, period of pause in, 83 ; sucking-movements, 34
Deafness, and babbling, 60 ; physiological, 38
Declarative function, 148, 150, 151, 157, 158, 194, 202, 203, 205, 208, 209, 221–2, 228
Delacroix, H., emmagasinement, 96 ; language in society, 16 ; response to intonational form, 48 ; vocal response to speech, 76, 139 ; words, earliest ; comprehension of, 105 ; —, meaning of, 143

De Laguna, G. A., language in society, 16, 224
Delayed imitation, see Metalalia
Dentals, see Consonants, front
Dempe, H., on Bühler, K., 14
De Saussure, F., language in society, 16
Descoeudres, A., conventional words, occurrence of, 125
Deville, G., assimilation, 181–4, 287–9 ; comprehension, observations of, 106 ; elision, 174–7, 271–3, 275–6 ; phonetic development, study of, 168, 262–5 ; reduplication, 182, 295 ; substitution, 177–81, 279–88, 294 ; words, earliest, 255
Dewey, J., language as an instrument, 6 ; reference in language, 14 ; similarity, functional, 197, 199
Differentiation, of expression, 21–2 ; — of intonation, 151
Discomfort, expression of, 21 ; cries, babbling transformation of, 57–64 ; cries, nasalisation, 28 ; cries, pitch, 28
Discrimination, affective, 219, 227 ; functional, 220–1 ; objective, 211, 217–19
Discriminative response to speech, 52
Disintegration, 227–30
Drever, J., play instinct, 62

Echolalia, 89, 100–2, 136
Eduction, 227–30
Elision, 174–7, 183–4, 186, 270–7
Emmagasinement, 96
Emotion, æsthetic, 67–8
Emotive function of language, 10, 13, 17
Evocation in language, 15, 17, 158
Expansion, of response to a word, 160, 200–2 ; of use of a word, 149, 155, 160, 189–209, 211–23, 228–9 ; of use of conventional act, 204
Experience, pattern of, 65, 139
Expression, and babbling, 55, 65, 135 ; of satisfaction, 33 ; theories of, 12
Expressive, cries of children, 17 ; features of speech, 28–37, 115–18, 128, 129–35, 138, 140–2, 154 ; response to speech, 41, 77, 87, 109, 120

Familiar sounds, imitation of, 80, 93–4 ; speech, dominance of, 158–9, 176, 179–81, 182–4, 187, 210, 215, 219–20

Fiji Islanders, 223
Form, and function in language, 17 ; intonational, see Intonational form ; phonetic, see Phonetic form
Fox, C., response to speech, 122
Freud, S., origin of repetition, 58 ; repetition of unpleasant experience, 64
Front-consonants, see Consonants, front
Fronting, 175–6
Function and form in language, 17
Functional discrimination, see Discrimination ; similarity, see Similarity

Galton, F., on Müller, 5
Gardiner, A. H., language and situations, 10 ; language in society, 16
Generalisation of meaning, 190
Gestures, rôle of, 48, 110, 116, 119, 121, 137
Gheorgov, I. A., earliest words, 255
Grammont, M., onomatopœia, 118
Grégoire, A., back comfort-sounds, 31
Groos, K., play instinct, 61
Guernsey, M., imitation and meaning, 91 ; — of intonational form, 94 ; — of pitch, 94 ; —, rôle of attention in, 74 ; metalalia, 96 ; patterns in babbling, 65 ; repetition of unpleasant experience, 64 ; vocal response to voice, 41
Guillaume, P., adult intervention in babbling, 88 ; back comfort-sounds, 31 ; Circular Reaction, 79 ; comprehension, observations of, 161 ; echolalia, 101 ; expansion of word's use, 189, 199, 208 ; imitation, intonational form in, 75 ; —, observations of, 245–6 ; —, period of pause in, 83 ; —, phonetic form in, 75, 80 ; —, rôle of interest in, 91 ; observations of smiling, 40, 78 ; repetition of unpleasant experience, 64 ; response to voice, 39, 41, 76–7

Head, H., aphasia and children's speech, 186–7 ; conceptual thinking, 225 ; schema, 187–8 ; symbolic formulation in language, 14
Hetzer, H., and Reindorf ; conventional words, occurrence of, 125 ; and Tudor-Hart ; early response

Hetzer, H.,—contd. to voice, 39 ; — response to noise, 38 ; see also Bühler, C., and Hetzer, H.
Hocart, A. M., language in society, 16, 223–4
Hoyer, A. and G., back comfort-sounds, 31–2 ; early utterance, 237–8 ; early response to voice, 39, 41, 73, 77 ; hunger cry, 22, 237 ; imitation, intonational form in, 75, 94 ; — of pitch, 95 ; —, observations of, 244 ; — period of pause in, 83 ; —, phonetic form in, 75 ; nasalisation, 25 ; repetitive babbling, 56
Hunger cry, 22, 34–5

i, words ending with, 182
Idelberger, H., earliest words, 254 ; expansion of a word's use, 192, 195, 199, 205, 206, 315
Imitation, 243–52 ; and babbling, 99, 140 ; and front-consonants, 35 ; and instrumental use of words, 90, 98, 100, 102 ; and meaning, 83–6, 91, 101, 130, 135–8, 139–40 ; as play, 92, 100 ; beginning of, 72–82 ; criterion of, 70, 72, 81 ; delayed, see Metalalia ; growth of awareness in, 89–90 ; in child's speech, origin of, 76–82 ; instinct of, 76, 100 ; intonational and phonetic form in, 75, 80, 94, 171–4 ; of familiar sounds, 80, 93–4 ; of pitch, 94–5 ; of unfamiliar acts, 99 ; of unfamiliar sounds, 98 ; period of pause in, 82–8 ; rôle of interest in, 74, 91 ; stages of development in, 71
Inhibition, affective, 155, 161, 212 ; of acts by speech, 109, 120, 146
Instinct, of imitation, 76, 100 ; to conform, 100 ; play, 61–2
Instrumental, function of language, 6, 8 ; use of words, 148, 158, 159, 184, 187, 190, 199, 200–9, 221–3 ; — and imitation, 90, 98, 100, 102
Intention in play, 63 ; in speech, 148
Interest in imitation, 74, 91
Intonation, differentiation of, 23, 151 ; response to, 43–4, 48, 113–15
Intonational patterns, 9, 17, 43, 48, 52, 112–16, 120–2, 151, 162, 171, 186, 191, 201, 203 ; — in imitation, 75, 94, 171–4

Jackson, H., emotional and propositional functions, 11

Jespersen, O., echolalia, 101 ; expansion of word's use, 189 ; front-consonants in blind children, 35 ; sucking and front-consonants, 33, 128, 132

Jones, D., consonants, 29–30

Jones, H. E., theory of training process, 51

K., affective inhibition, 155, 161 ; animals, names of, 215, 219, 221, 227, 320 ; assimilation, 181–2, 299 ; comprehension, observations of, 107–9, 121, 149, 160–1, 189, 200, 300–1, 304, 316–21 ; early utterance, 239–42 ; echolalia, 101 ; elision, 174–7, 274–5, 277 ; expansion of word's use, 189, 192, 195, 197, 198, 206–8, 215–16, 219, 221–2, 316–21 ; imitation, and meaning, 84 ; — as play, 92 ; —, observations of, 249–52 ; — of intonational form, 94 ; —, period of pause in, 83 ; —, phonetic form in, 80 ; inhibition of act, 121, 146 ; intonation, differentiation of, 151 ; *mama*, use of, 154, 161, 212, 228 ; manipulative function, 148, 151, 158, 207–8, 222 ; negative, response to, 107, 109, 121 ; phonetic development, study of, 169–84, 266–9 ; purposive movement, 112 ; reduplication, 170, 182, 296 ; reference, growth of, 122, 146–7, 149, 152–7, 161–2, 191–2 ; repetitive babbling, 56 ; resistance to change, 158, 177, 179, 184, 215 ; response to speech, wide range of, 200 ; similarity, affective, 197 ; —, functional, 198 ; —, objective, 195 ; substitution, 177–81, 288–94 ; sucking movements, 34 ; utterance, observations of, 146, 151–7, 302–3, 305–13, 316–21 ; wide use of sounds, 191 ; words, conventional, adoption of, 153, 191–3 ; —, earliest, 255

Kampik, A., deafness and babbling, 60

Keller, Helen ; objective discrimination, 217–18

Kenyeres, E., expansion of word's use, 189

Kinæsthetic sensation in babbling, 59–60

Koffka, K., Circular Reaction, 79 ; meaning and imitation, 101 ; pattern of experience, 65 ; training process, 51 ; vocal response to speech, 76

Köhler, W., chimpanzees, 202

Kussmaul, A., back comfort-sounds, 31

Labials, *see* Consonants, front

Lallen, meaning of term, 55, 57, 129 *n.* ; *see* Babbling

Language, and situations, 10 ; and speech, 7 ; communication in, 15, 222 ; emotive function, 10, 13, 17 ; evocative function, 15, 17, 158 ; function and form in, 17 ; in society, 16 ; instrumental function of, 6, 8 ; *langage, langue,* 7 ; patterns of spoken, 8–9, 17 ; propositional function of, 11 ; referential function, 14, 15, 17, 143 ; representation in, 113, 115–16 ; signs of thoughts, 9, 10 ; symbolisation in, 15

Le Dantec, F., emmagasinement, 96

Lindner, G., expansion of word's use, 189, 207 ; onomatopœia, 141–2 ; words, use of early, 160, 253

Lorimer, F., aphasia and children's speech, 186 ; babbling and meaning, 135 ; Circular Reaction, 79 ; echolalia, 101 ; emmagasinement, 96 ; expansion of word's use, 192 ; imitation of intonational form, 94 ; nasalisation, 25 ; origin of repetition, 59 ; vocal play, 56 ; words, earliest ; meaning of, 143

Löwenfeld, B., response to intonation, 43

Major, D. R., expansion of word's use, 189 ; hunger cry, 22 ; words, earliest, 255

Malinowski, B., language in society, 16, 224

Mama, development of use of, 125–9, 144, 154–5, 160–1, 212, 219–20, 227–9, 308–11

Manipulative function, 148, 150, 151, 157, 158, 194, 202, 203, 206–9, 222, 228 ; movements, 119

Marichelle, H., vocal response to speech, 76

Markey, J. F., Circular Reaction, 79; utterance and response, relation between, 16, 158

McDougall, W., Circular Reaction, 79; origin of repetition, 58; play, 60–2; vocal response to speech, 76

Meaning, and babbling, 135, 140; and expression, 87; and imitation, 83–6, 91, 101, 130, 135–8, 139–40; and metalalia, 95; and society, 134, 158, 212–13, 222; and vocal response to voice, 86–7; expansion of, *see* Expansion; generalisation of, 190; of earliest words, 125–9

Memory of speech, 97

Meringer, R., earliest words, 254

Metalalia, 89, 95–8

Metalepsis, 183

Meumann, E., affective speech, response to, 43, 48; assimilation, 183; early comprehension, 47–8; early response to voice, 38; reference, growth of, 143, 145, 147; similarity, affective, 196, 199, 205; words, earliest; meaning in, 129

Middle-consonants, *see* Consonants, middle

Mother, concept of, 225, 228–9; *see also, Mama*

Movement, conventional, expansion of use of, 204

Movements, maturation of purposive, 111–12, 119

Müller, M., 5

Names, growth of, 147, 159–62, 193, 209

Nasalisation, 25, 28

Nasals, 24, 26, 57, 129–30, 133

Negative, response to, 107, 109, 121

Nice, M. M., words, early use of, 160, 189

Noise, earliest response to, 38

Object, recall of, 150

Objective discrimination, *see* Discrimination; reference, *see* Reference; similarity, *see* Similarity

Ogden, C. K., and *Richards, I. A.*, 14

Oltuscewski, W., earliest words, 254

Onomatopœia, 115, 118, 135, 141, 154, 156

O'Shea, M. V., early response to voice, 38; hunger cry, 22

Paget, R., nasalisation, 28; onomatopœia, 118

papa, 98–9, 125–9, 160–1, 185, 226, 241

Patterns, in babbling, 65; intonational, *see* Intonational patterns; of experience, 65, 139; phonetic, *see* Phonetic patterns

Pause, period of, in imitation, 82–8

Pavlovitch, H., observations, 48, 255

Pelsma, J. P., expansion of word's use, 189

Perseveration, 96, 183

Phonetic patterns, in imitation, 75, 80, 171–4; in language, 8–9, 17; of earliest words, 125–9, 167, 171, 203; response to, 48, 111, 114–16, 118, 121–2, 150, 191

Piaget, J., 16

Pitch, of discomfort-cries, 28; imitation of, 94–5

Play, and babbling, 60–3; instinct, 61–2; intention in, 63; mastery in, 64–5; vocal, 56

Preyer, W., aphasia and children's speech, 186; back comfort-sounds, 31–2; hunger cry, 22; early utterance, 233–4; early words, 253; echolalia, 100; expansion of word's use, 189; imitation of intonational form, 94; — of pitch, 95; —, period of pause in, 83; repetitive babbling, 56

Propositional function of language, 11

Prolepsis, 183

Rasmussen, V., earliest words, 255

Recall, of an object, 150

Reduplication in earliest words, 125, 169–71, 181–2, 183–4, 256, 295–6

Reference, development of, 122, 131, 143, 146–7, 149–50, 152, 154–6, 159, 161–2; 191, 209, 217–18; in language, *see* Language

Repertory of sounds, the child's, 168–74

Repetition, and babbling, 56–8; in speech, origin of, 58–9; of unpleasant experience, 64–5, 68

Representation in language, 13, 115–16

Resistance by child to change, 158–9, 176, 179–81, 182–4, 187, 210, 215, 219–20

Response, by child to another's cry, 36–9; — to noise, 38; to affect, *see* Affect; to intonation, 43–4,

Response—contd.
48, 113–15 ; to speech, expansion of, 160, 200–2 ; —, expressive, 41, 77, 87, 109, 120 ; —, relation to utterance, 16, 157–8 ; —, stages of development, 46 ; —, training of, see Training ; vocal, to voice, 41, 76, 139
Romanes, G. J., expansion of word's use, 189, 195 ; on *Müller*, 5

Sander, H., earliest words, 254
Satiety, and comfort-sounds, 32
Satisfaction, expression of, 33
Schäfer, P., conventional act, expansion of use of, 204, 322 ; onomatopœia, 118 ; purposive movements, 111–12, 119 ; resistance to change, 159 ; response to intonational form, 48, 113–15 ; words, earliest, comprehension of, 105
Schema, 187–8
Schneider, O., earliest words, 254
Sigismund, B., expansion of word's use, 189
Signs, of thoughts, language as, 7, 10 ; nature of, 13
Similarity, affective, 157, 191, 196–7, 199, 201, 205, 208, 219–20, 227–8 ; functional, 197–9, 201, 208, 219, 228 ; objective, 156–7, 190, 193, 194–6, 199, 200, 208, 219, 228
Situation, reference to, 159, 163, 190
Situations, relation to speech, 10, 49, 194–9, 224 ; similarity of, see Similarity, objective.
Smiling, in response to voice, 40, 78 ; response to, 73, 82
Society, effect on growth of meaning, 134, 158, 212–13, 222 ; language in, 16, 223–5
Solomon Islanders, 224
Sound-change, see Assimilation, elision, substitution
Sounds, child's repertory of, 168–74 ; wide use of, 149, 151–3, 191–4
Spearman, C., conceptual thinking, 225, 226–30
Speech, and language, 7 ; child's response to, 38 ; conventional patterns of, 118 ; development of discriminative response to, 52 ; expressive features of, see Expressive features ; expressive response to, 41, 77, 87, 109, 120 ; familiar, see Familiar speech ;

Speech—contd.
inhibition of acts by, 109, 120, 146 ; memory of, 97 ; response to, by acts, 109 ; theories of training of response to, 50 ; uniformity of children's, 183–4 ; vocal response to, 41, 73–4, 76, 82, 83, 86–7, 91, 97, 135–9 ; see also Language
Stabilisation of meaning, see Words, earliest
Stern, W., affect in speech, 162, 196, 211 ; assimilation, 181–3 ; babbling, 56, 58, 60, 235–6 ; Circular Reaction, 79 ; comfort-sounds, 25, 31–2 ; comprehension, training in, 110, 138–40, 160 ; —, observations of, 106, 160 ; conceptual thinking, growth of, 225–6 ; differentiation of expression, 21 ; early utterance, 235–6 ; echolalia, 101 ; elision, 174–6, 270, 275 ; expansion of word's use, 189–91, 211, 212, 226 ; gestures, rôle of, 48, 110, 116, 121 ; imitation, and meaning, 91 ; —, beginning of, 72 ; —, form of the child's response in, 75 ; —, instinct of, 76 ; —, observations of, 234 ; — of intonational form, 94 ; — of *papa*, 98 ; — of pitch, 94–5 ; — phonetic form in, 75 ; —, period of pause in, 83 ; Lallen, 55, 129 *n.* ; metalalia, 95, 96 ; onomatopœia, 118, 141 ; phonetic development, 260–2 ; play, 60 ; similarity, affective, 196 ; —, functional, 198 ; —, objective, 194–6 ; substitution, 177–81, 278–9, 294 ; vocabulary, study of, 168 ; vocal response to speech, 41, 74 ; words, earliest, comprehension of, 105 ; —, meaning of, 128–9, 133, 143, 160, 253 ; —, occurrence, 124–5
Stout, G. F., kinds of signs, 13 ; language in society, 224
" Strong " consonants, 128, 133
Strümpell, E., earliest words, 254
Stumpf, C., earliest words, 354
Substitution in phonetic form, 177–181, 183, 186, 278–94
Sucking, anticipatory movements, 34 ; movements and front-consonants, 33, 127–35
Sully, J., expansion of word's use, 189
Symbolisation in language, 15

Taine, H., expansion of word's use, 189

Tappolet, E., experiment, 47

Thinking, conceptual, *see* Conceptual thinking

Tögel, H., earliest words, 254

Tone, *see* Intonation

Tracy, F., vocabulary, study of, 168

Tradition and earliest words, 131, 134

Training, of response to speech, 110, 130, 137, 138–40 ; —, theories of, 50

Uniformity of children's speech, 183–5

Unfamiliar sounds, imitation of, 98

Unpleasant experience ; repetition of, 64–5, 68

Utterance, meaningful ; growth of, 105, 146–7, 151–7 ; — relation to response, 16, 157–8

Valentine, C. W., early smiling, 40 ; imitation, observations of, 247–8 ; —, period of pause in, 83 ; —, phonetic form in, 75, 80 ; —, rôle of interest in, 74, 91

Verbal aphasia, 184–8

Vocabulary, study of, 168

Vocal play, 56 ; response to speech, *see* Speech

Voice, *see* Speech

Vowels and consonants, distinction between, 26

Ward, J., language in society, 16 ; theory of training process, 50

Watson, J. B., child's response to noise, 38 ; theory of training process, 51, 116

" Weak " consonants, 128–33

Werner, H., onomatopœia, 118

Whitehead, A. N., reference in language, 14

Whitney, W. D., on *Müller*, 5 ; language in society, 16 ; " strong " and " weak " consonants, 128 *n.*

Words, conventional, adoption of, 153, 158–9, 167–88, 191, 193, 202–5, 213–23 ; —, natural features of, 202–3 ; —, response to, 154 ; —, superior efficiency of, 159 ; earliest, analysis of, 256 ; — and tradition, 131, 134 ; —, meanings of, 125–9, 253–5 ; —, occurrence of, 124–5 ; —, phonetic form of, 125–9, 167, 171, 203 ; —, reduplication in, 125, 169–71, 181–2, 183–4 ; —, stabilisation of, 129–42 ; —, stabilisation of meaning of, 129, 153 ; instrumental use of, *see* Instrumental ; of conventional origin, 154, 157

Wundt, W., repetition in speech, 58 ; rhythmical utterance, 30 ; sucking and front-consonants, 33, 127–8, 133 ; words, form of earliest, 125, 127